# Immunology of the Lymphomas

Editor

## Simon B. Sutcliffe, M.D., M.R.C.P., F.R.C.P. (C)

Staff Radiation Oncologist
Senior Scientific Staff Member
Princess Margaret Hospital
Ontario Cancer Istitute
Toronto, Ontario, Canada

CRC Series in Immunology and Lymphoid Cell Biology

Editor-in-Chief

## A. Arthur Gottlieb, M.D.

Professor and Chairman
Department of Microbiology and Immunology
School of Medicine
Tulane University
New Orleans, Louisiana

CRC Press, Inc.
Boca Raton, Florida

Library of Congress Cataloging in Publication Data
Main entry under title:

Immunology of the lymphomas.

(CRC series in immunology and lymphoid cell biology)
Bibliography: p.
Includes index.
1. Lymphoma — Immunological aspects.   2. Hodgkin's
disease — Immunological aspects.   I. Sutcliffe, Simon B.,
1946—   II. Series.   [DNLM: 1. Lymphoma — Immunology.
WH 525 I33]
RC280.L9I44   616.99'446      84-1776
ISBN 0-8493-6371-3

This book represents information obtained from authentic and highly regarded sources. Reprinted material is quoted with permission, and sources are indicated. A wide variety of references are listed. Every reasonable effort has been made to give reliable data and information, but the author and the publisher cannot assume responsibility for the validity of all materials or for the consequences of their use.

All rights reserved. This book, or any parts thereof, may not be reproduced in any form without written consent from the publisher.

Direct all inquiries to CRC Press, Inc., 2000 Corporate Blvd., N.W., Boca Raton, Florida, 33431.

© 1985 by CRC Press, Inc.

International Standard Book Number 0-8493-6371-3

Library of Congress Card Number 84-1776
Printed in the United States

# PREFACE

The purpose of this book is to review selected topics of current interest in Hodgkin's disease and other malignant lymphomas. By design, no attempt has been made to cover the entire spectrum of knowledge on the immunology of these disorders. The topics chosen for discussion represent areas of controversy, or areas where existing information is undergoing reorganization based on data resulting from technological developments. The clinical utility of such developments is unclear, however, their impact in both conceptual and clinical terms may be substantial. To this end it is hoped that discussion of the technical and practical aspects of these developments in relation to their contribution to the pathogenesis of lymphomas will be of benefit primarily to those interested in the clinical immunology of the lymphomas.

In a purely clinical setting it is difficult, at present, to make a strong argument for the acquisition of more information on the immunology of Hodgkin's disease, as that which we have makes relatively little contribution to our knowledge of the pathogenesis or management of patients with this disease. Also, it seems unlikely, given the high degree of success with current therapy, that immunological data will profoundly modify therapeutic strategy. Nevertheless, there is a major role for immunological approaches in the understanding of the disease. To this end the demonstration of a clonal origin of a malignant cell, and the relationship of this cell to the morphologically more numerous, and presumably reactive nonclonal cells would be of great importance. Furthermore the mechanism of disease spread, the selectivity for involvement of T dependent regions of lymphoid tissue, and the relationship between the cell of origin and the high endothelial venules in lymphoid tissue in determining patterns of disease spread are areas of biological importance which may be expected to impact on patient management. Finally, a means of prospectively identifying patients with a high risk of failure on primary therapy, and a method for establishing complete remission of disease activity in biological rather than the inherently inaccurate clinical terms, would permit direction in choice and amount of therapy. To achieve this objective would be of immense clinical importance in balancing disease control against treatment-induced morbidity in a patient population with a high expectation of long-term survival.

The situation in non-Hodgkin's lymphoma is quite different, in that only a small proportion of the patient population may expect cure as a result of therapy. The majority have generalized disease, and have a survival largely uninfluenced by therapy. Despite this lack of clinical success, the clonality, lineage, and degree of differentiation of the malignant cell is generally available by use of morphology, and phenotypic, karyotypic, or molecular probes. Much attention is being directed to the incorporation of such data into new prognostic classifications which may direct therapy. The ultimate utility of such approaches will become evident only when sufficient time has elapsed to permit meaningfull survival analysis. If our treatment philosophy remains as in the past, however, it seems unlikely that re-classification will influence treatment sufficiently to contribute to improvements in survival.

Despite the multiplicity of surface components characterizing lymphoma cells, the functional nature of the majority of these markers, and the relationship of phenotypic expression to critical events in the genome is unknown. It is not clear whether maturation arrest within a cell lineage is the fundamental event, or whether these are disorders of a stem cell with variable phenotypic expressions. Although clonality is demonstrable for the major population, are the minor populations "normal"?

The ability to characterize the dominant cell should permit a more perceptive approach to staging of disease, and provide a better opportunity to define the nature of lymphoid infiltrates particularly in extranodal sites such as bone marrow or liver. In addition, the factors that determine lymphoma cell "traffic" routes and result in patterns of spread may be explored.

The availability of monoclonal reagents to cell surface components has permitted serologic monitoring of disease burden with therapy, and has opened the door for the investigation of monoclonal serotherapy. Such developments run in parallel with efforts to explore the use of bone marrow transplantation in non-Hodgkin's lymphoma.

One may anticipate that increased efforts to correlate phenotype with karyotype will ensue, with subsequent exploration of the molecular events underlying karyotypic, biochemical, and phenotypic expression. In short, while the clinical utility of such approaches is not yet apparent, the potential for expansion of knowledge concerning the biology of these disorders is great, and this may be a necessary step in determining more effective therapy.

Simon B. Sutcliffe<br>
May 1983

# CONTRIBUTORS

Ram Prakash Agarwal, Ph.D.
Section of Medical Oncology
Evans Memorial Department of Clinical
  Research
Boston University Medical Center
Boston, Massachusetts

Richard Bell, M.B., B.S., F.R.A.C.P.,
  F.R.C.P.A.
Section of Medical Oncology
Evans Memorial Department of Clinical
  Research
Boston University Medical Center
Boston, Massachusetts

H. S. Dhaliwal, M.B., Ch.B.,
  M.R.C.P.
Research Fellow
Honorary Senior Registrar
ICRF Department of Medical Oncology
St. Bartholomew's Hospital
West Smithfield, London, England

J. A. Habeshaw, M.D., Ph.D.
ICRF Medical Oncology Unit
St. Bartholomew's Hospital
London, England

David Rael Katz, M.B., Ch.B., Ph.D.,
  M.R.C.Path.
Senior Lecturer in Pathology
Middlesex Hospital Medical School
London, England

John R. Krause, M.D.
Associate Professor of Pathology
University of Pittsburgh School of
  Medicine; and Director
Central Hematology Laboratories
Health Center Hospitals
University of Pittsburgh
Pittsburgh, Pennsylvania

T. A. Lister
ICRF Department of
  Medical Oncology
St. Bartholomew's Hospital
West Smithfield, London, England

Anne Lillquist, B.S.
Section of Medical Oncology
Evans Memorial Department of Clinical
  Research
Boston University Medical Center
Boston, Massachusetts

Ronald McCaffrey, M.D.
Section of Medical Oncology
Evans Memorial Department of Clinical
  Research
Boston University Medical Center
Boston, Massachusetts

Peter C. Nowell, M.D.
Department of Pathology
School of Medicine
University of Pennsylvania
Philadelphia, Pennsylvanvia

David Osoba, M.D., F.R.C.P.(C)
Asssociate Professor
University of Toronto; and Head,
  Medical Oncology
Toronto-Bayview Clinic and
  Sunnybrook Medical Centre
Toronto, Ontario, Canada

John M. Pesando, M.D., Ph.D.
Divisions of Medical and Pediatric
  Oncology
Fred Hutchinson Cancer Research
  Center
Seattle, Washington

David T. Rowlands, Jr., M.D.
Department of Pathology
College of Medicine
University of South Florida
Tampa, Florida

Simon B. Sutcliffe, M.D., M.R.C.P.,
  F.R.C.P.(C)
Staff Radiation Oncologist
Senior Scientific Staff Member
Princess Margaret Hospital and Ontario
  Cancer Institute
Toronto, Ontario, Canada

# TABLE OF CONTENTS

Chapter 1
Hodgkin's Disease: A Review of the Clinical Immunology ................................... 1
Simon B. Sutcliffe

Chapter 2
Hodgkin's Disease: The Role of the Lymphocyte and Monocyte ........................ 33
David R. Katz and J. A. Habeshaw

Chapter 3
Non-Hodgkin's Lymphoma: Concepts of Classification .................................... 65
John R. Krause

Chapter 4
Immune Dysfunction in Non-Hodgkin's Lymphoma ........................................ 81
H. S. Dhaliwal and T. A. Lister

Chapter 5
Clinical Utility of Monoclonal Antibodies .................................................. 107
John M. Pesando

Chapter 6
The Spectrum of T Cell Neoplasms ......................................................... 133
David T. Rowlands, Jr. and Peter C. Nowell

Chapter 7
Biochemical Markers in Neoplastic Lymphoid Cells ....................................... 153
Richard Bell, Ram Prakash Agarwal, Anne Lillquist, and Ronald McCaffrey

Chapter 8
The Major Histocompatibility Complex and Lymphomas ................................ 167
David Osoba

Index .............................................................................................. 193

Chapter 1

# HODGKIN'S DISEASE: A REVIEW OF THE CLINICAL IMMUNOLOGY

Simon B. Sutcliffe

## TABLE OF CONTENTS

I. Introduction ................................................................................................ 2

II. Hodgkin's Disease: An Immunodeficiency State ................................... 2
    A. Clinical Observations of Cellular Immunity ................................... 2
        1. Susceptibility to Infection ........................................................ 2
        2. Delayed Hypersensitivity Skin Tests ...................................... 3
        3. Lymphocyte Transfer; Homograft Rejection; Bone Marrow Transplantation ........................................................................ 4
        4. Immune Modulation ................................................................. 4
    B. Clinical Observations of Humoral Immunity ................................... 5
    C. In Vitro Observation of Cellular Immunity ..................................... 6
        1. Peripheral Blood Lymphocytes ................................................ 6
        2. Tissue Lymphocyte Populations .............................................. 6
        3. Lymphocyte Proliferation in Response to Antigen and Mitogen ...................................................................................... 7
        4. Lymphokine Production ............................................................ 8
        5. Mixed Leukocyte Reaction (MLR) and Autologous Mixed Leukocyte Reaction (AMLR) ................................................... 8
        6. Mechanisms of Impaired Lymphocyte Reactivity ................... 9
            a. Monocyte-Mediated Suppression ................................ 9
            b. Lymphocyte-Mediated Suppression ......................... 10
        7. Natural Killing (NK) and Antibody-Dependent Cellular Cytotoxicity (ADCC) ............................................................... 10
        8. Macrophage Function ............................................................. 10
        9. In Vitro Antibody Synthesis ................................................... 11
        10. Other Factors ......................................................................... 11

III. Hodgkin's Disease, Autoimmunity and Nephrosis ................................ 11
    A. Autoimmune Disease ........................................................................ 12
        1. Systemic Lupus Erythematosus (SLE) ................................. 12
        2. Sjögren's Syndrome .............................................................. 12
        3. Dermatomyositis .................................................................... 13
        4. Immune Thrombocytopenic Purpura (ITP) ......................... 13
        5. Autoimmune Hemolytic Anemia ........................................... 14
        6. Autoimmune Neutropenia ...................................................... 14
    B. The Nephrotic Syndrome and Hodgkin's Disease ........................ 14

IV. Hodgkin's Disease, Immunodeficiency States, and Malignancy ........ 16
    A. Immunodeficiency States and Malignancy .................................... 16
        1. Primary Immunodeficiency States ........................................ 16
        2. Acquired Immunodeficiency States ...................................... 16
            a. The Existence of Intrinsic Defects in Lymphoid Cells ... 16
            b. The Role of Exogenous or Endogenous Viruses .......... 17
            c. Impaired Immunoregulation ....................................... 17
            d. Chronic Antigen Stimulation ...................................... 18

B. Hodgkin's Disease and Malignancy ............................................. 18

V. Concluding Remarks............................................................... 19

References ................................................................................. 20

## I. INTRODUCTION

Hodgkin's disease occupies a unique position in clinical medicine providing controversy both to its status as a malignant disease and also to the nature of the accompanying immunodeficiency state.

The disease is characterized initially by uncontrolled proliferation of cellular elements in affected tissues. Subsequent spread to other sites occurs and, untreated, the disease eventually has a fatal outcome. These characteristics, however, have certain deficiencies in defining this to be a "malignant" disease. The initial cellular proliferation is pleomorphic rather than monomorphic and progressive disease activity is characterized by cellular depletion rather than proliferation. The patterns of spread are often predictable, extralymphatic spread usually occurs late, and extracapsular invasion is unusual. Attempts to define a clonal cell population in phenotypic, karyotypic, or culture terms have been fraught with difficulties.

It would not be surprising that a disease originating in, and effacing the morphology of lymphoreticular tissue, might also affect the function of that tissue. Evidence for immunodeficiency in untreated and treated disease is abundant, however this poses more questions than answers. If immunodeficiency is a consequence of Hodgkin's disease, why is it so evident even in early stages of disease? Although impairment of immune function is a characteristic of other malignant tumors, it is usually evident only with advanced disease. What is the evidence that the immunodeficiency state is improved by therapeutic control of the disease? Certain studies indicate continued immunodeficiency despite complete remission of disease activity. Is it possible that immunodeficiency antedates the histological changes that we recognize to be Hodgkin's disease? Are the tissues morphologically unaffected by Hodgkin's disease immunologically "normal"?

In discussing the immunological aspects of Hodgkin's disease, consideration will be given initially to the clinical and in vitro evidence indicating immune dysfunction, and this will then be discussed in terms of the interrelationship between immunodeficiency, autoimmune disease, and neoplasia.

## II. HODGKIN'S DISEASE: AN IMMUNODEFICIENCY STATE

### A. Clinical Observations of Cellular Immunity
*1. Susceptibility to Infection*

Considerable attention has been focused upon the fact that infections known to be associated with immunoincompetence occur also in patients with Hodgkin's disease.

Sternberg[1] and Reed[2] reported the association of Hodgkin's disease and tuberculosis at the beginning of this century, and the observation was expanded by Jackson and Parker with the demonstration of active tuberculosis in approximately one-third of autopsies performed on deceased patients who had suffered from Hodgkin's disease.[3] So frequent was the association that for many years tuberculosis was considered to be of etiological significance.[4]

In 1940, Wise and Poston reported the isolation of brucella strains from node biopsies of patients with Hodgkin's disease living in an endemic area despite the frequent absence of a serologically detectable immune response.[5] Subsequent reports indicated that approximately 5 to 11% of cases of cryptococcosis occurred in patients with Hodgkin's disease, that the infection was more frequently disseminated, and that disseminated infection occurred in both treated and untreated patients.[6-9] A fulminant course has also been characteristic of the reports of listeriosis in patients with Hodgkin's disease.[10-12]

Goffinet reported herpes zoster infection in 15% of patients with Hodgkin's disease, noting that advanced stage, prior splenectomy, and therapy, all appeared to increase the incidence.[13] Zoster accounted for almost 50% of viral infections in Hodgkin's disease in the report of Casazza.[14]

The literature also contains case report association of Hodgkin's disease and histoplasma,[15] pneumocystis,[16,17] toxoplasma,[18,19] aspergillosis,[20] nocardia,[14] and salmonella.[21] However, despite the attention given to uncommon infections by organisms of relatively low virulence, termed opportunistic infections, the majority of infections are caused by common virulent pathogenic bacteria.[14-22] This has become more apparent with intensive treatment and consequent myelosuppression, and although the overall mortality from infection is low, infection remains an important cause of morbidity and mortality particularly in those with advanced and progressive disease.[22-23]

*2. Delayed Hypersensitivity Skin Tests*

In 1902 Reed noted that five of eight patients with Hodgkin's disease were unreactive to skin testing with tubercle bacilli.[2] The high incidence of anergy to strains of mycobacteria giving strong positive reactions in sensitized guinea pigs and patients with tubercle was confirmed in Hodgkin's disease by Jackson and Parker,[24] and Steiner.[25] Subsequent studies have noted a correlation between skin test anergy and the physical condition of the patient,[26] the extent of disease,[27,28] the activity of Hodgkin's disease,[29,31] the histological subtype,[27,28] the absolute lymphocyte count,[28] and the number of antigens used.[28,32] This literature indicates a disproportionate degree of skin test hyporeactivity in patients with Hodgkin's disease compared with normal subjects and patients with non-Hodgkin lymphoma or other forms of cancer.[26,30,33] Certain aspects of this extensive literature deserve attention:

1. Hyporeactivity is seen in untreated as well as treated patients,[28,30,35] and applies equally to microbial antigens and primary skin sensitizing chemicals.
2. Immediate hypersensitivity reactions[36] and a normal response to intradermal histamine are seen in patients with Hodgkin's disease.[26,36,37]
3. The true incidence of anergy depends on the number of antigens used and the dosage of antigen applied.[38] Using 2% DNCB, Eltringham et al. achieved a response in approximately 50% of their patients, whereas only 26% produced a response to 0.5% strength, and no responses were seen with 0.1% DNCB.[34]
4. Failure to elicit a positive skin response does not necessarily signify a defect in lymphocyte-mediated immunity. Johnson et al. performed DNCB skin testing with simultaneous croton oil skin application. All normal subjects reacted to DNCB and mounted an inflammatory response to croton oil; however, in patients with cancer there was a clear correlation between a negative DNBC response and the failure to produce an inflammatory response.[39] The failure of croton oil to produce a response in patients with Hodgkin's disease was noted by Goasguen, but only a quarter of such patients were anergic to microbial antigens.[27] The production of an inflammatory response has been shown by skin window technique to be abnormal, both quantitatively and qualitatively, in patients with Hodgkin's disease.[40]

5. Modification of the mode of presentation of antigen, e.g., tubercle protein emulsified in paraffin oil has not resulted in a higher incidence of positive responses,[41] nor has the use of systemic steroids at the time of challenge with antigen demonstrated more positive results as in sarcoidosis.[42,43]
6. The effect of leukocytosis at the time of skin testing may modify the number of positive responses. Heiss noted an increased incidence of anergy, reduced mitogen-induced lymphocyte blastogenesis, lymphopenia, and failure to mount an inflammatory response to croton oil in patients without cancer who had a peripheral leukocytosis ($> 15 \times 10^9/1$). In two of four patients studied following resolution of the leukocytosis, previous abnormalities had resolved. As noted previously, leukocytosis in Hodgkin's disease, particularly in advanced stages, is not uncommon.[44]
7. Although it is apparent that skin test hyporeactivity reflects disease extent and activity, and thus inferentially might be prognostically useful, this has not been borne out in studies undertaken at a time when chemotherapy was able to influence profoundly the natural history of disease.[45]

*3. Lymphocyte Transfer; Homograft Rejection; Bone Marrow Transplantation*

The intradermal injection of normal homologous human lymphocytes into recipient skin was developed as an assay of donor/recipient compatibility for organ transplantation.[46] Using this assay, lymphocytes from patients with Hodgkin's disease were noted to produce an evanescent response in normal recipient skin, thus implying poorer stimulation of response; in addition, a protracted response to injection of normal lymphocytes into patient skin was noted, thereby suggesting a weakened rejection reaction.[47] A failure of lymphocytes from patients with Hodgkin's disease to induce graft vs. host reaction following subcapsular placement in immunosuppressed rats has been described.[48]

Calciati and Fazio demonstrated reproducible transfer of tuberculin response by passive transfer of sensitized leukocytes in normal individuals, however, they failed to demonstrate transfer of antigen sensitivity despite production of lymphocyte transfer reaction in patients with Hodgkin's disease.[41] Similar results have been noted in treated and untreated patients with Hodgkin's disease.[32,49]

Delayed rejection or acceptance of homo- or heterograft skin has been reported in treated patients with Hodgkin's disease.[50,51] These studies indicate delayed rejection in patients with retained skin test reactivity to recall antigen, and suggest a correlation with stage of disease,[50] but no correlation with type of therapy.[51]

Two reports document unrelated donor bone marrow engraftment in patients with extensively treated Hodgkin's disease.[52,53] In both circumstances transfusion of homologous marrow was given for severe drug-induced marrow hypoplasia and donor markers established successful engraftment in each case.

Studies of this type indicating abnormal cell-mediated immunity gave rise to the theory that Hodgkin's disease might represent an autoimmune reaction of lymphoid cells against the host.[54] This was supported by the similarities of progressive Hodgkin's disease to homologous disease in mice, an experimentally induced graft vs. host reaction.

*4. Immune Modulation*

Vaccination of anergic patients with localized asymptomatic lymphoma with BCG has been reported to delay and reduce the recurrence rate, particularly in those remaining reactive on serial vaccination.[55]

Transfer factor has been used by several groups to attempt reversal of skin test anergy.[56-60] Rarely has there been a correlation with clinical improvement,[56] most authors addressing the question of production of skin test response and the specificity of the transfer-factor preparation. Although skin test conversions,[56-59] and in one case an in vitro correlation of antigen transfer[60] have been noted, the reproducibility and the specificity of transfer of reactivity remains unclear.

B. Clinical Observations of Humoral Immunity

Studies in the mid-1940s demonstrated that patients with Hodgkin's disease frequently had no serologically detectable antibody response to brucella despite active infection with the organism.[61,62] Low agglutination titers for typhoid, brucella, tularemia, and proteus X-19, and lower positive serology rates for syphilis in patients with Hodgkin's disease in comparison with area average figures were also noted.[62] These results could not be explained on the basis of low serum proteins. Other reports indicate impaired antibody response to histoplasmin,[63] pneumococcal polysaccharide[64,66] and poliovaccination,[67] while others reported normal antibody responses to typhoid/paratyphoid[67,68] and mumps.[67,69]

Some of the apparent confusion in these results stems from the heterogeneity of the patient population, which included all stages of disease, and also patients who had undergone extensive treatment. Furthermore, no distinction was made as to whether impairment of humoral immunity existed at the level of primary or secondary antibody response.

Impairment of primary antibody response has been reported using tetanus toxoid,[70,71] tularemia,[72,73] keyhole limpet hemocyanin,[74] and $\emptyset \times 174$ as antigens.[75] The latter study is of particular interest as the impaired response was documented in a normal volunteer who subsequently developed Hodgkin's disease, 4 years later. A normal response has been noted, using the $\alpha$ hemocyanin of helixpomatia.[76]

Normal secondary antibody response has been seen using tetanus-toxoid,[71] tularemia,[72,73] and red blood group A and B antigens.[77]

The relationship of impaired primary and secondary responses to other prognostic variables is difficult to determine. Certain authors have indicated that treatment has no effect on antibody response,[68,72,78] while others note impaired response with combined modality therapy.[79] Controversy also exists as to the influence of stage of disease.[65,66,68,73,76] While the influence of treatment cannot be clearly determined, the report of Brown et al. indicates that impaired primary antibody response does not exist in untreated patients.[73] A possible genetic component in the determination of antibody response to type A Hong Kong influenza vaccine has been noted by Sybesma et al.[78]

Splenectomy in patients with Hodgkin's disease has been stated to have no influence on antibody response,[79] and in terms of response to pneumococcal vaccination this is true for patients undergoing splenectomy for trauma.[80,81] However, splenectomy, when combined with active Hodgkin's disease and cytotoxic therapy, is a situation associated with impaired pneumococcal vaccine response and probably reduction in antibody duration. Recommendations for use of pneumococcal vaccine in patients with Hodgkin's disease have included pretherapy vaccination and revaccination after therapy if titers fall to nonprotective levels.[82]

Immunoglobulin levels have been studied by many groups, and no consistent features are observed. Although Aisenberg and Leskowitz noted hypogammaglobulinemia in three of five patients with advanced disease who failed to mount an antibody response to pneumococcal polysaccharide,[66] normal immunoglobulins,[76,78,83] or a polyclonal increase in IgG have been most frequently recorded.[84-86] Decreased IgM levels were noted in half the patients studied by Goldman and Hobbs, and this appeared to be associated with advanced stage.[84] Although splenectomy was not implicated in this series, Steidle noted a consistent reduction of IgM following splenectomy.[87] Normal and increased levels of IgM have also been recorded.[76,78,86] IgD levels have been reported to be reduced,[84] normal,[78] or elevated.[88] Increased levels of IgE have been noted,[89-91] although the relationship of this increase to the incidence of atopy is controversial.[89,91] Amlot and Green relate the presence of atopy to certain types of clinical presentation of Hodgkin's disease and also to the effect of treatment on IgE levels.[91]

C. In Vitro Observation of Cellular Immunity

*1. Peripheral Blood Lymphocytes*

In 1914 Bunting drew attention to changes in peripheral blood cell populations in Hodgkin's disease.[92] An initial lymphocytosis and basophilia was followed by lymphopenia and eosinophilia, with late cases being characterized by neutrophil leukocytosis and monocytosis. Lymphopenia and monocytosis were similarly documented by Wiseman,[93] and subsequent records indicated lymphopenia to be a function of untreated disease, irradiation or chemotherapy,[94-96] and to bear a relationship to disease extent and activity, and survival.

Crowther et al. reported increased periodic-acid Schiff positivity of peripheral blood lymphocytes in a third of untreated patients, this figure rising to 50% in posttreatment samples. This finding showed no correlation with delayed hypersensitivity skin test reactivity.[98]

An increase in spontaneous DNA synthesis,[99-102] and an inverse correlation between spontaneous and mitogen-stimulated uptake has been noted.[101,102] Two reports have documented the prognostic significance of immunocompetence as assessed by spontaneous and mitogen-stimulated lymphocyte DNA synthesis,[102,103] and while both agree that survival is strongly correlated with immunocompetence in multifactorial analysis, the methodological approaches place different emphasis on the exact interpretation of both basal and stimulable lymphocyte response.

The above findings are consistent with in vivo lymphocyte stimulation but the mechanism and relevance of this finding in the pathogenesis of Hodgkin's disease is unclear. The correlation with survival suggests, however, the immunocompetence as determined by these assays is a risk factor in discriminant analysis of prognosis.

Analysis of B and T lymphocyte populations in peripheral blood has not shown marked differences from normal distribution patterns,[104-109] although a reduction of T cells in untreated disease[110] and in advanced disease are recorded,[111] particularly when expressed in absolute values. Treatment reduces both the proportion and absolute numbers of circulating T cells,[105-107] but this has been reported to normalize in patients achieving durable remission.[111] Romagnani et al. have reported a decrease in E rosette receptor positive lymphocytes [E.R.+] expressing receptors for IgM (T$\mu$), with an increase in E. R. + IgG (T$\gamma$) lymphocytes implying a functional imbalance of helper to suppressor T cell ratio.[112] An aberrant ratio of T$\mu$:T$\gamma$ has also been noted by Gupta et al.[113] This result has not been confirmed using monospecific anti T-cell antibodies.[108]

*2. Tissue Lymphocyte Populations*

Detailed histological studies have shown that the earliest morphological lesion of Hodgkin's disease occurs in the paracortical areas of the lymph node and in the periarteriolar lymphoid sheath region of the spleen,[114] areas known to be T-dependent.[115]

Studies of lymphoid cell suspensions from node or spleen suffer from many complexities in their interpretation as manifest by potential selection artifacts in their preparation, expression of proportions or absolute numbers, the appropriate definition of the "normal" control, and the admixture of "involved" and "noninvolved" areas in diseased spleens. Results range from increased T cell proportions in involved spleens,[104,113,116-118] normal T cell proportions irrespective of involvement,[110] increased T cell proportions in noninvolved spleen,[119] reduced total T cell numbers irrespective of involvement,[108] an abnormally high T$\mu$T$\gamma$ ratio,[113] and a helper to suppressor ratio of 1:1 compared to 3:4:1 in blood and lymph node.[108]

While T cell proportions have generally been reported to be increased in involved lymph nodes,[100,119-122] the range of normal is wide. Subpopulation studies have indicated a predominance of helper phenotype in both suspension[108] and tissue section studies[123] (see Chapter 2).

Utilizing monoclonal reagents in an immunoperoxidase technique on tissue frozen sections, Poppema et al. have demonstrated that the majority of lymphocytes in the Hodgkin's disease lesion are T cells expressing $T_1$, $T_3$, and $T_{10}$ specificities without expression of $T_6$. Ia antigen was present on a minority of T cells and the $T_4$ (helper) phenotype was in excess of the $T_{5/8}$ (suppressor) phenotype.[123] T cells are clustered around large stellate cells bearing Ia antigen but not T or B cell surface markers or antimacrophage serum reactivity — this latter cell morphologically resembling a Reed-Sternberg (R.S.) cell.[123] Considerable attention is now being directed to the relationship between the R.S. cell and the interdigitating reticulum cell, the latter cell bearing morphological resemblance to the R.S. cell in metallophil preparations, and being ideally suited to undertake cooperative interactions with lymphocytes in T cell dependent areas of lymphoid tissue[124] (see Chapter 2).

*3. Lymphocyte Proliferation in Response to Antigen and Mitogen*

Lymphocyte proliferation assays have been employed by a number of investigators as an in vitro tool for exploring the nature of impaired immune response. Depressed recall responses have generally been recorded with vaccinia,[125] PPD[126,127] candida,[128] and tetanus toxoid.[129] The relationship of depressed responsiveness to stage of disease and in vivo parameters of immune response has not been readily apparent.

Initial studies with mitogens also indicated depressed blastoid transformation as assessed visually or by label uptake.[125,126] These studies included treated patients, thus introducing additional factors into the interpretation, as both radiation and chemotherapy are recognized to affect mitogen-induced transformation response.[100,130-136] Further studies with single dose-standard culture time assays have revealed a multiplicity of controversial findings bearing on correlation with symptoms of disease,[125,137-139] stage of disease,[125,138,140,141] activity of disease,[136-139,141] skin test reactivity,[28,125,136] histological type,[136,140] and survival and relapse risk.[140] In addition, variable effects were noted by addition of patient serum to the culture system.[125,137,139,142]

A more discrete interpretation of mitogen response has been afforded by utilization of variable dose-time assays to assess the kinetics and quantitation of PHA response.[143-145] Abnormalities of mitogen response have been demonstrated in untreated patients with limited disease[100,143,146] and also in those in long-term remission following therapy.[100,131-133,147] Correlation of response pattern to PHA with skin test anergy and lymphocyte depletion has been documented,[146] and quantitative and qualitative PHA response has been proposed as a powerful indicator of survival in Hodgkin's disease.[103]

Limited data are available on tissue leukocyte PHA response, one study indicating normal response of splenic leukocytes while lymph node leukocyte responses paralleled those of peripheral blood.[130]

Several possible mechanisms have been advanced to explain the defective mitogen response in Hodgkin's disease. Serum factors inhibiting leukocyte response to PHA have been noted.[148-150] Their relationship to clinical prognostic factors is controversial.[149-150] Although partial characterization has been undertaken, the exact nature of the relevant components remains unclear.[148,149]

Defective movement of receptors on lymphocytes from patients with Hodgkin's disease has been demonstrated as assessed by failure of con A cap formation using fluorescein-conjugated lectin.[151-153] Other studies imply that the lectin response is not a defect intrinsic to the lymphocyte, but a defect reflecting abnormal lymphocyte circulation patterns. Disparity of lectin response between peripheral blood lymphocytes, and thoracic duct[154] and splenic lymphocytes[143] has been noted, and this has generated hypotheses of defective lymphocyte traffic through the reticulo-endothelial system (ecotaxopathy) as the underlying disturbance in Hodgkin's disease.[154] The role of suppression as a mechanism of impaired lymphocyte response will be reviewed subsequently.

*4. Lymphokine Production*

Various lymphocyte-derived mediators involved in the inflammatory response have been studied. These include lymphocytotoxin,[156] macrophage migration inhibition factor (MIF),[157-158] leukocyte migration inhibition factor (LIF),[159-160] macrophage-aggregation factor (MAF),[128] interferon,[161,162] and leukocyte chemotaxis factor.[163] Serum-derived chemotactic factor inhibitors have also been described.[164] While increased basal levels with a reduced mitogen-induced increment are recorded frequently, the relationship of these observations to clinical parameters, skin test reactivity, and lectin-induced DNA synthesis is too variable for correlative interpretation.

*5. Mixed Leukocyte Reaction (MLR) and Autologous Mixed Leukocyte Reaction (AMLR)*

Stimulation and response to alloantigens have been employed in mixed leukocyte culture to assess immunological competence. Using peripheral blood leukocytes, variable deficits in stimulation capacity[165-168] and in response to alloantigens have been recorded.[145,167] Other studies demonstrate normal stimulation,[145] normal response,[169] or no evident abnormality.[170] A correlation between MLR response and delayed hypersensitivity skin test results has been noted.[17] Cell fractionation studies have subsequently been performed to further analyze the mechanism of impaired blastogenic response to mitogen or alloantigen — these studies are presented in Section II.C. 6.

The autologous MLR assesses the ability of T lymphocytes to respond to autologous non-T lymphocytes resulting in the generation of cytotoxic T cell, and also T cells associated with B cell regulation and cell-mediated immunity. While this phenomenon can be reliably demonstrated in normal individuals, Engleman et al. have shown that the AMLR is depressed in patients with Hodgkin's disease, and may be more consistently demonstrated than defects in allogeneic MLR.[172] This finding was not related to other clinical characteristics and persisted despite successful therapy. By studying the AMLR in HLA — A, B, and DR — identical siblings, one of whom had Hodgkin's disease and the other of whom was in normal health, the defect was shown to be due to a reduction of responder T cell activity rather than poor non-T cell stimulation. The reduced AMLR was unrelated to patient serum, however some contribution could be attributed to adherent cells in the stimulator population as indicated by partial amelioration of the deficit consequent on their removal.

Zarling et al. have demonstrated depressed cytotoxic T cell regeneration in allogeneic MLR in treated patients with Hodgkin's and non-Hodgkin's lymphoma.[173] Depletion of histamine-receptor-positive lymphocytes from the responding population resulted in enhanced generation of cytotoxic T cells, with the presence of a circulating histamine-receptor-positive suppressor cell in these patients being inferred.[173] Impaired PHA-induced cytotoxicity of leukocytes from patients with Hodgkin's disease has been reported previously.[174,175]

Characteristics of leukocytes derived from peripheral blood, spleen, and nodes removed from treated and untreated patients with Hodgkin's disease, have been studied in mixed leukocyte culture.[170] No abnormality of MLR was noted with peripheral blood leukocytes, however, leukocytes from histologically involved tissues demonstrated markedly depressed stimulation and response characteristics. This deficit was most pronounced in tissues demonstrating active disease after therapy. Interestingly, significant deficit was also noted in histologically normal tissues excised during staging laparotomy in patients with untreated disease. Leukocytes derived from tissues removed from patients in remission of disease demonstrated normal reactivity in MLR.

### 6. Mechanisms of Impaired Lymphocyte Reactivity

Based on the observations of impaired blastogenic responses of leukocytes from patients with Hodgkin's disease to mitogen, alloantigen (MLR), and autoantigen stimulation (AMLR), studies have been undertaken to define whether the observed defects are intrinsic to the responding lymphocyte population or are mediated through suppressor mechanisms. Such studies have usually employed selective depletion or enrichment techniques. In the author's studies, enrichment utilizing mononuclear cells from tissue cultures demonstrating impaired lymphoproliferative response in MLR has been employed to demonstrate functional suppression of blastogenesis.[170] A similar enrichment technique has been described by addition of autologous peripheral blood mononuclear cells in MLR.[176] In addition to previously mentioned uncharacterized inhibiting substances in patient serum, two mechanisms for cellular suppression of lymphocyte response have been defined.

#### a. Monocyte-Mediated Suppression

In vitro monocyte-mediated suppression has been documented in a number of animal systems and human disease states[177-184] and has been shown to contribute to depressed peripheral blood lymphoproliferative response in Hodgkin's disease.[176,185-189] Such studies have demonstrated that removal of adherent cells improves lymphoproliferative response and that partial or total amelioration of depressed lymphocyte blastogenesis can be achieved by addition of indomethacin to lymphocyte culture. Increased prostaglandin synthesis in leukocyte cultures from peripheral blood of patients with Hodgkin's disease has been documented.[188-190] Suppression of lectin-induced T lymphocyte proliferation and also B cell antibody synthesis is also apparent.[191]

Although this phenomenon is readily reproducible, the question of its in vivo relevance is germane. It is clearly dependent on monocyte density in leukocyte culture and, under circumstances of isopyknic flotation for mononuclear cell preparation, preferential monocyte enrichment appears to occur with peripheral blood from patients with Hodgkin's disease.[185,191] By adjustment of the adherent mononuclear cell density, a graded response of a superimposed MLR can be achieved, with marked suppression of blastogenesis by monocyte enrichment.[170,176,192] This phenomenon is not genetically restricted and has been described with leukocyte cultures from normal donors,[192] Hodgkin's disease patients, and from patients with other disease states, e.g., systemic lupus erythematosus.[193,194] Thus the abnormality is not specific for Hodgkin's disease and it remains to be established whether a quantitative and/or qualitative monocyte abnormality underlies in vivo expression of impaired immune response.

Interestingly, while monocyte-mediated suppression of lymphoproliferation has been consistently demonstrated in peripheral blood leukocyte culture, adherent cell depletion of tissue leukocyte cultures did not improve depressed lymphoproliferative response,[170] suggesting differing mechanisms for suppression in blood and tissue. Bukowski et al., utilizing a nylon-wool column technique have, however, demonstrated augmented lymphoproliferation in spleen cell culture.[189]

Bockman et al. have studied PHA-induced peripheral blood T cell colony formation in patients with Hodgkin's disease.[190] They note a stage-related reduction in T cell colonies, and elevated prostaglandin synthesis by mononuclear cell cultures. While prostaglandin-inhibitors caused augmentation of T cell colony formation, blockade of prostaglandin synthesis did not fully reverse the stage-dependent effect, thus suggesting mechanisms in addition to monocyte elaboration of prostaglandin E.

### b. Lymphocyte-Mediated Suppression

The evidence for lymphocyte-mediated suppression is both direct and inferential. The admixture experiments of Hillinger et al. indicated that while monocyte-mediated suppression was apparent in certain cultures, in other experiments abrogation of impaired lymphoproliferation was achieved by selective T cell depletion.[176] Lymphocyte-mediated suppression has been inferred by the failure of indomethacin to reverse impaired PHA-induced blastogenesis,[191] and by the failure of adherent cell depletion to reverse the reduced MLR noted with leukocytes from involved tissues.[170]

Activation of suppressor cells with con A was normal in monocyte-depleted leukocyte cultures from patients with Hodgkin's disease;[191] however Schulof et al. have indicated deficient con A suppressor activity in one-third of patients studied.[195] The role of monocyte-mediated suppression in the latter study is unclear.

A histamine-receptor-positive mononuclear cell giving rise to suppression of cytotoxic effector cell generation in MLR has been described.[173] While this cell was reportedly not a macrophage, its exact characterization was not defined.

A functional T cell defect is implied in the MLR[196] and AMLR[172] studies of Engleman et al. in which impaired lymphoproliferation could not be reversed by adherent cell depletion, and purified T cell response of a histoidentical sibling to patient non-T cell was normal in comparison to an impaired response with patient purified T cells.[172]

### 7. Natural Killing (NK) and Antibody-Dependent Cellular Cytotoxicity (ADCC)

Gupta et al. have studied peripheral blood T cell and non-T cell spontaneous (NK) and ADCC in patients with Hodgkin's disease.[197] No abnormality of spontaneous (NK) or ADCC was noted with purified non-T cell populations, however T cell spontaneous and ADCC were abnormal in the majority of patients, although in a manner unrelated to known clinical prognostic factors. In related studies the same authors noted increased proportions of T$\gamma$ (suppressor) lymphocytes in peripheral blood leukocyte populations compared to spleen where T$\mu$ (helper) populations were in excess. Despite the increased proportion of T$\gamma$ cells in peripheral blood and the demonstration that T$\gamma$ cells are the effector cells of spontaneous and ADCC, no correlation was observed between the two parameters.[197]

### 8. Macrophage Function

Increased macrophage clearance of radiolabeled aggregated albumin has been demonstrated in patients with Hodgkin's disease and this correlates with advanced stage, symptoms of disease, and remission of disease activity.[198] Increased monocyte glucose metabolism reflected by Krebs cycle activity, glycolysis, and hexose monophosphate shunt activity is seen in male patients with lymphoma,[199] and an increased uptake and killing of facultative intracellular organisms has been described.[200,201]

Macrophage augmentation of lymphocyte PHA response has been studied using adherent cells from patients with Wiskott-Aldrich Syndrome (WAS) and Hodgkin's disease. In these experiments, the deficient PHA response of purified normal lymphocyte populations could be restored with WAS or Hodgkin's disease monocytes, but normal monocytes could not restore PHA reactivity to purified lymphocytes from purified lymphocytes from WAS or Hodgkin's disease patients.[202]

The possibility of a monocyte:macrophage as the underlying "malignant" cell of Hodgkin's disease has been inferred by two sets of observations — first, the in vitro studies indicating monocyte-mediated suppression of mitogen or alloantigen-induced lymphoproliferation[176,185-189] and second, the tissue culture studies indicating the growth of a cell line from Hodgkin's tissue having the characteristics of a macrophage.[202] This interpretation is now further complicated by the recognition of subtypes of histiocytic cells, some of which appear to be structural or phagocytic, while others appear to serve immunoregulatory function in B and T cell-dependent areas in tissue.[204] Attention is now being focused on the interdigitating reticulum cell in the T-dependent areas of reticuloendothelial tissue as the Reed-Sternberg or classical pathognomonic cell of Hodgkin's disease, however, it is not clear that this cell has been described in the previously mentioned tissue culture studies.

*9. In Vitro Antibody Synthesis*

Longmire et al. noted increased basal and stimulated immunoglobulin synthesis from known volumes of leukocyte suspension from involved or noninvolved spleens from patients with Hodgkin's disease.[205] The mechanism of increased production incorporated both an increased cellular synthesis in small or minimally involved spleens, compared with an increased net synthesis due to splenomegaly with gross disease.

Immunoglobulin synthesis in response to stimulation with pokeweed mitogen is decreased in Hodgkin's disease peripheral blood mononuclear cells. Mononuclear cells from patients with Hodgkin's disease depressed mitogen-induced Ig synthesis by normal mononuclear cells suggesting the presence of suppressor cells in Hodgkin's disease leukocyte populations. Removal of adherent cells increased the mitogen-induced Ig response in patient mononuclear cell populations, and also alleviated the suppression in admixture experiments with normal leukocyte populations.[191]

*10. Other Factors*

Several serum factors of potential relevance in in vitro immunological assay have been studied. These include complement, immune complexes, PHA-binding substances, lymphocytoxins, and ferritin. Their role, and the interpretation of the observed phenomena, is conjectural at present and they will not be discussed further.

The preceding evidence derived from clinical observation and in vitro data clearly imply that impaired cellular immunity is a feature of untreated Hodgkin's disease. It appears disproportionate to the degree of illness, being more profound than the deficit noted with other advanced malignancies. Furthermore, it is curious that the abnormalities are not reversed by successful therapy if they are assumed to be a feature of disease activity. This raises the question of the immunodeficiency being a state underlying the development of Hodgkin's disease. There is no evidence to support this argument other than the anecdotal observation of Jones et al.,[75] and the in vitro data indicating abnormal MLR reactivity in morphologically normal tissues removed from untreated patients undergoing staging investigations.[170] Either model of Hodgkin's disease — an underlying immunodeficiency state giving rise to a malignancy, or a malignancy giving rise to an immunodeficiency state — by analogy, with experience accrued from patients with primary or acquired immunodeficiency, would carry implications in terms of associated autoimmune disorders and an increased risk of subsequent malignancy. Accordingly, the information pertinent to these two points will now be discussed.

## III. HODGKIN'S DISEASE, AUTOIMMUNITY, AND NEPHROSIS

Fudenberg et al. have drawn attention to the association between human genetically determined immunodeficiency (adult onset hypogammaglobulinemia) and autoimmune phenomena,[206,207] and the subsequent development of lymphoma. The evidence for immunodeficiency being a feature of Hodgkin's disease has been discussed. Attention is now directed to the association of autoimmune phenomena and lymphoma, and immunodeficiency and the subsequent development of neoplasia, particularly lymphoma. This is discussed in terms of the association of both conditions with Hodgkin's disease, a condition accompanied by immunodeficiency.

## A. Autoimmune Disease

### 1. Systemic Lupus Erythematosus (SLE)

Approximately 20 cases of SLE preceding, occurring simultaneously with, or following the diagnosis of lymphoma are recorded. The majority of reports describe non-Hodgkin's rather than Hodgkin's lymphoma and detail lymphoma evolving up to 15 years (median 4 years) after the onset of SLE. However, four cases of simultaneous development and two cases of lymphoma preceding SLE are noted.[208-214]

The reports are quite heterogeneous, however, two points are noteworthy. Frequently the manifestations of SLE are protean and include ITP and nephrotic syndrome and respond variably to steroids and/or azathioprine. There appears to be a correlation between exacerbation of SLE and the presence of adenopathy demonstrated to be lymphoma. More striking is the often reported complete remission of both diseases when effective treatment for lymphoma is offered — this including regional irradiation. In fact, the use of combination chemotherapy for SLE in the absence of lymphoma has been discussed based on complete clinical and serological control of chronic active disease in a patient treated with chemotherapy following diagnosis of lymphoma.[214]

Although the number of case associations of lymphoma and SLE would not preclude coincidence, the relationship between the two diseases is of interest. Hodgkin's disease is associated with other autoimmune phenomena, and frequently the activity of the lymphoma and autoimmune disease bear a striking temporal relationship. The relationship between genetically determined immunodeficiency, viral infection autoimmunity, and malignancy has been noted in New Zealand black mice[215,216] and Aleutian mink disease.[217] Immune deficiency in terms of delayed hypersensitivity response, and in vitro measurements of T and B cell function have been recorded in SLE, some studies indicating aberrant suppressor T cell function,[218,219] while others note monocyte-mediated[220,221] and serum factor inhibition of lymphocyte function.[222]

The role of a virus in the etiology of SLE has been discussed by Schwartz both for a canine model and for human disease, and evidence brought forward for a role of a C-type RNA virus, in association with a preexisting genetic predisposition or state of aberrant immunological regulation.[223]

Two studies discuss the development of malignancy in patients with SLE, or similar disorders requiring therapeutic immunosuppression. In Penn's series, 70 such patients were identified and 28% of the tumors were lymphomas.[224] Canoso et al. reported 8 of 70 patients with SLE developing malignancies after a median interval of 6 years and 8 months.[225] The malignancies recorded were lymphoma (two), skin carcinoma (one), and five cases of carcinoma of the cervix. The role of steroids and other immunosuppressives in the development of malignancy in addition to any preexisting immunological due to SLE is impossible to define.

### 2. Sjögren's Syndrome

The association between Sjögren's syndrome and lymphoreticular disorders is well described.[226-230] Most commonly reticulum cell sarcoma, Waldenstrom's macroglobulinemia, and pseudolymphoma are reported following an initial diagnosis of Sjögren's syndrome. Hodgkin's disease has been recorded during the course of Sjögren's syndrome and, more recently, Sjögren's syndrome and pseudolymphoma have been recorded 13 years after successful treatment for Hodgkin's disease.[227] Features characterizing the case reports include an unusual degree of persistent or recurrent lymphadenopathy, splenomegaly, lymphopenia, purpura or vasculitis, and gammopathy.

*3. Dermatomyositis*

Approximately 15 to 34% of cases of dermatomyositis are associated with an underlying malignancy.[231,232] The most common sites recorded are stomach, breast, lung, ovary, lymphoma, and leukemia. In 80% of cases, dermatomyositis precedes the diagnosis of malignancy.

Polymyositis is recorded in association with Hodgkin's disease.[233,234] One case report documents Hodgkin's disease, Coomb's-positive autoimmune hemolytic anemia, and dermatomyositis occurring during remission of Hodgkin's disease; it should be noted, however, that recurrent Hodgkin's disease was apparent 22 months later.[234]

In general terms, there appears to be no correlation between the severity of the myositis and the extent of malignancy. Improvement of the myositis, however, is contingent upon control of the associated tumor. The mechanism underlying the association of the two diseases is unknown.

*4. Immune Thrombocytopenic Purpura (ITP)*

The association of Hodgkin's disease and ITP is well recorded, although to date, only 27 well-documented cases exist in the literature.[223,235-242] The diagnosis of ITP has not been uniformly stringent and in many cases it cannot be considered idiopathic but should rather be considered immune; in most cases, however, thrombocytopenia has existed in the presence of normal numbers of megakaryocytes in the bone marrow and in the absence of splenomegaly. Some authors have demonstrated an absence of disseminated intravascular coagulation, and a shortened survival of transferred homologous platelets. One report indicates high levels of platelet-associated IgG prior to, and in greater amount, following splenectomy.[240] The mechanism of immune-mediated thrombocytopenia in this study was unclear — the levels of platelet-associated IgG in the patient being greatly in excess of those measured in patients with Hodgkin's disease without thrombocytopenia, and in normal controls or patients with primary ITP. The authors favored a mechanism involving phagocytosis of immune complexes, based on similar platelet asociated IgG levels in diseases associated with circulating immune complexes, e.g., SLE, however, they could not exclude the possibility of a platelet autoantibody, or an antibody response to a tenaciously absorbed antigen. Further studies on the specificity of such antibodies are required.

The spectrum of clinical features surrounding the association of Hodgkin's disease and ITP is broad. ITP more commonly occurred in patients previously treated for Hodgkin's disease, although in five cases the diagnosis either preceded, or was made concurrently with, the diagnosis of Hodgkin's disease. Males were more commonly affected than females, in contradistinction to primary ITP. No specific histologic subtype was incriminated although an association with lymphocyte predominant disease has not been recorded. All ages including adolescents were represented and, where recorded, all stage IA to IVB were represented. The mean interval from the diagnosis of Hodgkin's disease to ITP was 52 months (range 1 month to 12 years). Platelet counts were most commonly ≤ 10,000/mm³. In approximately half the patients, Hodgkin's disease was active when ITP was diagnosed. The remainder were in complete remission of disease with follow-up durations of 3 to 120 months. The majority of patients developing ITP following a diagnosis of Hodgkin's disease had undergone splenectomy as a staging procedure. Concurrent autoimmune hemolytic anemia or positive Coomb's test was occasionally recorded.

In terms of response of ITP to therapy, certain features of clinical relevance can be defined. Those patients in whom ITP occurred during remission of Hodgkin's disease and who had a previous splenectomy, had a high response rate with corticosteroids. Those with active Hodgkin's disease or those with an intact spleen did not respond to steroids, even when that organ showed no evidence of active Hodgkin's disease. Patients failing to respond to steroids often responded following splenectomy, even when active disease was evident at sites other than the spleen.[239,241]

In practical terms, the occurrence of ITP in a patient with Hodgkin's disease does not necessarily mean that relapse of Hodgkin's disease has occurred,[238] however, all attempts must be made to demonstrate that complete remission continues. Furthermore, the presence of ITP does not carry an adverse prognostic implication. Palpable lymphadenopathy per se is insufficient for a diagnosis of relapse, as biopsies have demonstrated benign lymphoid hyperplasia.[238] Furthermore, thrombocytopenia may occur with nodal relapse in previously splenectomized patients.[236]

The mechanism of thrombocytopenia is unclear. Hypersplenism can rarely be invoked and, where measured, antibodies to platelets have not usually been identified. The possibility of viral infection as a possible etiologic factor has been raised.[242]

### 5. Autoimmune Hemolytic Anemia (AIHA)

AIHA occurring in adults is associated with malignancy in approximately 50 to 60, of cases and reticuloendothelial malignancy is particularly associated with this complication. A Coomb's-positive hemolytic anemia occurs in appoximately 1 to 3.0% of patients with Hodgkin's disease.[243-247] AIHA may rarely antedate the diagnosis of lymphoma,[248-250] both sexes are affected, there is no age predilection, all histological subtypes other than lymphocyte depletion are recorded, and all stages are represented. The association of AIHA with ITP either coincident or temporarily unrelated, has been recorded in patients with Hodgkin's disease. Measured hemoglobin has usually been 90 g/$\ell$ or less. The antibody is usually a warm or gamma Coomb's-positive type, although cold antibodies have been recorded. Splenomegaly has variably been present but the enlarged spleen has not necessarily been involved by Hodgkin's disease.[247] Furthermore, while splenectomy or splenic irradiation (either with or without steroids) has usually been beneficial, response has also been noted with abdominal radiation not encompassing the spleen.

In the majority of cases, AIHA has occurred at times of activity of Hodgkin's disease, either at initial presentation or at subsequent relapse. It has not been considered an adverse prognostic factor, but its amelioration has been dependent on control of the lymphoma. AIHA has persisted in the presence of active Hodgkin's disease despite prior splenectomy.

### 6. Autoimmune Neutropenia

Neutropenia in a patient presenting with Hodgkin's disease without evidence of splenomegaly or bone marrow infiltration has been noted by Hunter et al.[251] Serum granulocyte-binding antibodies were assessed by two methods and were shown to be elevated in the patient's serum, but not in serum from patients with Hodgkin's disease without neutropenia. The antibody was directed at both patient and normal donor granulocytes. Prompt resolution of the granulocytopenia was evident with steroid administration, and remission of both neutropenia and Hodgkin's disease was achieved with systemic therapy.

## B. The Nephrotic Syndrome and Hodgkin's Disease

Nephritis or nephrosis as a manifestation of immune complex disease is well recognized, hence the association of the nephrotic syndrome and Hodgkin's disease has provided additional stimulus for the belief that immunological aberrations are a component of the etiology or pathogenesis of Hodgkin's disease. The nephrotic syndrome is but one of the renal complications of lymphoma,[252] and it may result from a number of causes including renal vein thrombosis, renal vein obstruction by adenopathy[253] amyloidosis, as well as by immunological phenomena.

Nephrotic syndrome has been reported in association with both age peaks for Hodgkin's disease. It is more common in males than females, and mixed cellularity is the most frequent histological type. The syndrome bears a close temporal relationship to the activity of the lymphoma, either preceding or occurring simultaneously with the diagnosis of lymphoma, remitting with control of disease, and recurring with subsequent relapse of lymphoma. It may be manifest with discrete adenopathy remote from the kidneys and may be controlled with localized irradiation therapy to remote nodal sites,[254,255] or even surgical excision of adenopathy.[256]

The interest for an immunological basis for development of nephrosis is based upon:

1. The temporal relationship with disease activity despite spatial separation between the involved nodal areas and the kidneys and subsequently applied localized therapy.[256-260]
2. The association between membranous nephropathy and immune complex deposition noted in disease such as systemic lupus erythematosus. Immune complexes have been demonstrated in the serum of patients with Hodgkin's disease.
3. The demonstration of immune-complex-mediated nephropathy in other malignancies and, more particularly, the demonstration of tumor-associated antigen within the immune complex.[261,262]

However, the association is not as straightforward in Hodgkin's disease. Several articles have collated the data pertinent to renal biopsy findings in patients with nephrosis and Hodgkin's disease.[263-267] Some 46 case reports are available and 17 have information regarding the light, electron, and immunofluorescent microscopy.[266] In approximately three-quarters of the reports, the renal lesion is of the minimal change (lipoid nephrosis) type with no evidence of amyloid or immune complex deposition. A proliferative glomerulonephritis with subepithelial deposition of electron-dense deposits and positive staining for immunoglobulin is rare, but has been recorded.

The lipoid nephrosis associated with Hodgkin's disease has been typical of that occurring in the absence of lymphoma. The proteinuria is highly selective, the light microscopic changes minimal, and the electron microscopic changes indicate effacement of epithelial cell foot-processes. The glomerular basement membrane appears normal and there is no deposition of electron-dense material. Furthermore the nephrosis has resolved rapidly with either radiation or chemotherapy, the latter usually incorporating corticosteroids.

The etiology of minimal change or lipoid nephrosis is unclear. Although immune complexes are not demonstrable in the glomerulus, several investigators have demonstrated their presence in the serum of patients with lipoid nephrosis by a variety of techniques.[268-270] It has been questioned whether the molecular size of the complex or the ability to bind complement affects the renal manifestation of disorders characterized by circulating immune complexes.[270] Other mechanisms that have been advanced include lymphocytotoxins,[271] lymphocyte response to fetal kidney antigens,[272] and a lymphokine demonstrated by culture of lymphocytes from patients with lipoid nephrosis that mediates increased vascular permeability.[273]

An hypothesis to unify these observations into an immunological mechanism has been proposed.[274] A T cell disorder supposedly results in lymphokine production which affects the competence of an "immunologically innocent" basement membrane. Ancillary support for the existence of a T cell disorder is provided by the susceptibility to pneumococcal and other bacterial infections, remission induced by measles, and the therapeutic benefits of steroids and immunosuppressive agents. The existence of lipoid nephrosis with Hodgkin's disease, a disorder associated with demonstrable abnormalities of T lymphocyte function, is cited as additional supportive evidence.

## IV. HODGKIN'S DISEASE, IMMUNODEFICIENCY STATES, AND MALIGNANCY

### A. Immunodeficiency States and Malignancy

#### 1. Primary Immunodeficiency States

The cancer mortality for patients with primary immunodeficiency syndromes has been reported to be 100-fold greater than that prevailing for the general population.[275]

Spector et al. have identified 227 patients with malignancy arising in association with genetically determined immunodeficiency states.[276] Lymphoreticular tumors constituted over 50% of the total malignancies, being the most common tumors in all but IgA-deficiency and X-linked hypogammaglobulinemia. By comparison with age-matched population mortality statistics, deaths due to lymphoreticular neoplasms were greatly in excess. Although all types of lymphoma including Hodgkin's disease were recorded, by representation with the distribution of lymphoma in the general population of similar age, histiocytic lymphomas were greatly over-represented compared with other types of lymphoma.

#### 2. Acquired Immunodeficiency States

Patients undergoing organ transplantation are subjected to therapeutic immunosuppression to optimize engraftment of the donor organ. Penn has documented 31 patients developing a malignancy in a population of 556 recipients of a renal transplant. This incidence of 5.6% is approximately 100-fold greater than the incidence in the general population, a figure similar to that noted in primary immunodeficiency states.[277] The Denver Transplant Tumor Registry has provided data on 357 patients developing 375 tumors following organ transplantation.[278] Cancer of the skin and lip occurred most frequently (39%), followed by lymphoreticular malignancies (26%), and a variety of epithelial carcinomas. Leukemias and soft tissue sarcomas were infrequent, although 11 cases of Kaposi's sarcoma were recorded, but classified within lymphoreticular malignancies. Of the solid lymphomas, the majority (71%) were of reticulum cell sarcoma type (including histiocytic lymphoma, immunoblastic sarcoma, and cerebral microgliomata. Only one case of Hodgkin's disease was recorded.

Lymphomas following transplantation tended to occur in younger patients, and to occur sooner following transplantation than nonlymphomatous tumors (23 vs. 35 months). Approximately half the patients with lymphoma had disseminated disease, and of the remaining half with localized lymphoma, over 50% occurred within the central nervous system.

No clear relationship was apparent between the development of lymphoma and the type of immunosuppressive agents(s) employed.

Although lymphoma of donor origin has been recorded in animal transplantation experiments, in the three cases appropriately studied in human transplantation the lymphomas were of host origin.

Further evidence in this system of immune manipulation modifying the behavior of a transplanted neoplasm derives from the regression of graft-acquired metastases following cessation of immunosuppressive therapy,[279,280] and also the development of fatal metastases acquired from the donor organ following successful engraftment.[281,282]

Several hypotheses have been advanced to account for the predisposition for malignant lymphoreticular tumors in immunodeficiency states, which are discussed below.

#### a. The Existence of Intrinsic Defects in Lymphoid Cells

Lymphocytes from patients with ataxia-telangiectasia have demonstrable chromosomal instability with translocation, breakage, and deletion defect. Attention has been drawn to translocation involving chromosome 14 in this disorder.[283]

This is particularly relevant with regard to the expanding body of evidence indicating translocations involving chromosome 14 to be frequently associated with non-Hodgkin's lymphoma for both Burkitt and non-Burkitt type (Rowley,[284] Reeves[285]), T cell lymphoma (see Chapter 6), and with a lower frequency in Hodgkin's disease (Rowley[286]). They are also noted with B cell acute lymphoblastic leukemia (Rowley[287]) and multiple myeloma (Liang[288]). This would support the hypothesis that aberrations involving chromosome 14 provide a proliferative advantage for lymphoid cells.[283] It is noteworthy that translocations noted in Burkitt lymphoma (8;14, 2;8, and 8;22) involve chromosomes upon which immunoglobulin genes are located. That such translocations may be relevant to cellular transformation is supported by the expression of a novel oncogene following a DNA rearrangement involving chromosome 8 in the murine plasmacytoma system.[289]

DNA repair has also been shown to be impaired in patients with ataxia-telangiectasia.[290] A similar defect in fibroblasts has been noted in xeroderma pigmentosum, a genetically determined disorder associated with a predisposition to skin cancer.[291]

### b. The Role of Exogenous or Endogenous Viruses

Immunologically compromised individuals have a greater susceptibility to viral infections. BK virus (a papovavirus) has been demonstrated in the urine of renal transplant patients; it is implicated in the development of multifocal leukoencephalopathy, and a similar virus has been isolated from a cerebral lymphoma in a patient with Wiskott-Aldrich Syndrome.[292] A type C RNA virus plays some role in the autoimmune disease developing in New Zealand black mice, a disease state characterized by the subsequent development of lymphoma, and has been implicated in the canine homologue of systemic lupus erythematosus.

Although a viral etiology for human neoplasia is far from established, it is notable that the viral infections commonly seen in immunosuppressed individuals are associated with E-B virus, herpes, and polyoma viruses. These viruses are considered potentially oncogenic, herpes virus being associated with lymphomas in primates, and cervical carcinomas in humans, and E-B virus being implicated in African Burkitt's lymphoma and nasopharyngeal carcinoma.

### c. Impaired Immunoregulation

The immune system is characterized by regulatory circuits which govern its normal functioning. Examples of perturbed immunoregulation characterized by lymphoproliferation, autoimmune phenomena, and subsequent lymphoma are seen in New Zealand black mice,[215,216] Aleutian mink disease,[217] and Allogeneic disease.[293] All three demonstrate some overlap of genetic, viral, and immunologic factors in the pathogenesis of disease, and it is unclear whether a disturbance of immunoregulation leads to lymphoproliferation and thus an increased risk of lymphoma or whether activation of latent viruses occurs as a result of immunological aberration. In NZB mice the incidence of lymphoma is increased when therapeutic immunosuppression with azathioprine is used to control the immune complex nephritis.[216] In this system, a defect in suppressor T cell function has been described. In Aleutian mink disease a virus has been implicated, and the autoimmune phenomena and lymphoproliferation in this disease are believed to result from a persistent host antiviral immune response. Of further interest is that susceptibility of mink to the disease, the severity of the renal lesions, the time of death, and the mortality, are all considerably greater in those animals with aa (Chediak-Higashi syndrome genotype) compared with the heterozygote aA or AA genotypes.[217] Furthermore, immunosuppression may prevent the development of the disease syndromes.

*d. Chronic Antigen Stimulation*

Chronic stimulation with foreign antigens may give rise to a high incidence of lymphoma. Whether this occurs by stimulation of latent viruses or by induced lymphoproliferation and subsequent neoplasia is unknown. Consistent with this theory would be the high incidence of "immunoblastic" malignancies in individuals with immunodeficiency.

The alternatively proposed mechanism to account for the development of malignancy in immunodeficient individuals is the "failure of immune surveillance" theory. Although such a theory is plausible it would fail to account for the high incidence of lymphomas compared with all other possible malignancies, and it would not explain why immunodeficient individuals get one malignancy rather than multiple diseases.

B. Hodgkin's Disease and Malignancy

The occurrence of other malignant tumors in patients with Hodgkin's disease is a topic that has assumed considerable importance in the past decade. However, a key point is to what extent Hodgkin's disease is itself a predisposing factor to the development of malignancy, and is this predisposition altered either by intensity of treatment or treatment-induced longevity?

In 1957, Moertel and Hagedorn reviewed the world literature and the Mayo Clinic experience of coexistent primary malignancies occurring in patients with lymphoma and leukemia.[294] They found 13 reported instances of coexistent Hodgkin's disease and other malignancies [Kaposi's sarcoma (6), skin (2), lung (2), larynx (1), melanoma (1), and myeloma (1)]. From the 10-year Mayo experience (January 1944 to December 1953) they identified 13 clinical cases of coexisting malignancy from a total of 826 patients with Hodgkin's disease (1.6%). This figure increased to 5.4% if necropsy data were included. Two additional cases of Kaposi's sarcoma were identified in the Mayo series. Several points should be noted in this study — coexistent malignancies included those diagnosed before, concurrent with, and following the diagnosis of lymphoma; the average age at diagnosis of lymphoma was 57 years; the series was selected; and no adequate control group was studied in parallel to allow a comparison of incidence.

Razis et al. reported other malignant neoplasms in 2.2% of their Hodgkin's disease patients (24 cases in 1102 patients).[295] No note was made as to the inclusion of lesions antedating Hodgkin's disease or autopsy data, documenting incidental malignancies. In this report, two cases of Kaposi's sarcoma were documented, and also two patients with subsequent acute leukemia (2 of 1102, 0.18%). In addition, two patients with Hodgkin's disease had necropsy findings indicating reticulum cell sarcoma.

Berg reported data from Memorial Hospital in 1967 confining his study to those cancers diagnosed after registration of lymphoma and excluding those detected consequent on care for lymphoma and those found incidentally at autopsy.[296] Twelve later clinical cancers were detected in 1028 patients with Hodgkin's disease with 3117 patient-years at risk. Three *in situ* and four autopsy cancers were recorded. Kaposi's sarcoma accounted for two of the malignancies. The excess risk for skin cancer was five times greater than expected using age-adjusted New York state figures as an approximate control. There was no excess risk for any other malignancy.

These three studies discuss second cancer incidence in the period from 1944 to 1962 — an era antedating the routine use of extended and prophylactic irradiation fields and the introduction of combination chemotherapy. The median survival for patients treated during this period was approximately 3 years. The association with Kaposi's sarcoma is clearly evident, and an excess risk for skin cancer is documented. However there was no excess risk for any other solid malignancy, and the development of leukemia was a rare event. Put in perspective with the primary immunodeficiency states, the risk for subsequent neoplasia appears less and the type of malignancy is different in patients with Hodgkin's disease; however, the age spectra are quite different. In comparison with organ transplantation data, again the risk of subsequent malignancy is much less in patients with Hodgkin's disease; however, both Kaposi's sarcoma and skin cancer are recorded in excess of the expected rate in both circumstances. The average period to development of malignancy in the transplant group was 35 months for nonlymphomatous tumors and 23 months for lymphomas, a time period within the median survival for patients with Hodgkin's disease studied between 1944 to 1962.

Following the use of intensive radiation therapy and chemotherapy, attention has focused on an apparent excess risk of second malignancy in patients successfully treated for Hodgkin's disease.

Arseneau et al. reported 12 of 425 patients developing second malignancies, a ratio of 3.5:1, observed to expected.[297] Within the subgroups designated by type of therapy a greatly increased ratio of 29:1, observed to expected, was demonstrated for 35 patients undergoing intensive irradiation and chemotherapy. This study was subsequently expanded and a ratio of 1.6:1, observed to expected, was given for patients receiving no intensive therapy (2 malignancies in 131 patients).[298] O/E ratios of 3.8:1 and 4.0:1 were noted for intensive radiation and intensive chemotherapy, respectively. The highest figures were noted for combined intensive therapy (6.3:1), and for combined therapy occurring around an intervening relapse of disease (18.4:1).[301] Two patients in the latter report developed acute myeloid leukemia, a situation recorded rarely prior to intensive therapy. In 1977, the Stanford group reported an actuarial probability of developing leukemia at 5 and 7 years of 1.5 and 2.0% for 680 patients treated intensively between 1968 and 1975, the actuarial survival for this group being approximately 80% at 7 years.[299] The 7-year risk figures were 3.9% ($\pm$ 1.5) for combined therapy; 3.2% ($\pm$ 1.6) when used in adjuvant mode; and 4.7% ($\pm$ 2.7) when applied for salvage. These figures represented an observed to expected ratio for development of leukemia of 1333 for patients treated with intensive radiation and chemotherapy. An update of this study has now put the 9-year actuarial leukemia risk as high as 17.6 $\pm$ 12.1%.[300] This group has also reported six patients treated with radiation and chemotherapy for Hodgkin's disease who developed a non-Hodgkin's lymphoma at a time when the primary disease was quiescent.[301] The actuarial risk for development of a second lymphoma was 4.4% at 10 years, a figure comparable to the risk of development of leukemia.

The risk of leukemia has been discussed in terms of the role of prior splenectomy, the role of irradiation and the types of tumor associated with radiation therapy, the influence of type of chemotherapy and the implication of nitrogen mustard as the principal offender,[302,303] and the importance of age at the time of treatment.[304]

It seems likely that Hodgkin's disease per se is a situation associated with a risk of second malignancy. The magnitude of risk can only be inferred as there can never be an untreated control group to derive accurate data. Furthermore the risk, as assessed in a group from the preintensive treatment era, cannot be used reliably for comparison with patients receiving current therapy as survival characteristics are quite different. However, given current 5-year actuarial risks in excess at 5%, it appears that intensive therapy has increased the risk of developing a subsequent malignancy, and in certain subgroups this increase may be very substantial as indicated by the figures of 20.3% ($\pm$ 6.4) and 32.5% for 7-year actuarial leukemia risk for patients over 40 years of age treated with chemotherapy or combined irradiation and chemotherapy, respectively.[304]

## V. CONCLUDING REMARKS

Considerable emphasis has been placed on the immunodeficiency state characterizing Hodgkin's disease. At the clinical level, immunodeficiency has been expressed in a number of ways — susceptibilty to infection, skin test hyporeactivity to primary and recall antigens, impaired lymphocyte transfer, delayed allograft rejection, and impaired primary antibody response. Most of these observations support the contention that a qualitative and quantitative defect in cellular immunity is present in untreated individuals with Hodgkin's disease, and that the extent of impairment appears disproportionate to the degree of illness.

The bulk of the in vitro work has been directed at assays of peripheral blood lymphocyte function. Again, in most assay systems, a qualitative and quantitative defect has been recorded. Several mechanisms (principally by means of monocyte-mediated suppression or by excessive lymphocyte-mediated suppression) have been proposed to account for the findings of impaired lymphocyte blastogenesis in response to stimulation by mitogen, antigen, or alloantigen. Monocyte:macrophage properties have been demonstrated for the cell demonstrating persistent growth in culture studies, and immunological studies on tissue have suggested identity between the interdigitating reticulum cell in the T cell zone and the Reed-Sternberg cell demonstrable in conventional histological preparations.

It is tempting to correlate the presence of immunodeficiency with the in vitro observation of suppression of lymphocyte response, and to link the phenomenon of monocyte-mediated suppression with the culture evidence for a monocytoid malignant cell, and the histochemical evidence of identity between the Reed-Sternberg cell and the reticulum cell of the T cell zone of lymphoid tissue. It is not yet clear, however, that such correlations would be correct. Furthermore, such speculation tends to focus attention on immunodeficiency and neoplasia each being a function of the same cell.

Of concern with this interpretation is the cellular pleomorphism of the diagnostic infiltrate, the failure to define a clonal cell population, and the lack of conclusive proof of the origin and the malignant nature of the Reed-Sternberg cell, the major diagnostic criterion for the presence of Hodgkin's disease in lymphoid tissue. It is also difficult to reconcile persisting immunodeficiency with sustained remission of disease if neoplasia and immune dysfunction have the same cellular origin.

The possibility exists that immune dysfunction may be a precedent for neoplasia, and hence a persisting feature following control of neoplasia. It might also represent a disturbance of regulation of immune response, perhaps as a reactive phenomenon, which is not necessarily reversed by control of the initial neoplastic event. Despite the paucity of data to support either suggestion, their consideration is relevant in relation to the recognized association of autoimmune disease, nephrosis, and malignancy, with both primary and acquired immunodeficiency states. These conditions are also features of Hodgkin's disease, an immunodeficiency state, and have thus been discussed in some detail as being representative of the spectrum of immune dysfunction in this disorder.

## REFERENCES

1. Sternberg, C., Uber eine Eigenartige unter dem bilde der Psuedoleukamie verlaufende Tuberculose des Lymphatischen Apparates, *Zeitschr F. Heilk,* 19, 21, 1898.
2. Reed, D. M., On the pathological changes in Hodgkin's disease with special reference to its relationship to tuberculosis, *Bull. Johns Hopkins Hosp.,* 10, 133, 1902.
3. Jackson, F. and Parker, H., Studies of disease of the lymphoid and myeloid tissues. V. The co-existence of tuberculosis with Hodgkin's disease and other forms of malignant lymphoma, *Am. J. Med. Sci.,* 184, 694, 1932.
4. Hoster, H. A. and Dratman, M. B., Hodgkin's disease. II, *Cancer Res.,* 8, 58, 1948.
5. Wise, N. B. and Poston, M. A., The co-existence of brucella infection and Hodgkin's disease, *JAMA,* 115, 1976, 1940.

6. Gendel, B. R., Ende, M., and Norman, S. L., Cryptococcosis — a review with special reference to apparent association with Hodgkin's disease, *Am. J. Med.,* 9, 343, 1950.
7. Benham, R. W., Cryptococci, their identification by morphology and serology, *J. Infect. Dis.,* 57, 255, 1935.
8. Collins, V. P., Gellhorn, A., and Trimble, J. R., The coincidence of cryptococcosis and diseases of the reticulo-endothelial and lymphatic systems, *Cancer,* 4, 883, 1951.
9. Zimmerman, L. E. and Rappaport, H., Occurrence of cryptococcosis in patients with malignant disease of reticulo- endothelial system, *Am. J. Clin. Pathol.,* 24, 1050, 1954.
10. Gray, M. L. and Killinger, A. H., *Listeria monocytogenes* and listeric injections, *Bacteriol. Rev.,* 30, 309, 1966.
11. Simpson, J. F., Leddy, J. P., and Hare, J. D., Listeriosis complicating lymphoma — report of four cases and interpretative review of pathogenetic factors, *Am. J. Med.,* 43, 39, 1967.
12. Louria, D. B., Hensle, T., Armstrong, D., Collins, H. S., Blevins, A., Krugman, D., and Buse, M., Listeriosis complicating malignant disease — a new association, *Ann. Intern. Med.,* 67, 261, 1967.
13. Goffinet, D., Glatstein, E. J., and Merigan, T. C., Herpes zoster-varicella infections and lymphoma, *Ann. Intern. Med.,* 76, 235, 1972.
14. Casazza, A. R., Duvall, C. P., and Carbone, P. P., Summary of infectious complications occurring in patients with Hodgkin's disease, *Cancer Res.,* 26, 1290, 1966.
15. Kauffman, C. A., Israel, K. S., Smith, J. W., White, A. C., Schwartz, J., and Brooks, G. F., Histoplasmosis in immunosuppressed patients, *Am. J. Med.,* 64, 923, 1978.
16. Rubin, E. and Zak, F. G., Pnuemocystis carinii pneumonia in the adult, *N. Engl. J. Med.,* 262, 1315, 1960.
17. White, W. F., Saxton, H. M., and Dawson, I. M. P., Pneumocystis pneumonia, *Br. Med. J.,* 2, 1327, 1961.
18. Cheever, A. W., Valsmais, M. P., and Rabson, A. S., Necrotising toxoplasmic encephalitis and herpetic pneumonia complicating treated Hodgkin's disease, *N. Engl. J. Med.,* 272, 26, 1965.
19. Connolly, C. S., Hodgkin's disease associated with *Toxopolasma gondii, Arch. Intern. Med.,* 112, 393, 1963.
20. Hutter, R. V. P., Lieberman, P. H., and Collins, H. S., Aspergillosis in a cancer hospital, *Cancer,* 17, 747, 1964.
21. Heinemann, H. S., Jensen, W. N., Cooper, W. M., and Braude, A.I., Hodgkin's disease and *Salmonella typhimurium* injection, *JAMA,* 188, 632, 1964.
22. Feld, R. and Bodey, G. P., Infections in patients with malignant lymphoma treated with combination chemotherapy, *Cancer,* 39, 1018, 1977.
23. Feld, R., Bodey, G. P., Rodriguez, V., and Luna, M., Causes of death in patients with malignant lymphoma, *Am. J. Med. Sci.,* 268, 97, 1974.
24. Parker, F., Jackson, H., Hugh, G. F., and Spies, T. D., Studies of disease of the lymphoid and myeloid tissues. IV. Skin reaction to human and avian tuberculin, *J. Immunol.,* 22, 277, 1932.
25. Steiner, P. E., Etiology of Hodgkin's disease. II. Skin reaction to avian and human tuberculin proteins in Hodgkin's disease, *Arch. Intern. Med.,* 54, 11, 1934.
26. Lamb, D., Pilney, F., Kelly, W. D., and Good, R. A., A comparative study of the incidence of anergy in patients with carcinoma, leukemia, Hodgkin's disease and other lymphomas, *J. Immunol.,* 89, 555, 1962.
27. Goasguen, J., Leblay, R., Guerin, D., LePrise, P.-Y., and Richier, J.-L., Maladie de Hodgkin: etude de l'hypersensibilite retardee de 64 malades non traites, *Semin. Hop. Paris,* 53, 219, 1977.
28. Brown, R. S., Haynes, H. A., Foley, T., Godwin, H. A., Berard, C. W., and Carbone, P. P., Hodgkin's disease — immunologic, clinical and histologic features of 50 untreated patients, *Ann. Intern. Med.,* 67, 291, 1967.
29. Aisenberg, A. C., Studies on delayed hypersensitivity in Hodgkin's disease, *J. Clin. Invest.,* 41, 1964, 1962.
30. Sokal, J. E. and Primikirios, N., The delayed skin test response in Hodgkin's disease and lymphosarcoma, *Cancer,* 14, 597, 1961.
31. Bastai, P., Ueber die Klinische bedeutung der Tuberkulin-anergie bei malignem Lymphogranulom, *Klin. Wochenschr.,* 7, 1606, 1928.
32. Kelly, W. D., Lamb, D. L., Vares, R. L., and Good, R. A., An investigation of Hodgkin's disease with respect to the problem of homotransplantation, *Ann. N. Y. Acad. Sci.,* 87, 187, 1960.
33. Levin, A. G., McDonough, E. F., Miller, D. G., and Southam, C. M., Delayed hypersensitivity response to DNFB in sick and healthy persons, *Ann. N.Y. Acad. Sci.,* 120, 400, 1964.
34. Eltringham, J. R. and Kaplan, H. S., Impaired delayed — hypersensitivity responses in 154 patients with untreated Hodgkin's disease, *Natl. Cancer Inst. Monogr.,* 36, 107, 1973.
35. Check, J. H., Damsker, J. I., Brady, L. W., and O'Neill, E. A., Effect of radiation therapy on mumps — delayed type hypersensitivity reaction in lymphoma and carcinoma patients, *Cancer,* 32, 580, 1973.

36. Schier, W. W., Cutaneous anergy and Hodgkin's disease, *N. Engl. J. Med.*, 250, 353, 1954.
37. Schier, W. W., Roth, A., Ostroff, G., and Schrift, M. H., Hodgkin's disease and immunity, *Am. J. Med.*, 20, 94, 1956.
38. Chase, M. W., Delayed-type hypersensitivity and the immunology of Hodgkin's disease, with a parallel examination of sarcoidosis, *Cancer Res.*, 26, 1097, 1966.
39. Johnson, M. W., Maibach, H. I., and Salmon, S. E., Skin reactivity in patients with cancer, impaired delayed hypersensitivity or faulty inflammatory response?, *N. Engl. J. Med.*, 284, 1255, 1971.
40. Rebuck, J. W., Monto, R. W., Monaghan, E. A., and Riddle, J. M., Potentialities of the lymphocyte, with an additional reference to its dysfunction in Hodgkin's disease, *Ann. N. Y. Acad. Sci.*, 73, 8, 1958.
41. Calciati, A. and Fazio, M., Delayed anergy in Hodgkin's disease, *Panminerva Med.*, 6, 156, 1964.
42. Fairley, G. H. and Matthias, J. G., Cortisone and skin sensitivity to tuberculin in reticuloses, *Br. Med. J.*, 2, 433, 1960.
43. Citron, K. M. and Scadding, J. G., The effect of cortisone upon the reaction of the skin to tuberculin in tuberculosis and in sarcoidosis, *Q. J. Med.*, 26, 277, 1957.
44. Heiss, L. I. and Palmer, D. L., Anergy in patients with leukocytosis, *Am. J. Med.*, 56, 323, 1974.
45. Young, R. C., Corder, M. P., Hayner, H. A., and DeVita, V. T., Delayed hypersensitivity in Hodgkin's disease, *Am. J. Med.*, 52, 63, 1972.
46. Gray, J. G. and Russell, P. S., Donor selection in human organ transplantation, *Lancet*, 2, 863, 1963.
47. Aisenberg, A. C., Studies of lymphocyte transfer reactions in Hodgkin's disease, *J. Clin. Invest.*, 44, 4, 555, 1965.
48. Shohat, B., Joshua, H., and Ben-Bassart M., Investigation of the cellular immunocompetence in chronic lymphatic leukemia and malignant lymphoma patients as assessed by the local graft versus host reaction in rats, *J. Reticuloendothel. Soc.*, 17, 276, 1974.
49. Muftuoglu, A. U. and Balkuv, S., Passive transfer of tuberculin sensitivity to patients with Hodgkin's disease, *N. Engl. J. Med.*, 277, 126, 1967.
50. Green, I. and Corso, P. F., A study of skin homografting in patients with lymphomas, *Blood*, 14, 235, 1959.
51. Miller, D. G., Lizardo, J. G., and Snyderman, R. K., Homologous and heterologous skin transplantation in patients with lymphomatous disease, *J. Natl. Cancer Inst.*, 26, 569, 1961.
52. Beilby, J. O. W., Cade, I. S., Jelliffe, A. M., Parkin, D. M., and Stewart, J. W., Prolonged survival of a bone marrow graft resulting in a blood-group chimera, *Br. Med. J.*, 1, 96, 1960.
53. Miller, D. G. and Diamond, H. D., The biological basis and clinical application of bone marrow transplantation, *Med. Clin. N. Am.*, 45, 711, 1961.
54. Kaplan, H. S. and Smithers, D. W., Auto-immunity in man and homologous disease in mice in relation to the malignant lymphomas, *Lancet*, 2, 1, 1959.
55. Sokal, J. E., Aungst, C. W., and Snyderman, M., Delay in progression of malignant lymphoma after BCG vaccination *N. Engl. J. Med.*, 291, 1226, 1974.
56. McIlvanie, S. K., Arrest of stage IVB Hodgkin's disease following combined BCG-transfer factor therapy, *Blood*, 42, 987, 1973.
57. Ng, R. P., Moran, C. J., Alexopoulos, C. G., and Bellingham, A. J., Transfer factor in Hodgkin's disease, *Lancet*, 2. 901, 1975.
58. Khan, A., Hill, J. M., MacLellan, A., Loeb, E., Hill, N. O., and Thaxton, S., Improvement in delayed hypersensitivity in Hodgkin's disease with transfer factor: lymphophoresis and cellular immune reactions of normal donors, *Cancer*, 36, 86, 1975.
59. Phillips, J., Boucheix, Cl., Pizza, G., Santorio, C., and Viza, D., Effect of in-vitro produced transfer factor on Hodgkin patients, *Br. J. Hematol.*, 38, 430, 1978.
60. Smith, R. A., Ezdinli, E., Bigley, N. J., and Han, T., Lawrence transfer factor and Hodgkin's disease, *Lancet*, 1, 434, 1973.
61. Forbus, W. D., Studies on Hodgkin's disease and its relation to infection by brucella, *Am. J. Pathol.*, 18, 745, 1942.
62. Dubin, I. N., The poverty of the immunological mechanism in patients with Hodgkin's disease, *Ann. Intern. Med.*, 27, 898, 1947.
63. Bunnell, I. L., and Furelow, M. L., Report on 10 proven cases of histoplasmosis, *Public Health Rep.*, 63, 299, 1948.
64. Gellar, W., A study of antibody formation in patients with malignant lymphomas, *J. Lab. Clin. Med.*, 42, 232, 1953.
65. Larson, D. L. and Tomlinson, L. J., Quantitative antibody studies in man. III. Antibody response in leukemia and other malignant lymphomata, *J. Clin. Invest.*, 32, 317, 1953.
66. Aisenberg, A. C. and Leskowitz, S., Antibody formation in Hodgkin's disease, *N. Engl. J. Med.*, 268, 1269, 1963.

67. Kelly, W. D., Good, R. A., Varco, R. L., and Levitt, M., The altered response to skin homografts and to delayed allergens in Hodgkin's disease, *Surg. Forum*, 9, 785, 1958.
68. Hoffman, G. T. and Rottino, A., Studies of immunologic reactions of patients with Hodgkin's disease, *Arch. Intern. Med.*, 86, 872, 1950.
69. Schier, W. W., Roth, A., Ostroff, G., and Schrifft, M. H., Hodgkin's disease and immunity, *Am. J. Med.*, 20, 94, 1956.
70. Greenwood, R., Smellie, H., Barr, M., and Cunliffe, A. C., Circulating antibodies in sarcoidosis, *Br. Med. J.*, 1, 1388, 1958.
71. Barr, M. and Fairley, G.H., Circulating antibodies in reticuloses, *Lancet*, 1, 1305, 1961.
72. Saslaw, S., Carlisle, N. H., and Bouroncle, B., Antibody responses in hemotologic patients, *Proc. Soc. Exp. Biol. Med.*, 106, 654, 1961.
73. Brown, R. S., Haynes, H. A., Foley, H. T., Godwin, H. A., Berard, C. W., and Carbone, P. P., Hodgkin's disease: immunologic, clinical and histologic features of 50 untreated patients, *Ann. Intern. Med.*, 67, 291, 1967.
74. Hersh, E. M., Kinetic approach to the study of cell-mediated immunity in Hodgkin's disease, *Natl. Cancer Inst. Monogr.*, 36, 123, 1973.
75. Jones, J. V., Peacock, D. B., Greenham, L. W., and Bullimore, J. A., Antibody production in preclinical Hodgkin's disease, *Lancet*, 1, 92, 1975.
76. DeGast, G. C., Halie, M. R., and Nieweg, H. O., Immunological responsiveness against two primary antigens in untreated patients with Hodgkin's disease, *Eur. J. Cancer*, 11, 217, 1975.
77. Fairely, G. H. and Akers, R. J., Antibodies to blood group A and B substances in reticuloses, *Br. J. Hematol.*, 8, 375, 1962.
78. Sybesma, J. P. H. B., Holtzer, J. D., Borst-Eilers, E., Moes, M., and Zegers, B. J. M., Antibody response in Hodgkin's disease and other lymphomas related to HLA antigens, immunoglobulin levels and therapy, *Vox Sang.*, 25, 254, 1973.
79. Weitzman, S. A., Aisenberg, A. C., Silber, G. R., and Smith, D. H., Impaired humoral immunity in treated Hodgkin's disease, *N. Engl. J. Med.*, 297, 245, 1977.
80. Sullivan, J. L., Ochs, H. D., Schiffman, G., Hammerschlag, M. R., Miser, J., Vichinsky, E., and Wedgewood, R. J., Immune response following splenectomy, *Lancet*, 1, 178, 1978.
81. Giebink, G. S., Foker, J. E., Kim, Y., and Schiffman, G., Serum antibody and opsonic response to vaccination with pneumonococcal capsular polysaccharide in normal and splenectomised children, *J. Infect. Dis.*, 141, 404, 1980.
82. Landesman, S. H. and Schiffman, G., Assessment of the antibody response to pneumococcal vaccine in high-risk populations, *Rev. Infect. Dis.*, Suppl. 3, 184, 1981.
83. Good, R. A., Kelly, W. D., Rotstein, J., and Varco, R. L., Hodgkin's disease and other lymphomas, *Prog. Allergy*, 6, 275, 1962.
84. Goldman, J. M. and Hobbs, J. R., The immunoglobulins in Hodgkin's disease, *Immunology*, 13, 421, 1967.
85. McKelvey, E. M. and Fahey, J. L., Immunoglobulin changes in disease, *J. Clin. Invest.*, 44, 1778, 1965.
86. Wagener, D. J. Th., Van Munster, P. J. J., and Haanen, C., The immunoglobulin in Hodgkin's disease, *Eur. J. Cancer*, 12, 683, 1976.
87. Steidle, C., Fatch-Moghadam, A., Lamerz, R., and Huhn, D., Quantitatives verhalten der Immunoglobuline bei Hodgkin-Patienten nach Splenectomie, *Blut*, 30, 331, 1975.
88. Burton, P., Guilbert, B., and Buffe, D., Deux cas de myeloma a immunoglobuline D, *Bull. Cancer (Paris)*, 53, 57, 1966.
89. Waldmann, T. A., Bull, J. M., and Bruce, R. M., Serum immunoglobin E levels in patients with neoplastic disease, *J. Immunol.*, 113, 379, 1974.
90. Thomas, M. R., Steinberg, P., Votan, M. L., and Bayne, N. K., IgE levels in Hodgkin's disease, *Ann. Allergy*, 37, 416, 1976.
91. Amlot, P. L. and Green, L. A., Atopy and immunoglobulin E concentrations in Hodgkin's disease and other lymphomas, *Br. Med. J.*, 1, 327, 1978.
92. Bunting, C. H., The blood-picture in Hodgkin's disease, 2nd Paper, *Bull. Johns Hopkins Hosp.*, 25, 173, 1914.
93. Wiseman, B. K., The blood pictures in the primary disease of the lymphatic system, their character and significance, *JAMA*, 107, 2016, 1936.
94. Aisenberg, A. C., Lymphocytopenia in Hodgkin's disease, *Blood*, 25, 1037, 1965.
95. Crowther, D., Fairley, G. H., and Sewell, R. L., The periodic acid-Schiff reaction of lymphocytes in human malignant disease, *Br. J. Hematol.*, 16, 389, 1969.
96. Swan, H. T. and Knowelden, J., Prognosis in Hodgkin's disease related to the lymphocyte count, *Br. J. Hematol.*, 21, 343, 1971.
97. Meytes, D. and Modan, B., Selected aspects of Hodgkin's disease in a whole community, *Blood*, 34, 91, 1969.

98. Crowther, D., Fairley, G. H., and Sewell, R. L., Lymphoid cellular responses in the blood after immunization in man, *J. Exp. Med.*, 129, 849, 1969.
99. Huber, C., Huber, H., Schmaltzl, F., Lederer, B., Butterich, D., and Braunsteiner, H., DNS — syntheses in Blut-lymphozyten beim malignen Lymphogranulom, *Acta Hematol.*, 44, 222, 1970.
100. Levy, R. L. and Kaplan, H. S., Impaired lymphocyte function in untreated Hodgkin's disease, *N. Engl. J. Med.*, 290, 181, 1974.
101. Shiftan, T. A., Caviles, A. P., Jr., and Mendelsohn, J., Spontaneous lymphocyte proliferation and depressed cellular immunity in Hodgkin's disease, *Clin. Exp. Immunol.*, 32, 144, 1978.
102. Wedelin, C., Björkholm, M., Holm, G., Ogenstad, S., Johansson, B., and Mellstedt, H., Lymphocyte function in untreated Hodgkin's disease: an important predictor of prognosis, *Br. J. Cancer*, 45, 70, 1982.
103. Faguet, G. B. and Davis, H. C., Survival in Hodgkin's disease: the role of immunocompetence and other major risk factors, *Blood*, 59, 938, 1982.
104. Kaur, J., Catovsky, D., Spiers, A. S. D., and Galton, D. A. G., Increase of T lymphocytes in the spleen in Hodgkin's disease, *Lancet*, 2, 800, 1974.
105. Huber, C., Michlmayr, G., Falkensamer, M., Fink, U., Zur Nedden, G., Braunsteiner, H., and Huber, H., Increased proliferation of T lymphocytes in the blood of patients with Hodgkin's disease, *Clin. Exp. Immunol.*, 21, 47, 1975.
106. Hunter, C. P., Tannenbaum, H., Churchill, W. H., Moloney, W. C., and Schur, P. H., Immunologic abnormalities in patients with malignant lymphoproliferative disease, *J. Natl. Cancer Inst.*, 58, 1185, 1977.
107. Cohnen, G., Augener, W., Konig, E., Brittinger, G., and Douglas, S. D., B lymphocytes in Hodgkin's disease, *N. Engl. J. Med.*, 288, 161, 1973.
108. Dorreen, M. S., Habeshaw, J. A., Wrigley, P. F. M., and Lister, T. A., Distribution of T lymphocyte subsets in Hodgkin's disease characterised by monoclonal antibodies, *Br. J. Cancer*, 45, 491, 1982.
109. Gupta, S., Subpopulation of human T lymphocytes. XVI. Maldistribution of T cell subsets associated with abnormal locomotion of T cells in untreated adult patients with Hodgkin's disease, *Clin. Exp. Immunol.*, 42, 186, 1980.
110. Bukowski, R. M., Noguchi, S., Hewlett, J. S., and Deodhar, S., Lymphocyte subpopulations in Hodgkin's disease, *Am. J. Clin. Pathol.*, 65, 31, 1976.
111. Swain, A. and Trounce, J. R., Rosette formation in Hodgkin's disease, *Oncology*, 30, 449, 1974.
112. Romagnani, S., Maggi, E., Biagiotti, R., Guidizi, M. G., Amadori, A., and Ricci, M., Altered proportion of the Tμ and Tγ cell subpopulations in patients with Hodgkin's disease, *Scand. J. Immunol.*, 7, 511, 1978.
113. Gupta, S. and Tan, C., Subpopulations of human T lymphocytes. XIV. Abnormality of T cell locomotion and of distribution of subpopulations of T and B lymphocytes in peripheral blood and spleen from children with untreated Hodgkin's disease. *Clin. Immunol. Immunopathol.*, 15, 133, 1980.
114. Berard, C. W., Reticuloendothelial system: an overview of neoplasia; the reticuloendothelial system, *Int. Acad. Pathol. Monogr. No. 16*, The Williams and Wilkins Co., Baltimore, 1975, 310.
115. Gowans, J. L. and Knight, E. J., The route of recirculation of lymphocytes in the rat, *Proc. R. Soc. Lond. (Biol.)*, 159, 257, 1964.
116. Belpomme, D., Joseph, R. R., Navares, L., Gerard-Marchant, R., Huchet, R., Botto, I., Grandjon, D., and Mathe, G., T lymphocytes and Reed-Sternberg cells in spleen of Hodgkin's disease, *N. Engl. J. Med.*, 291, 1417, 1974.
117. Hunter, C. P., Pinkers, G., Woodward, L., Moloney, W. C., and Churchill, W. H., Increased T lymphocytes and IgMEA — receptor lymphocytes in Hodgkin's disease spleens, *Cell Immunol.*, 31, 193, 1977.
118. Kaur, J., Spiers, A. S. D., and Galton, D. A. G., T and B lymphocytes in spleens of patients with malignant disease, *Lancet*, 1, 747, 1975.
119. Payne, S. V., Jones, D. B., Haegert, D. G., Smith, J. L., and Wright, D. H., T and B lymphocytes and Reed-Sternberg cells in Hodgkin's disease lymph nodes and spleens, *Clin. Exp. Immunol.*, 24, 280, 1976.
120. Habeshaw, J. A., Stuart, A. E., Dewar, A. E., and Young, G., IgM receptors on cells in Hodgkin's disease, *Lancet*, 1, 916, 1976.
121. Aisenberg, A. C. and Long, J. C., Lymphocyte surface characteristics in malignant lymphoma, *Am. J. Med.*, 58, 300, 1975.
122. Braylan, R. C., Jaffe, E. S., and Berard, C. W., Surface characteristics of Hodgkin's lymphoma cells, *Lancet*, 2, 1328, 1974.
123. Poppema, S., Bhan, A. K., Reinherz, E. L., Posner, M. R., and Schlossman, S. F., *In-situ* immunologic characterisation of cellular constituents in lymph nodes and spleens involved by Hodgkin's disease, *Blood*, 59, 226, 1982.

124. Kadiu, M. E., Possible origin of the Reed-Sternberg cell from an interdigitating reticulum cell, *Cancer Treat. Rep.*, 66, 601, 1982.
125. Hersh, E. M. and Oppenheim, J. J., Impaired in-vitro lymphocyte transformation in Hodgkin's disease, *N. Engl. J. Med.*, 273, 1006, 1965.
126. Aisenberg, A. C., Quantitative estimation of the reactivity of normal and Hodgkin's disease lymphocytes with thymidine-2-14C, *Nature (London)*, 4977, 1233, 1965.
127. Holm, G., Mellstedt, H., Bjorkholm, M., Johansson, B., Killander, D., Sundblad, R., and Soderberg, G., Lymphocyte abnormalities in untreated patients with Hodgkin's disease, *Cancer*, 37, 751, 1976.
128. Gotoff, S. P., Lolekha, S., Lopata, M., Kopp, J., Kopp, R. I., and Malecki, T. J., The macrophage aggregation assay for cell-mediated immunity in mass studies of patients with Hodgkin's disease and sarcoidosis, *J. Lab. Clin. Med.*, 82, 682, 1973.
129. Fuks, Z., Strober, S., and Kaplan, H. S., Interaction between serum factors and T lymphocytes in Hodgkin's disease, *N. Engl. J. Med.*, 295, 1273, 1976.
130. Millard, R.E., Effect of previous irradiation on the transformation of blood lymphocytes, *J. Clin. Pathol.*, 18, 783, 1965.
131. Fuks, Z., Strober, S., Bobrove, A. M., Sasazuki, T., McMichael, A., and Kaplan, H. S., Long term effects of radiation on T and B lymphocytes in peripheral blood of patients with Hodgkins disease, *J. Clin. Invest.*, 58, 803, 1976.
132. Stjernsward, J., Jonadal, M., Vanky, F., Wigzell, H., and Sealy, R., Lymphopenia and change in distribution of human B and T lymphocytes in peripheral blood induced by irradiation for mammary carcinoma, *Lancet*, 1, 1352, 1972.
133. Björkholm, M., Holm, G., and Mellstedt, H., Persisting lymphocyte deficiencies during remission in Hodgkin's disease, *Clin. Exp. Immunol.*, 28, 389, 1977.
134. Hersh, E. M. and Oppenheim, J. J., Inhibition of in-vitro lymphocyte transformation during chemotherapy in man, *Cancer, Res.*, 27, 98, 1967.
135. Cheema, A. R. and Hersh, E. M., Patient survival after chemotherapy and its relationship to invitro lymphocyte blastogenesis, *Cancer*, 28, 851, 1971.
136. Han, T. and Sokal, J. E., Lymphocyte response to phytohemagglutinin in Hodgkin's disease, *Am. J. Med.*, 48, 728, 1970.
137. Trubowitz, S., Masek, B., and DelRosario, A., Lymphocyte response to phytohemagglutinin in Hodgkin's disease, lymphatic leukemia and lymphosarcoma, *Cancer*, 19, 2019, 1966.
138. Jackson, S. M., Garret, J. V., and Craig, A. W., Lymphocyte transformation changes during the clinical course of Hodgkin's disease, *Cancer*, 25, 843, 1970.
139. Thomas, J. W., Boldt, W., Horrocks, G., and Low, B., Lymphocyte transformation by phytohemagglutinin. I. In Hodgkin's disease, *Can. Med. Assoc. J.*, 97, 832, 1967.
140. Corder, M. P., Young, R. C., Brown, R. S., and DeVita, V.T., Phytohemagglutinin-induced lymphocyte transformation: the relationship to prognosis of Hodgkin's disease, *Blood*, 39, 595, 1972.
141. Braeman, J. and Cottam, P., The PHA response in Hodgkin's disease, *Eur. J. Cancer*, 11, 879, 1975.
142. Han, T., Effect of sera from patients with Hodgkin's disease on normal lymphocyte response to phytohemagglutinin, *Cancer*, 29, 1626, 1972.
143. Matchett, K. M., Huang, A. T., and Kremer, W. B., Impaired lymphocyte transformation in Hodgkin's disease — evidence for depletion of circulating T lymphocytes, *J. Clin. Invest.*, 52, 1908, 1973.
144. Ippoliti, G., Marini, G., Ascari, E., and Casirola, G., The influence of repeated and prolonged stimulation on the PHA - response of lymphocytes in Hodgkin's disease, *Acta Hematol. (Basel)*, 51, 266, 1974.
145. Ruhl, H., Vogt, W., Bochert, G., Schmidt, S., Moelle, R., and Schaoua, H., Mixed lymphocyte culture stimulating and responding capacity of lymphocytes from patients with lymphoproliferative diseases, *Clin. Exp. Immunol.*, 19, 55, 1975.
146. Zeigler, J. B., Hansen, P., and Penny, R., Intrinsic lymphocyte defect in Hodgkin's disease: analysis of the phytohemagglutinin dose-response, *Clin. Immunol. Immunopathol.*, 3, 451, 1975.
147. Case, D. C., Hansen, J. A., Corrales, E., Young, C. W., Dupont, B., Pinsky, C. M., and Good, R. A., Depressed in-vitro lymphocyte response to PHA in patients with Hodgkin's disease in continuous long remissions, *Blood*, 49, 771, 1977.
148. Scheurlen, P. G., Schneider, W., and Pappas, A., Inhibition of transformation of normal lymphocytes by plasma factor from patients with Hodgkin's disease and cancer, *Lancet*, 2, 1265, 1971.
149. Amlot, P. L. and Unger, A., Binding of phytohemagglutinin to serum substances and inhibition of lymphocyte transformation in Hodgkin's disease, *Clin. Exp. Immunol.*, 26, 520, 1976.
150. Zorini, C. O., Neri, A., Comis, M., Mannella, E., and Paciucci, P. A., Influence of Hodgkin's serum on PHA stimulation of normal lymphocytes, *Lancet*, 1, 745, 1974.
151. Mintz, U. and Sachs, L., Changes in the surface membrane of lymphocytes from patients with chronic lymphocytic leukemia and Hodgkin's disease, *Int. J. Cancer*, 15, 253, 1975.

152. Ben-Bassat, H. and Goldblum, N., Concanavalin A receptors on the surface membrane of lymphocytes from patients with Hodgkin's disease and other malignant lymphomas, *Proc. Natl. Acad. Sci. U.S.A.*, 72, 1046, 1975.
153. Aisenberg, A. C., Weitzman, S., and Wilkes, B., Lymphocyte receptors for concanavalin A in Hodgkin's disease, *Blood*, 51, 439, 1978.
154. Benninghoff, D. L. and Girardet, R., Lymphocyte function in Hodgkin's disease, *Lymphology*, 9, 39, 1976.
155. DeSousa, M., Yang, M., Lopes-Corrales, E., Tan, C., Hansen, J. A., Dupont, B., and Good, R. A., Exotaxis: the principle and its application to the study of Hodgkin's disease, *Clin. Exp. Immunol.*, 27, 143, 1977.
156. Savel, H. and Moehring, T., Lymphotoxin production in human neoplasia, *Proc. Soc. Exp. Biol.*, 137, 374, 1971.
157. Churchill, W. H., Rocklin, R. R., Moloney, W. C., and David, J. R., In-vitro evidence of normal lymphocyte function in some patients with Hodgkin's disease and negative delayed cutaneous hypersensitivity, *Natl. Cancer Inst. Monogr.*, 36, 99, 1973.
158. Cohen, S., Fisher, B., Yoshida, T., and Bettigole, R. E., Serum migration-inhibitory activity in patients with lymphoproliferative diseases, *N. Engl. J. Med.*, 290, 882, 1974.
159. Hancock, B. W., Bruce, L., and Richmond, J., Cellular immunity to Hodgkin's splenic tissue measured by leukocyte migration inhibition, *Br. Med. J.*, 1, 556, 1976.
160. Golding, B., Golding, H., Lomnitzer, R., Jacobson, R., Koornhof, H. J., and Rabson, A. R., Production of leukocyte inhibitory factor (LIF) in Hodgkin's disease, *Clin. Immunol. Immunopathol.*, 7, 114, 1977.
161. Pidot, A. L. R. and McIntrye, O. R., In-vitro leukocyte interferon production in patients with Hodgkin's disease, *Cancer Res.*, 34, 2995, 1974.
162. Chisholm, M. and Cartwright, T., Interferon, production in Hodgkin's disease, *Clin. Exp. Immunol.*, 20, 419, 1975.
163. Ruhl, H., Vogt, W., Bochert, G., Schmidt, S., Schaoua, H., and Moelle, R., Lymphocyte transformation and production of a human mononuclear leukocyte chemotactic factor in patients with Hodgkin's disease, *Clin. Exp. Immunol.*, 17, 407, 1974.
164. Ward, P. A. and Berenberg, J. L., Defective regulation of inflammatory mediators in Hodgkin's disease, *N. Engl. J. Med.*, 290, 76, 1974.
165. Tworney, J. J., Douglass, C. C., and Morris, S. M., Inability of leukocytes to stimulate mixed leukocyte reactions, *J. Natl. Cancer Inst.*, 51, 345, 1973.
166. Tworney, J. J., Douglass, C. C., and Morris, S. M., Failure of leukocytes in Hodgkin's disease to stimulate a mixed leukocyte reaction (MLR), *Proc. 7th Leukocyte Culture Conf.*, Daguillard, F., Ed., Academic Press, New York, 1973, 627.
167. Kasakura, S., MLS stimulatory capacity and production of a blastogenic factor in patients with chronic lymphatic leukemia and Hodgkin's disease, *Blood*, 45, 823, 1975.
168. Björkholm, M., Holm, G., Mellsedt, H., and Pettersson, D., Immunological capacity of lymphocytes from untreated patients with Hodgkin's disease evaluated in mixed lymphocyte culture, *Clin. Exp. Immunol.*, 22, 373, 1976.
169. Lang, J. M., Tongio, M. M., Oberling, F., Mayer, S., and Wattz, R., Mixed lymphocyte reaction as assay for immunological competence of lymphocytes from patients with Hodgkin's disease, *Lancet*, 1, 1261, 1972.
170. Sutcliffe, S. B., Studies on the Mechanism of Immunodeficiency in Hodgkin's Disease, M. D. thesis, University of London, 1978.
171. Graze, P. R., Perlin, E., and Royston, I., In-vitro lymphocyte dysfunction in Hodgkin's disease, *J. Natl. Cancer Inst.*, 56, 239, 1976.
172. Engleman, E. G., Benike, C. J., Hoppe, R. T., and Kaplan, H. S., Autologous mixed lymphocyte reaction in patients with Hodgkin's disease, evidence for a T cell defect, *J. Clin. Invest.*, 66, 149, 1980.
173. Zarling, J. M., Berman, C., and Raich, P. C., Depressed cytotoxic T cell responses in previously treated Hodgkin's disease and non-Hodgkin's lymphoma patients, *Cancer Immunol. Immunother.*, 7, 243, 1980.
174. Holm, G., Perlmann, P., and Johansson, B., Impaired phytohemagglutinin induced cytotoxicity in-vitro of lymphocytes from patients with Hodgkin's disease or chronic lymphatic leukemia, *Clin. Exp. Immunol.*, 2, 351, 1967.
175. Thomas, J. W., Boldt, W., and Horrocks, G., Lymphocyte transformation by phytohemagglutinin. III. In-vitro cytotoxicity, *Can. Med. Assoc. J.*, 99, 303, 1968.
176. Hillinger, S. M. and Herzig, G. P., Impaired cell-mediated immunity in Hodgkin's disease mediated by suppressor lymphocytes and monocytes, *J. Clin. Invest.*, 61, 1620, 1978.

177. Kirchner, H., Muchmore, A. V., Chused, T. M., Holden, H. T., and Herberman, R. B., Inhibition of proliferation of lymphoma cells and T lymphocytes by suppressor cells from spleens of tumour-bearing mice, *J. Immunol.*, 114, 206, 1975.
178. Pope, B. L., Whitney, R. B., Levy, J. G., and Kilburn, D. G., Suppressor cells in the spleens of tumour bearing mice: enrichment by centrifugation on hypaque-ficoll and characterization of the suppressor population, *J. Immunol.*, 116, 1342, 1976.
179. Elgert, K. D. and Farrar, W. L., Suppressor cell activity in tumour-bearing mice. I. Dualistic inhibition by suppressor T lymphocytes and macrophages, *J. Immunol.*, 120, 1345, 1978.
180. Weiss, A. and Fitch, F. W., Macrophages suppress CTL generation in rat mixed leukocyte cultures, *J. Immunol.*, 119, 510, 1977.
181. Oehler, J. R., Herbergman, R. B., Campbell, D. A., Jr., and Djeu, J. Y., Inhibition of rat mixed lymphocyte cultures by suppressor macrophages, *Cell. Immunol.*, 29, 238, 1977.
182a. Baird, L. G. and Kaplan, A. M., Macrophage regulation of mitogen-induced blastogenesis. I. Demonstration of inhibitory cells in the spleens and peritoneal exudates of mice, *Cell. Immunol.*, 28, 22, 1977.
182b. Baird, L. G. and Kaplan, A. M., Macrophage regulation of mitogen-induced blastogenesis. II. Mechanism of inhibition, *Cell. Immunol.*, 28, 36, 1977.
183. Berlinger, N. T., Lopez, C., and Good, R. A., Facilitation or attenuation of mixed leukocyte culture responsiveness by adherent cells, *Nature (London)*, 260, 145, 1976.
184. Zembala, M., Mytar, B., Popiela, T., and Asherson, G. L., Depressed in-vitro peripheral blood lymphocyte response to mitogens in cancer patients: the role of suppressor cells, *Int. J. Cancer*, 19, 605, 1977.
185. Schecter, G. P. and Soehnlen, F., Monocyte-mediated inhibition of lymphocyte blastogenesis in Hodgkin's disease, *Blood*, 52, 261, 1978.
186. Tworney, J. J., Laughter, A. H., Farrow, S., and Douglass, C. C., Hodgkin's disease, an immunodepleting and immunosuppressive disorder, *J. Clin. Invest.*, 56, 467, 1975.
187. Sibbitt, W. L., Jr., Bankhurst, A. D., and Williams, R. C., Jr., Studies of cell subpopulations mediating mitogen hyporesponsiveness in patients with Hodgkin's disease, *J. Clin. Invest.*, 61, 55, 1978.
188. Goodwin, J. S., Messner, R. P., Bankhurst, A. D., Peake, G. T., Saiki, J. H., and Williams, R. C., Prostaglandin-producing suppressor cells in Hodgkin's disease, *N. Engl. J. Med.*, 297, 963, 1977.
189. Bukowski, R. M., Hewlett, J. S., and Deodhar, S., PHA and mixed leukocyte culture (MLC) reactivity in Hodgkin's disease, *Proc. Am. Assoc. Cancer Res.*, 17, (Abstr.,) 323, 1976.
190. Bockman, R. S., Stage-dependent reduction in T colony formation in Hodgkin's disease, coincidence with monocyte synthesis of prostaglandins, *J. Clin. Invest.*, 66, 523, 1980.
191. Tworney, J. J., Laughter, A. H., Rice, L., and Ford, R., Spectrum of immunodeficiencies with Hodgkin's disease, *J. Clin. Invest.*, 66, 629, 1980.
192. Laughter, A. H. and Tworney, J. J., Suppression of lymphoproliferation by high concentrations of normal human mononuclear leukocytes, *J. Immunol.*, 119, 173, 1977.
193. Markenson, J. A., Morgan, J. W., Lockshin, M. D., Joachim, C., and Winfield, J. B., Responses of fractionated cells from patients with systemic lupus erythematosus and normals to plant mitogen: evidence for a suppressor population of monocytes, *Proc. Soc. Exp. Biol. Med.*, 158, 5, 1978.
194. Breshnihan, B. and Jasin, H. E., Suppressor function of peripheral blood mononuclear cells in normal individuals and in patients with systemic lupus erythematosus, *J. Clin. Invest.*, 59, 106, 1977.
195. Schulof, R. S., Lee, B. J., Lacher, M. J., Straus, D. J., Clarkson, B. D., Good, R. A., and Gupta, S., Concanavalin-A-induced suppressor cell activity in Hodgkin's disease, *Clin. Immunol. Immunopathol.*, 16, 454, 1980.
196. Engleman, E. G., McMichael, A. J., Batey, M. E., and McDevitt, H. O., Suppressor T cell of the mixed lymphocyte reaction in man specific for the stimulating alloantigen: evidence that identity at HLA-D between suppressor and responder is required for suppression, *J. Exp. Med.*, 147, 137, 1978.
197. Gupta, S. and Good, R. A., Spontaneous and antibody-dependent cellular cytotoxicity by lymphocyte subpopulations in peripheral blood and spleen from adult untreated patients with Hodgkin's disease, *Clin. Exp. Immunol.*, 45, 205, 1981.
198. Sheagren, J. N., Block, J. B., and Wolff, S. M., Reticulo-endothelial system phagocytic function in patients with Hodgkin's disease, *J. Clin. Invest.*, 46, 855, 1967.
199. King, G. W., Lobuglio, A. F., and Sagone, A. L., Human monocyte glucose metabolism, in lymphoma, *J. Lab. Clin. Med.*, 89, 316, 1977.
200. Steigbigel, R. T., Lambert, L. H., and Remington, J., Polymorphonuclear leukocyte, monocyte, and macrophage bactericidal function in patients with Hodgkin's disease, *J. Lab. Clin. Med.*, 88, 54, 1976.
201. King, G. W., Bain, G., and Lobuglio, A. F., The effect of tuberculosis and neoplasia on human monocyte staphylocidal activity, *Cell. Immunol.*, 16, 389, 1975.

202. Blaese, R. M., Oppenheim, J. J., Seeger, R. C., and Waldmann, T. A., Lymphocyte macrophage interaction in antigen induced in-vitro lymphocyte transformation in patients with the Wiskott-Aldrich syndrome and other diseases with anergy, *Cell. Immunol.*, 4, 228, 1972.
203. Kaplan, H. S., and Gartner, S., "Sternberg-Reed" giant cells of Hodgkin's disease: cultivation in-vitro, heterotransplantation, and characterisation as neoplastic macrophages, *Int. J. Cancer*, 19, 511, 1977.
204. Lennert, K., Stationary elements of the lymph node, in *Malignant Lymphomas Other Than Hodgkin's Disease,* Part VII, Springer-Verlag, Basel, 1978, 51.
205. Longmire, R. L., McMillan, R., Yelenosky, R., Armstrong, S., Lang, J. E., and Craddock, C. G., In-vitro splenic IgG synthesis in Hodgkin's disease, *N. Engl. J. Med.*, 289, 763, 1973.
206. Fudenberg, H. and Solomon, A., "Acquired aggammaglobulinemia" with auto-immune hemolytic disease: graft-versus-host reaction?, *Vox Sang.*, 6, 68, 1961.
207. Fudenberg, H., German, J. L., III, and Kunkel, H. G., The occurrence of rheumatoid factor and other abnormalities in families of patients with agammaglobulinemia, *Arthritis Rheum.*, 5, 565, 1962.
208. Andreev, V. C. and Zlatkov, N. B., Systemic lupus erythematosus and neoplasia of the lymphoreticular system, *Br. J. Dermatol.*, 80, 503, 1968.
209. Harvey, A. M., Schulman, L. E., Tumulty, P. A., Conley, C. L., and Schoenrich, E. H., Systemic lupus erythematosus: review of the literature and clinical analysis of 138 cases, *Medicine (Baltimore)*, 33, 291, 1954.
210. Camerata, R. J., Rodnan, G. P., and Jensen, W. N., Systemic rheumatic disease and malignant lymphoma, *Arch. Intern. Med.*, 3, 330, 1963.
211. Nilsen, L. B., Missah, M. E., and Condemi, J. J., Appearance of Hodgkin's disease in a patient with systemic lupus erythematosus, *Cancer*, 20, 1930, 1967.
212. Green, J. A., Dawson, A. A., and Walker, W., Systemic lupus erythematosus and lymphoma, *Lancet*, 2, 753, 1978.
213. Blanc, A. P., Gastaut, J. A., Lefevre, P., Tubiana, N., Favre, R., and Carcassonne, Y., Association lupus — maladie de Hodgkin, *Sem. Hop. Paris*, 56, 477, 1980.
214. Goodwin, J. S., Remission in systemic lupus erythematosus after combination chemotherapy for Hodgkin's Disease, *JAMA*, 244, 1962, 1980.
215. Mellors, R. C., Autoimmune disease in NZB/BL mice. II. Autoimmunity and malignant lymphoma, *Blood*, 27, 435, 1966.
216. Casey, T. P., The development of lymphomas in mice with autoimmune disorders treated with Azathioprine, *Blood*, 31, 396, 1968.
217. Ingram, D. G. and Cho, H. Y., Aleutian disease in mink: virology, immunology, and pathogenesis, *J. Rheumatol.*, 1, 74, 1974.
218. Abdou, N. I., Sagawa, A., Pascual, E., Hebert, J., and Sadeghee, S., Suppressor T cell abnormality in idiopathic systemic lupus erythematosus, *Clin. Immunol. Immunopathol.*, 6, 192, 1976.
219. Fauci, A. S., Sternberg, A. D., Haynes, B. F., and Whalen, G., Immunoregulatory aberrations in systemic lupus erythematosus, *J. Immunol.*, 121, 1473, 1978.
220. Markenson, J. A., Morgan, J. W., Lockshin, M. D., Joachin, C., and Winfield, J. B., Responses of fractionated cells from patients with systemic lupus erythematosus and normals to plant mitogen: evidence for a suppressor population of monocytes, *Proc. Soc. Exp. Biol. Med.*, 158, 5, 1978.
221. Breshnihan, B. and Jasin, H. E., Suppressor function of peripheral blood mononuclear cells in normal individuals and in patients with systemic lupus erythematosus, *J. Clin. Invest.*, 59, 106, 1977.
222. Tworney, J. J., Laughter, A. H., and Sternberg, A. D., A serum inhibitor of immune regulation in patients with systemic lupus erythematosus, *J. Clin. Invest.*, 62, 713, 1978.
223. Schwartz, R. S., Viruses and systemic lupus erythematosus, *N. Engl. J. Med.*, 293, 132, 1975.
224. Penn, I., Cancer associated with immunosuppression, *Handbook of Clinical Immunology,* Baumgarten, A. and Richards, F. F., Eds., CRC Press, Boca Raton, Fla., 1978.
225. Canoso, J. J. and Cohen, A. S., Malignancy in a series of 70 patients with systemic lupus erythematosus, *Arthritis Rheum.*, 17, 383, 1974.
226. Rothman, S., Block, M., and Hauser, F. V., Sjogren's syndrome associated with lymphoblastoma and hypersplenism, *Arch. Derm. Syph.*, 63, 642, 1951.
227. Kennealey, G.T., Kaetz, H. W., and Walker-Smith, G. J., Sjogren's syndrome with psuedolymphoma 13 years after Hodgkin's disease, *Arch. Intern. Med.*, 138, 635, 1978.
228. Anderson, L. G. and Talal, N., The spectrum of benign to malignant lymphoproliferation in Sjogren's syndrome, *Clin. Exp. Immunol.*, 9, 199, 1971.
229. Talal, N., Sokoloff, L., and Barth, W. F., Extrasalivary lymphoid abnormalities in Sjogren's syndrome (reticulum cell sarcoma, "psuedolymphoma", macroglobulinemia), *Am. J. Med.*, 43, 50, 1967.
230. Talal, N. and Bunim, J. J., The development of malignant lymphoma in the course of Sjogren's syndrome, *Am. J. Med.*, 36, 529, 1964.

231. Williams, R. C., Dermatomyositis and malignancy: a review of the literature, *Ann. Intern. Med.*, 50, 1174, 1959.
232. Bohan, A. and Peter, J. B., Polymyositis and dermatomyositis, *N. Engl. J. Med.*, 292, 344, 1975.
233. Kadar, A., Khan, A. B., Mattern, J. Q. A., Fisher, J., Thomas, P. R. M., and Freeman, A. I., Autoimmune disorders complicating adolescent Hodgkin's disease, *Cancer*, 44, 112, 1979.
234. Bosly, A., Isaac, G., Salamon, E., and Fievez, C., Dermatomyosite revelatrice d'une maladie de Hodgkin, *Nouv. Rev. Fr. Hematol. Blood Cells*, 18, 164, 1977.
235. Rudders, R. A., Autoimmune thrombocytopenic purpura in Hodgkin's disease, *N. Engl. J. Med.*, 291, 49, 1975.
236. Fink, K., Al-Mondhiry, H., Idiopathic thrombocytopenic purpura in Hodgkin's disease, *Cancer*, 37, 1999, 1976.
237. Weitzman, S., Dvilansky, A., and Yanai, I., Thrombocytopenic purpura as the sole manifestation of recurrence in Hodgkin's disease, *Acta Hematol.* 58, 129, 1977.
238. Cohen, J. R., Idiopathic thrombocytopenic purpura in Hodgkin's disease, *Cancer*, 41, 743, 1978.
239. Waddell, C. C. and Cimo, P. L., Idiopathic thrombocytopenic purpura occurring in Hodgkin's disease after splenectomy, *Am. J. Hematol.*, 7, 381, 1979.
240. Hassidim, K., McMillan, R., Conjalka, M. S., and Morrison, J., Immune thrombocytopenic purpura in Hodgkin's disease, *Am. J. Hematol.*, 6, 149, 1979.
241. Kirschner, J. J., Zamkoff, K. W., and Gottlieb, A. J., Idiopathic thrombocytopenic purpura and Hodgkin's disease: report of two cases and a review of the literature, *Am. J. Med. Sci.*, 280(1), 21, 1980.
242. Duhamel, G., Moise, A., Najman, A., Gorin, N., Mayaud, Ch., Chatelet, F., and Burguière, A. M., Maladie de Hodgkin, purpura thrombopénique, polyradiculonevrite et penumopathie à cytomegalovirus, *Ann. Med. Interne. (Paris)*, 130, 449, 1979.
243. Kübböck, J., Von., Aiginger, P., Pötzi, P., and Smolen, J., Hämolytische anämie bei morbus Hodgkin, *Acta Med. Austriaca*, 6, 186, 1979.
244. Andrieu, J. M., Youinou, P., and Marcelle, A., Anémie hémolytique autoimmune associée à la maladie de Hodgkin, *Nouv. Presse Med.*, 10, 2951, 1981.
245. Lanier, R. L. and Amare, M., Autoimmune cytopenias in Hodgkin's disease, *Rocky Mountain Med. J.*, 76, 165, 1979.
246. Eisner, E., Ley, A. B., and Mayer, K., Coomb's-positive hemolytic anemia in Hodgkin's disease, *Ann. Intern. Med.*, 66, 258, 1967.
247. Case records of the Massachusetts General Hospital, case 24 — 1978, *N. Engl. J. Med.*, 298, 1407, 1978.
248. Bowdler, A. J. and Glick, I. W., Autoimmune hemolytic anemia as the herald state of Hodgkin's Disease, *Ann. Intern. Med.*, 65, 761, 1966.
249. Cazenave, J. P., Autoimmune hemolytic anemia terminating 7 years later in Hodgkin's disease, *Can. Med. Assoc. J.*, 109, 748, 1973.
250. Björkholm, M., Holm, G., and Merk, K., Cyclic autoimmune hemolytic anemia as a presenting manifestation of splenic Hodgkin's disease, *Cancer*, 49, 1702, 1982.
251. Hunter, J. D., Logue, G. L., and Joyner, J. T., Autoimmune neutropenia in Hodgkin's disease, *Arch. Int. Med.*, 142, 386, 1982.
252. Kiely, J. M., Wagoner, R. D., and Holley, K. E., Renal complications of lymphoma *Ann. Int. Med.*, 71, 1159, 1969.
253. Piessens, W. F., and Zercher, M., Hodgkin's disease causing a reversible nephrotic syndrome by compression of the inferior vena cava, *Cancer*, 25, 880, 1970.
254. Bichel, J. and Jensen, K. B., Nephrotic syndrome and Hodgkin's disease, *Lancet*, 2, 1425, 1971.
255. Hansen, H. E., Skov, P. E., and Askjaer, S. A., Hodgkin's disease associated with nephrotic syndrome without kidney lesion, *Acta Med. Scand.*, 191, 307, 1972.
256. Froom, D. W., Franklin, W. A., Hans, J. E., and Potter, E. V., Immune deposits in Hodgkin's disease with nephrotic syndrome, *Arch. Pathol. Lab. Med.*, 94, 547, 1972.
257. Plager, J. and Stuzman, L., Acute nephrotic syndrome as a manifestation of active Hodgkin's disease, *Am. J. Med.*, 50, 56, 1971.
258. Szabó, J., Lustyik, Gy., Szabó, T., Erdei, I., and Szegedi, Gy., Glomerulonephritis of immune-complex origin associated with Hodgkin's disease, *Acta Med. Acad. Sci. Hung.*, 31, 187, 1974.
259. Berthoux, F.-C., Zech, P.-Y., Blanc-Brunat, N., Colon, S., Ducnet, F., and Traeger, J., Association syndrome nephrotique — maladie de Hodgkin, *Nouv. Presse Med.*, 5, 255, 1976.
260. Hyman, L. R., Burkholder, P. M., Joo, P. A., and Segar, W. E., Malignant lymphoma and nephrotic syndrome, *J. Pediatr.* 82, 207, 1973.
261. Loryhridge, L. W. and Lewis, M. G., Nephrotic syndrome in Hodgkin's disease, *Lancet*, 1, 1127, 1971.

262. Costanza, M. E., Pinn, V., Schwartz, R. S., and Nathanson, L., Carcinoembryonic antigen-antibody complexes in a patient with colonic carcinoma and nephrotic syndrome, *N. Engl. J. Med.*, 289, 520, 1973.
263. Moorthy, A. V., Zimmerman, S. W., and Burkholder, P. M., Nephrotic syndrome in Hodgkin's disease, evidence for pathogenesis alternative to immune complex deposition, *Am. J. Med.*, 61, 471, 1976.
264. Sherman, R. L., Susin, M., Weksler, M. E., and Becker, E. L., Lipoid nephrosis in Hodgkin's disease, *Am. J. Med.*, 52, 699, 1972.
265. Capra, Marzani, M., La sindrome nefrosica nel morbo di Hodgkin, *Arch. Sci. Med.*, 138, 543, 1981.
266. Shitara, T., Kohl, S., Sullivan, M. P., Richie, E., Brewer, E. D., and Butler, J. J., Hodgkin's disease complicated by nephrotic syndrome, *Am. J. Pediatr. Haematol. Oncol.*, 3, 177, 1981.
267. Kramer, P., Sizoo, W., and Twiss, E. E., Nephrotic syndrome in Hodgkin's disease, report of five cases and review of the literature, *Neth. J. Med.* 24, 114, 1981.
268. Stuhlinger, W. D., Verroust, P. J., and Morel-Maroger, L., Detection of circulating immune complexes in patients with various renal diseases, *Immunology*, 30, 43, 1976.
269. Poston, R. N., Cerio, R., and Cameron, J. S., Circulating immune complexes in minimal-change nephritis, *N. Engl. J. Med.*, 298, 1089, 1978.
270. Levinsky, R. J., Malleson, P. N., Barratt, T. M., and Soothill, J. F., Circulating immune complexes in steroid-responsive nephrotic syndrome, *N. Engl. J. Med.*, 298, 126, 1978.
271. Ooi, B. S., Orlina, A. R., and Masaitis, L., Lymphocytotoxins, in primary renal disease, *Lancet*, 2, 1348, 1974.
272. Eyres, K. E., Mallick, N. P., and Taylor, G., Evidence for cell-mediated immunity to renal antigens in minimal change nephrotic syndrome, *Lancet*, 1, 1158, 1976.
273. Lagrue, G., Xheneumont, S., and Branellec, A., A vascular permeability, factors elaborated from lymphocytes. I. Demonstration in patients with nephrotic syndrome, *Biomedicine*, 23, 37, 1975.
274. Shalhoub, R. J., Pathogenesis of lipoid nephrosis: a disorder of T cell function, *Lancet*, 2, 556, 1974.
275. Kersey, J. H., Spector, B. D., and Good, R. A., Primary immunodeficiency disease and cancer: the immunodeficiency — cancer registry, *Int. J. Cancer*, 12, 333, 1973.
276. Spector, B. D., Perry, G. S., III, Good, R. A., and Kersey, J. H., Immunopathology of lymphoreticular neoplasms, in *Immunodeficiency Diseases and Malignancy*, Tworney, J. J. and Good, R. A., Eds., Plenum Medical Book Company, New York, 1978, 203.
277. Penn, I., *Malignant Tumors in Organ Transplant Recipients*, Springer-Verlag, Basel, 1970.
278. Penn, I., Immunopathology of lymphoreticular neoplasms, in *Immunosuppression and Malignant Disease*, Tworney, J. J. and Good, R. A., Eds., Plenum Medical Book Company, New York, 1978, 223.
279. Wilson, R. E., Hager, E. B., Hampers, C. L., Corson, J. M., Merrill, J. P., and Murray, J. E., Immunologic rejection of human cancer transplanted with a renal allograft, *N. Engl. J. Med.*, 278, 479, 1968.
280. Matter, B., Zukoski, C. F., and Killen, D. A., Transplanted carcinoma in an immuno-suppressed patient, *Transplantation*, 9, 71, 1970.
281. Martin, D. C., Rubini, M., and Rosen, V. J., Cadaveric renal homotransplantation with inadvertent transplantation of carcinoma, *JAMA*, 192, 752, 1965.
282. McPhaul, J. J. and McIntosh, D. A. Tissue transplantation still vexes, *N. Engl. J. Med.*, 272, 105, 1965.
283. Kaiser-McCain, B., Hecht, F., and Harnden, D. G., Somatic rearrangement of chromosome 14 in human lymphocytes, *Proc. Natl. Acad. Sci. U.S.A.*, 72, 207, 1975.
284. Rowley, J. D. and Fukuhara, S., Chromosome changes in non-Hodgkin's lymphomas, *Semin. Oncol.*, 7, (3), 255, 1980.
285. Reeves, B. R. and Pickup, V. L., The chromosome changes in non-Burkitt lymphomas, *Hum. Genet.*, 53, 349, 1980.
286. Rowley, J. D., Chromosomes in Hodgkin's disease, *Cancer Treat. Rep.*, 66, (4), 639, 1982.
287. Rowley, J. D., Chromosomal changes in acute lymphoblastic leukemia, *Cancer Genet., Cytogenet.*, 1, 263, 1980.
288. Liang, W., Hopper, J. E., and Rowley, J. D., Karyotypic abnormalities and clinical aspects of patients with multiple myeloma and related paraproteinemic disorders, *Cancer*, 44, 630, 1979.
289. Shen-Ong, G. L. C., Keath, E. J., Piccoli, S. P., and Cole, M. D., Novel MYC oncogene RNA from abortive immunoglobulin-gene recombination in mouse plasmacytomas, *Cell*, 31, 443, 1982.
290. Paterson, M. C., Smith, B. P., Lohman, P. H. M., Anderson, A. K., and Fishman, L., Defective excision repair of gamma ray damaged DNA in human (ataxia-telangiectasia) fibroblasts, *Nature (London)*, 260, 444, 1976.
291. Cleaver, J. E., Defective repair replication of DNA in xeroderma pigmentosum, *Nature (London)*, 218, 652, 1968.

292. Takemoto, K. K., Rabson, A. S., Mullarkey, M. F., Blaese, R. M., Garon, C. F., and Nelson, D., Isolation of papovavirus from brain tumor and urine of a patient with Wiskott-Aldrich syndrome, *J. Natl. Cancer Inst.*, 53, 1205, 1974.
293. Schwartz, R. S. and Beldotte, L., Malignant lymphomas following allogenic disease: transition from immunological to a neoplastic disorder, *Science,* 149, 1511, 1965.
294. Moertel, C. G. and Hagedorn, A. B., Leukemia or lymphoma and coexistent primary malignant lesions: a review of the literature and a study of 120 cases, *Blood,* 12, 788, 1957.
295. Razis, D. V., Diamond, H. D., and Craver, L. F., Hodgkin's disease associated with other malignant tumors and certain non-neoplastic disease, *Am. J. Med. Sci.,* 238, 327, 1959.
296. Berg, J. W., The incidence of multiple primary cancers. I. Development of further cancers in patients with lymphomas, leukemias and myeloma, *J. Natl. Cancer Inst.,* 38, 741, 1967.
297. Arseneau, J. C., Sponzo, R. W., Levin, D. L., Schnipper, L. E., Bonner, H., Young, R. C., Canellos, G. P., Johnson, R. E., and DeVita, V. T., Non-lymphomatous malignant tumours complicating Hodgkin's disease, *N. Engl. J. Med.,* 287, 1119, 1972.
298. Canellos, G. P., DeVita, V. T., Arseneau, J. C., Whang-Peng, J., and Johnson, R. E. C., Second malignancies complicating Hodgkin's disease in remission, *Lancet,* 1, 947, 1975.
299. Coleman, C. N., Williams, C. J., Flint, A., Glatstein, E. J., Rosenberg, S. A., and Kaplan, H. S., Hematologic neoplasia in patients treated for Hodgkin's disease, *N. Engl. J. Med.,* 297, 1249, 1977.
300. Coleman, C. N., Burke, J. S., Varghese, A., Rosenberg, S. A., and Kaplan, H. S., Secondary leukemia and non-Hodgkin's lymphoma in patients treated for Hodgkin's disease, in *Advances In Malignant Lymphomas, Etiology, Immunology, Pathology and Treatment,* Kaplan, H. S. and Rosenberg, S. A., Eds., Academic Press, New York, 1982, 259.
301. Krikorian, J. G., Burke, J. S., Rosenberg, S. A., and Kaplan, H. S., Occurrence of non-Hodgkin's lymphoma after therapy for Hodgkin's disease, *N. Engl. J. Med.,* 300, 452, 1979.
302. Nelson, D. F., Cooper, S., Weston, M. G., and Rubin, P., Second malignant neoplasms in patients treated for Hodgkin's disease with radiotherapy or radiotherapy and chemotherapy, *Cancer,* 48, 2386, 1981.
303. Valagussa, P., Santoro, A., Kenda, R., Fossati-Bellani, F., Franchi, F., Banfi, A., Rilke, F., and Bonadonna, G., Second malignancies in Hodgkin's disease: a complication of certain forms of treatment, *Br. Med. J.,* 1, 216, 1980.
304. Coltman, C. A. and Dixon, D. O., Second malignancies complicating Hodgkin's disease, *Cancer Treat. Rep.,* 66, 1023, 1982.

Chapter 2

# HODGKIN'S DISEASE: THE ROLE OF THE LYMPHOCYTE AND MONOCYTE

D. R. Katz and J. A. Habeshaw

## TABLE OF CONTENTS

| | | |
|---|---|---|
| I. | Introduction | 34 |
| II. | Structure of Normal Lymphoid Tissue | 34 |
| III. | What is Hodgkin's Disease? | 36 |
| IV. | Hodgkin's Disease Compared to Other Lymphomas | 38 |
| | A. Histology | 38 |
| | B. Immunohistology | 39 |
| | C. In Vitro Analysis | 41 |
| | D. Conclusions | 41 |
| V. | Immune Mechanisms in the Etiology of Hodgkin's Disease | 42 |
| | A. Epidemiology | 43 |
| | B. Virology | 43 |
| | C. Pathogenesis | 44 |
| | D. Conclusions | 45 |
| VI. | Hodgkin's Disease Tissue | 45 |
| | A. Histology | 46 |
| | B. Immunohistology | 47 |
| | C. In Vitro Analysis | 48 |
| | D. Conclusions | 49 |
| VII. | Peripheral Blood Cells in Hodgkin's Disease | 50 |
| | A. T Lymphocytes | 50 |
| | B. B Lymphocytes | 52 |
| | C. Monocytes | 52 |
| | D. Conclusions | 53 |
| VIII. | Immunological Deficiency in Hodgkin's Disease | 53 |
| | A. Histological Aspects | 53 |
| | B. Clinical Aspects | 54 |
| | C. Tumors | 55 |
| IX. | Treatment Effects in Hodgkin's Disease | 55 |
| X. | Future Trends in Hodgkin's Disease Research | 56 |
| XI. | Summary and Conclusions | 57 |
| References | | 57 |

## I. INTRODUCTION

Compared to the analysis of the immunology of other lymph node malignancies, the immunology of Hodgkin's disease represents a minefield into which only the most foolhardy are prepared to tread; nonetheless, "foolhardiness" is appropriate because the immunological aspects of Hodgkin's disease represent a fascinating unresolved problem in human biology and because they also represent an instructive example of some general principles about human disease mechanisms.

First, to view any disease process from one vantage point — be it diagnostic, cell biological, clinical, therapeutic, or epidemiological — may give a misleading impression that there is a static fixed point from which the disease can be examined. The histological diagnosis of Hodgkin's disease has by convention been regarded as such a fixed point but like all such fixed points, it is in fact only a transient morphological moment in a welter of immunologic activity which may extend for years.

Second, while cellular interactions and interrelationships involved in the immune response have been explored extensively in recent years there remain areas of uncertainty. One of these is the cell lineage of inducer cells in immunity and another is the relationship between transformation and neoplasia. Both these questions are central in Hodgkin's disease cell biology. Thus the lack of conclusive data about Hodgkin's disease tissue immunology may reflect these basic uncertainties rather than problems about Hodgkin's disease in particular.

Third, while Hodgkin's disease represents a relative modern therapeutic triumph, the empiricism upon which this is based can only go so far and no further without a clearer understanding of pathogenetic and immunologic mechanisms.

The easy way to approach this subject would be to take the diagnosis of Hodgkin's disease as given and then to analyze only the immune disturbances which happen en route, bearing in mind the immunomodulatory role of therapy and considering primarily the clinical and peripheral blood findings associated with the disease. Resisting that option, it is proposed here that the immunology of the disease be examined from the point of view of the tissue specimen as well as the blood, and from the point of view of pathogenesis as well as established pathology.

The nomenclature in this brief carries with it a problem: while the term lymphocyte is relatively clearly defined, the term monocyte is less so particularly when dealing with the interface between blood cells, definitely monocytes, and tissue cells which could be monocytic but could also be categorized as macrophages, histiocytes, or mononuclear phagocytes. A contentious issue is how to classify other marrow-derived stromal components of a node which may act accessory to lymphoid cells such as the dendritic cells. Here, the term monocyte is interpreted in its widest sense and the subdivisions are ignored except where appropriate in the context of the discussion and where other work is being quoted which refers specifically to subcategories.

Another problem of this brief is that some of the guidelines of discussion need to be formulated in a rather unusual fashion. It becomes essential to ask whether or not there are substantive differences between Hodgkin's disease and other lymphomas, and to use quantitative methods of looking at lymphocytes and monocytes in relationship to immunodeficiency to try to explain how specific cellular changes are related to the subtle cell-mediated immune defect. One inevitably becomes involved in the problem of whether or not the Reed-Sternberg cell/Hodgkin cell is in fact representative of any known cell lineage.

## II. STRUCTURE OF NORMAL LYMPHOID TISSUE

Before discussing the immunology of altered lymphoid tissue as seen in Hodgkin's disease it is important to examine briefly normal lymphoid tissue structure, taking cognizance in particular of functional markers and surface antigens identified by monoclonal reagents.

Normal lymphoid tissues are composed of relatively fixed polymorphous structural elements (reticular cells, interdigitating cells, dendritic cells, and endothelium) which serve as a framework within which lymphoid cells are organized to form functional compartments such as the primary follicles, germinal centers, and periarteriolar lymphocytic sheath of the spleen. These functional units are identifiable morphologically and have important associations with subsets of lymphoid cells which belong either to the B or T cell class.

The normal T lymphocytes develop from bone marrow lymphoid stem cells and migrated via the thymic cortex where they proliferate and undergo a process of selection in which T lymphocytes acquire the ability to distinguish between self and nonself major histocompatibility antigens.[1] The human cortical T cell expresses terminal deoxynucleotidyl transferase enzyme[2] and has been characterized by monoclonal antibodies as bearing the antigens Leu 1, OKT 6, and either OKT 4 or 8.[3] Usually this cell will rosette with sheep erythrocytes at 4°C. In fetal life and sometimes in the T cell lymphomas this cell will also express complement receptors on its surface. After release from the thymus, T lymphocytes migrate to the periphery where they become functionally competent T cells. This peripheralization process occurs largely in the spleen and results in either T helper/inducer cells or T suppressor/cytotoxic cells. As a general rule the T helper cell expresses the phenotype Leu 1, OKT 3, and OKT 4, lacks terminal deoxynucleotidyl transferase, and may have Fc receptors. The T suppressor subset also has Leu 1 and OKT 3 and lacks terminal deoxynucleotidyl transferase but expresses OKT 8 rather than OKT 4. Common to both subsets are the sheep erythrocyte rosetting and the pan T cell antigen OKT 11.[4] Recently, further subsets of T cells have been identified including the neutral T cell which has all the other T cell features but lacks both OKT 4 and OKT 8.

B lymphocytes also originate from bone marrow stem cells and characteristically express immunoglobulin determinants.[5] The earliest B cell component is identified as the pre-B cell, which has on its surface the common ALL antigen and antigens coded for by the major histocompatibility complex such as HLA-DR. The pre-B cell may have small amounts of cytoplasmic immunoglobulin which is usually of $\mu$ heavy chain class. No light chain is expressed. This cell may also have some surface terminal deoxynucleotidyl transferase activity in the early stages of development but this is lost with the beginning of immunoglobulin synthesis.[6] The B cell matures first to an IgM and light chain expressing B cell and in this form may retain expression of cytoplasmic IgM and common ALL antigen.[7] The question as to whether or not there is a human bursa equivalent for B cell processing has never been fully clarified, but at the periphery various forms of B cell do exist. Broadly the B cell bifurcation is into those cells which produce immunoglobulin of various types and those cells which act as controlling cells retaining immunological memory.[8] In the germinal centers there are B cells which stain weakly for surface IgM, and express Leu 1; and there are other cells which are expressors of various immunoglobulin subclasses, are reactive with peanut agglutinin, and resemble the common ALL positive precursors. The coronal B cells which are present around the germinal centers express surface IgM and IgD and are strongly HLA-DR positive.[9]

There are also circulating small B lymphocytes which have some features in common with the coronal B cell but which can express multiple heavy chain isotypes in addition to IgM and IgD. Proplasma cells and plasma cells are the cells which express single specific immunoglobulin isotypes; HLA-DR is less strongly expressed than in the precursors.[10]

The null cell population is a third population of cells found in blood and lymph nodes and is heterogeneous. Included in this population are cells which express both Leu 1 and HLA-DR;[10] these may be either B or T cells. There are also natural killer cells which are identified by the marker Leu 7.[11] These cells will sometimes form sheep erythrocyte rosettes and may react with OKM 1, a monocyte specific marker, but concordance with rosetting, marker, and functional data is rarely absolute in the null cell population. The tissue localization of Leu 7 positive null cells is to the germinal center region of the lymph node.[12]

The monocytes are bone-marrow-derived cells, and in the blood and tissues the numbers of cells belonging to this group is frequently underestimated. The promonocytic form of these cells is also sometimes encountered in periphery samples. The monocyte expresses receptors for the Fc portion of IgG and for complement, is weakly peanut agglutinin positive, and has OKM 1 on its surface.[13] The promonocyte has similar features but may lack the Fc and complement receptors. There is considerable overlap between the promonocyte and natural killer populations but formal proof of their relationship is lacking.

The distribution of all these cells is highly organized in the tissues. The lymph node cortex consists mainly of B cells aggregated in primary follicles and germinal centers. The core of each B cell aggregate is the follicular dendritic cell[14] which shares intimate contact with the surrounding B cells and by means of its dendritic processes creates a syncytium with the denser reticular structure of the deeper cortex and paracortex. In the primary follicles B cells express IgM; in germinal centers different kinds of B cell occupy different zones.[15] The peanut lectin reactive B cells are located towards the coronal pole and the weak IgM expressing B cells are situated adjacent to the paracortex. The coronal B lymphocyte cuff is often thicker in the region overlying the denser staining pole of the germinal center. This coronal region stains for IgM and IgD and contains many double staining cells for both IgM and IgD. Plasma cells can be quite numerous in the follicles and are present in the area adjacent to the corona. The normal follicle also contains macrophages of the tingible body type which gather the debris of the reactive events.

The paracortical region[13] is distinguished by the presence of interdigitating dendritic cells and there may be islands of small lymphocytes which have IgM and IgD admixed. The predominant cell is the T cell with both helper and suppressor subsets.

In the spleen the B cell area is distributed peripherally in the white pulp, occupying a compact zone inwards of the marginal sinus. These cells express surface IgM.[16] B cells of coronal type are rare except when there is a germinal center formation. Germinal centers develop eccentric to the periarteriolar lymphoid sheath between the sheath and the B cell zone. First IgM and IgD expressing B cells develop followed by the coronal cuff. Plasma cells are scattered in the red pulp and in the vicinity of the marginal sinus. The natural killer component is randomly distributed as judged by the expression of Leu 7 but these cells are probably most numerous in the red pulp cords rather than the white pulp.[17] The main T cell region is the periarteriolar lymphoid sheath itself and in this there are both T helper and T suppressor cells; T suppressor cells are more numerous in the spleen than in lymph nodes. However, the T suppressor marker OKT 8 also stains the endothelium of splenic sinuses making the precise localization of these cells diffucult.

## III. WHAT IS HODGKIN'S DISEASE?

At the outset it must be made clear that the argument that Hodgkin's disease represents a malignancy on the one hand or is an immunological disorder on the other is quite artificial to the clinician. Treatment for Hodgkin's disease is effective and it matters little whether Hodgkin's disease is one or the other. The convenience of the label malignancy is to proffer the diagnostic pathologists's reassurance to the clinician that if he does not actively treat the patient the disease will progress inexorably to a fatal conclusion. Thus in fact, by these criteria Hodgkin's disease is a malignant neoplasm.

From the academic vantage point such simplistic definitions of malignancy are philosophically unsound and leave one with the disquieting feeling that the late effects of current treatment might be somehow avoided if alternative and better methods both of definition and of treatment could be devised. In order to achieve this the search to understand the basic nature of Hodgkin's disease must continue.

In fact examining Hodgkin's disease highlights how little we know about the malignant process in general; not enough to define neoplasia itself, let alone complex interactive events such as must happen in Hodgkin's disease. The three basic tenets of our current thinking about malignancy are that malignancy is frequently a disease characterized by cells of single clonal derivation; that it is marked by progressive expansion of these cells in the absence of effective treatment and that this expansion leads to metastasis; and that untreated, the condition is invariably fatal.

Following on this much of the research work into the nature of malignancy has concentrated on demonstrating one feature that a malignant cell has in common with another malignant cell and that normal cells do not have. Examples are specific chromosomal translocations[18] or oncogenes[19] related in the genome to the functional and specific effects of such translocations. However much work is done on these malignant cells it is important to remember that in all neoplasia there is an area of possibly greater significance which emphasizes not the nature of the malignant cell itself but the important relationship between that cell and the host or patient in which it grows. If a cell is altered or expresses an inherited or acquired change which could be classified as malignant (that is, is shared by other malignant cells) the presence of that cell in an intact host still only constitutes malignancy of the cell itself when the cell follows this by growing in the particular fashion regarded as malignant. This altered emphasis switches the important question from the cells to the relationship between the cell and the host in which it grows. Cells which are otherwise normal can be made to grow in a malignant fashion if transformed or if present in an abnormal host. An example of this is in graft vs. host disease[20] where the graft proliferates and may become both expanded and fatal. This type of "malignant" potential can also be seen in hosts less severely modified than the immunosuppressed host that is killed by the graft: the classic examples are that T cell leukemia does not develop in thymectomized host A/JAX mice and that teratomas from transplanted embryos also do not develop if thymectomy has been performed on the recipients.[21]

For the clinical oncologist it is important to remember some of these philosophical considerations while he is treating the patient because the aim of eliminating the malignant cell often masks the fact that interference cannot alter some of the basic events which act at the single-cell level to induce either premalignant or malignant changes. The relationship between the malignant cell and the host is always accessible to manipulation provided that this occurs within the limits which do not destroy the host, and this may in the future be a fruitful line of clinical research.

In analyzing Hodgkin's disease it makes far more sense to use the philosophically sound and therapeutically advantageous definition of cancer or malignancy. This defines the malignant process as an abnormal interaction between a cell/cell mass and the host in which it grows, such that the normal processes of growth control and differentiation cannot occur either because of a primary defect within a component of the neoplasm or because of some intrinsic or acquired abnormality of the host. For therapeutic interference to be totally effective in this process requires elimination of the cell mass as one stage. The abnormality in the host must also be corrected and/or the relationship between the host and the cell mass must be altered so as to curtail the progressive expansion of the cell mass.

If one then examines Hodgkin's disease more closely, one finds a disease characterized by the presence of a cellular component (the Reed-Sternberg and Hodgkin cells). This cell is probably related to a normal class of nonlymphoid cell found in association with germinal centers. Both in vivo and in vitro, these cells have features which they share with the related group of cells which interact with lymphocytes. These cells are variably described as dendritic cells,[22] dendritic reticulum cells,[23] follicular dendritic cells,[24] interdigitating reticular cells,[25] Langerhans cells,[26] veil cells,[27] and the perifollicular fuchsinophilic cell.[28] The tumor mass in Hodgkin's disease does not contain more than a small fraction of these cells, but their presence is associated with a marked host reaction characterized by influx and sequestration of T cells, chiefly of T helper phenotype, and a failure of skin-related T cell immune functions, such as delayed type hypersensitivity and homograft rejection. This cellular picture is accompanied by B cell changes relating morphologically particularly to the formation of germinal centers in affected tissues and the disorganization of the normal anatomical arrangements between B and T cell areas. At the same time the T cells are activated with HLA-DR and OKT 10 surface expression, and spontaneous high levels of tritiated thymidine incorporation.

A model of this type places the common link between Hodgkin's disease immunity and neoplasia at a slightly different site from the conventional. While malignant cell definition studies remain necessary at both cellular and subcellular levels, and the oncogenes need to be identified, it is not essential that the relationship between Hodgkin's disease and other neoplasia in general should lie at that level. Rather, it is in the common immune deficiency and defective immunoregulation which antecede the malignant state. In this model Hodgkin's disease differs in that the tissue evidence of the immune dyscrasia remains more visible than it does in other tumors.

## IV. HODGKIN'S DISEASE COMPARED TO OTHER LYMPHOMAS

We have suggested that Hodgkin's disease differs from other neoplasia and that immunological factors play a central role in this. In practical terms the widespread use of the term non-Hodgkin's lymphomas for other lymph node malignancies indicates that it is in this context that it is most essential to separate Hodgkin's disease as a separate entity. Viewed immunologically Hodgkin's disease is clearly different from other lymph node neoplasms. To understand why requires background knowledge of the comparative histology of the disease incorporating modern techniques of immunology, and also some knowledge of recent studies on tumor cell pathology.

### A. Histology

The diagnostic morphology of conventional lymphomas incorporates information about gland structure with loss of normal architecture and/or a follicular pattern. The cellular features are categorized using criteria which grade lymphocytes in various ways but which are all broadly related to cell size, pleomorphism, and growth pattern. This type of analysis is confused by a bewildering range of terminology,[29-32] but there is a general consensus that a monomorphic or rather "monotonous pleomorphic" appearance is an important distinguishing feature.

In Hodgkin's disease normal functional units of diagnostic morphology in both lymph node and spleen are distorted with replacement by Hodgkin's disease tissue containing the Reed-Sternberg cell. There is disorganization of the expected relationships between the different subsets of T and B lymphocytes as a consequence of the

Hodgkin's disease process in sites involved by the disease. However, despite the cellular confusion, similar confusion of terminology has been avoided in Hodgkin's disease by the widespread adoption of a uniform classification system[33] which has outlasted previous such attempts.[34] It is significant that the choice of words used in this classification is purely descriptive: "lymphocyte predominant" and "mixed cellularity" are two examples. The nature of these terms compared with "diffuse immunoblastic" or even "centrocytic/centroblastic" indicates the difference of approach. The Hodgkin's disease classification describes the tissue responses, how many lymphoid cells are present, and what other cells or tissues are mixed with the tumor, and does not describe the tumor cells themselves. The opposite also applies: the notion that the scar tissue, the eosinophil and granulocyte infiltrate, or even the lymphoid cells, are part of the neoplastic component of the disease is a notion that is not regarded as tenable today, but it is on these components that the classification rests.

The dominance of the other cell types in the histology plays a part in making it difficult to identify the neoplastic element and differentiate what is neoplastic from what is either immune response to tumor or tumor-associated infiltrate. Certainly the neoplastic cells do have morphological variation: the two best known are the mononuclear Hodgkin cell[35] and the lacunar cell,[36] Even in mixed cellularity Hodgkin's disease where Reed-Sternberg cells and other associated neoplastic cells are common these cells rarely form more than 10% of the total cellular content of the involved node. Pathologists will often refer to a "cellular depletion of nodules" in nodular sclerosing disease which is usually regarded as meaning that there are more atypical cells and less reactive cells, but even this interpretation does not say the converse: that the atypical cells can be categorized by conventional means to yield useful prognostic implications.

Thus the paradox of Hodgkin's disease is highlighted: a disease which requires morphologic criteria for diagnosis does not conform to the morphologic norms for analysis, and a condition which is at least some of the time neoplastic has tumors which consist primarily of nonneoplastic cells.

B. Immunohistology

As in routine histology so in immunohistology Hodgkin's disease differs from other lymph node malignancies. To understand why this difference is important it is necessary to recapitulate briefly the current viewpoint as to the histogenesis of the lymphomas. Using modern technology most of these tumors in Western countries are derived from B cells. This can be shown by a variety of techniques to demonstrate the presence of unique determinants by marking them with an immunologic second label.[37] These methods will also show that the tumor cells may not express surface immunoglobulin but may nonetheless represent a B cell population at an earlier stage of development and that the follicular center cell origin of many of these tumors may be masked by a diffuse morphology.[38] The clonal origin of many of these tumors can also be shown by the same techniques[39] since only a particular heavy chain isotype and only a particular light chain will be synthesized by the tumor cells, compared with the polyclonality of a reactive cell population. Individual tumors will remain true to type in this respect: an IgA-secreting tumor will remain so;[40] an IgG kappa tumor likewise.

Such phenotyping also reveals a range of variability in cell type other than just the cloned B cell. There are T cell lymphomas[41] whose clonality is more difficult to establish using these techniques, and there are lymphomas in which none of the conventional lineages predominates.[42] The clonal origin of what, by morphology are clearly follicular lymphomas can only be demonstrated in about 75% of tumors.[43] The perifollicular region in some of these tumors contains an excess of cells which are probably reactive and thus make it impossible to identify any clones lurking beneath. The only instance in which the correlation between histology, immune markers, and clonality appears to be absolute is in the B lymphoblastic (Burkitt-like) lymphomas.[44]

Application of these methods to Hodgkin's disease tissue was an inevitable area to study. Theoretically the presence of clonality could be examined in the atypical element, in the related surrounding cells, and possibly in both. This would resolve the problem of which are the neoplastic cells and could possibly lead to a reevaluation of the relationship between tumor and responder.

The previous analyses before the advent of clonality as a concept in lymphomas had suggested a nonmacrophage neoplastic cell type based upon the enzyme histochemistry[45] and thus a B cell origin was a tenable proposition. However, no clear evidence for either B cell origin or clonality has been found.[46] Hodgkin's disease-associated B lymphocytes are virtually never restricted to a particular single light chain class. The exceptions constitute about 5% of all cases of Hodgkin's disease and these show borderline dominance of one or another isotype.[47]

While Reed-Sternberg cells themselves may contain immunoglobulin, more than one isotype and more than one light chain have been demonstrated in the same cell; this suggests an absorption rather than a secretion phenomenon. On the other hand, conventional accessory cell markers are not seen on these cells.[48] The optimum immunohistological definition on positive grounds is that these cells are clearly of bone marrow origin since they stain specifically with a monoclonal antibody aimed to identify just such a population (Dorreen and Habeshaw[175]). The theoretical conclusion reached on the basis of this type of analysis is that immunohistology could justify either a B cell or a myelomonocytic origin but that neither of the two could account for all the known characteristics of the neoplastic cell.

There are two recent reports which may have some bearing on these comments. One is that very small base modification in the DNA of an immunocompetent cell population can result in change from a B cell to a myelomonocytic phenotype.[49] The other suggests that there may be a Hodgkin's disease cell-specific monoclonal reagent which does not react with cells that belong to either of the normal phenotypes propounded.[50] The significance of both these reports to the understanding of Hodgkin's disease cell biology cannot be assessed as yet.

The typical Hodgkin's disease lymph node differs from normal and lymphoma nodes in having a T cell predominance which is also seen in immunohistology. This is neither unique nor invariable but is unusually common. There are two particular types of lymphoma with which this is often confused. In some follicular lymphomas as much as 30% of the total cell population can be T cells and in high grade tumors such as the centroblastic and immunoblastic forms, the T cell proportion can sometimes be as high as 60%,[51] but apart from these instances Hodgkin's disease is more commonly linked to a T cell preponderance than any other lymphoma. Occasionally these T cell infiltrates can be associated with expression of HLA-DR by T cells, suggesting that they are activated.

Thus in a given node immunohistology is probably most useful to allow for the identification of a monoclonal surface immunoglobulin despite a large background of T cells, and thus for the identification of "occult" B cell tumors when either Hodgkin's disease or a T cell lymphoma is suspected. The converse is also true: T cell lymphomas are usually of one phenotype (commonly a T helper cell) while a mixed T cell phenotype is more like Hodgkin's disease. It is interesting that there is one recorded example where phenotyping did raise the possibility of a T cell lymphoma rather than Hodgkin's disease in a child but this did not hold true,[53] highlighting the necessity of using more than one method of analysis.

A problem of phenotyping is that the mixed T cell predominance seen in Hodgkin's disease can be confused with lymphoma-like or lymphoma-related conditions. "Lennert's lymphoma" shows a T cell predominance in which one T cell type may predominate; this is usually a T suppressor cell and the associated epithelioid cells do not have surface immunoglobulin but do have HLA-DR. Another condition is angioimmunoblastic lymphadenopathy in which both T cell predominance and B cell polyclonality are seen. Here again the T cells are mostly of the suppressor rather than helper class.

What is clear from these findings is that unlike other lymph node malignancies, in Hodgkin's disease immunohistology has clarified neither the cell of origin nor the nature of the process involved. The main clarification has been in the area of the non-Reed-Sternberg cells where as a fringe benefit of attempts to clarify the histogenesis of the neoplastic cell, it has become clear that the lymphoid cell component is polyclonal.

## C. In Vitro Analysis

The same contrasts that apply in histology and immunohistology occur in the in vitro analysis of Hodgkin's disease vs. the other lymph node malignancies. Distinguishing between a lymph node involved by Hodgkin's disease and a reactive lymph node, particularly in conditions like toxoplasmosis or cat scratch disease, is not possible on an in vitro cell suspension; it would be irresponsible to base a diagnosis on this type of methodology.

For the lymphomas clonal origin has been established,[54] continuously proliferating cell lines have been established,[55] and transplantable tumors have been identified.[56] All these methods support the single cell origin of at least some of the lymphomas. Hodgkin's disease cell cultures do not demonstrate clonality; the one acceptable cell line so far maintained over long term has not been cloned; and the few continuous cell lines have not lasted indefinitely.[57]

These types of results are not conclusive evidence that such a clonable neoplastic element is absent from the Hodgkin's disease tumor sample. In vitro analysis of human tumor tissue is a complex subject and failure to produce a suitable line and clone may represent the inadequacy of specific aspects of the technology rather than absence of a clonable population.[58] Even if clonal origin is confirmed then there may be difficulty in satisfying the requirement of transplantation to nude mice.[56] Alternatively, clonality may not be an absolute in the confirmation of neoplastic disease. This is illustrated in the immune system by the failure of response to Epstein-Barr virus (EBV) seen in Duncan's disease[59] where the proliferative immune response may have all the features of neoplasia in terms of spread and rapid downhill progression, but in which all the evidence including in vitro studies suggests polyclonality.[60]

Since this aspect of comparative analysis between Hodgkin's disease and the conventional lymphomas has not yet been fully investigated under optimum conditions it is probably premature to draw conclusions. However, the short-term cultures raise interesting possibilities. Most of the successful short-term cultures to date have been from nodular sclerosing Hodgkin's disease rather than from other forms.[61] This could be due to heterogeneity in the disease itself: some examples being truly neoplastic, others being nonneoplastic and others being neoplastic but for which the technology is inadequate even for short-term analyses. If B cell lymphomas represent a failure to turn off unrestrained proliferation in the immune system and T cells are the controlling step in this, then in vitro analyses should examine the nonneoplastic element as well as the neoplastic in such derived populations.

## D. Conclusions

Current technology has succeeded in showing that Hodgkin's disease is clearly different from other lymphomas in several crucial respects. The Hodgkin's disease tumor cells are few and far between in a tumor sample, the response to these cells is polyclonal, pleomorphic and variable, and the tumor cells are more difficult to examine. The lymphomas which are difficult to differentiate using combined parameter analysis are those follicular lymphomas where polyclonal mantle-zone lymphocytes are identifiable as the predominant cell type and those high grade lymphomas in which the reactive component is excessively visible.

Viewed from the three vantage points considered, the conclusion is that to study Hodgkin's disease it is necessary to understand lymphocyte/monocyte interaction as well as neoplasia. To date the evidence for clonal origin and for other "Koch's postulates" of neoplasia have not been forthcoming in this disease.

## V. IMMUNE MECHANISMS IN THE ETIOLOGY OF HODGKIN'S DISEASE

The etiology of Hodgkin's disease is unknown. It is not even clear whether a single event is responsible for all examples of the disease, or whether the clinical syndrome with which we associate the disease is really the end stage of a number of processes, each of which has a different etiology.

As has already been suggested, the common denominator of most analysis of the etiology postulates an immune mechanism. The definition of this mechanism raises several problems, such as the starting point at which one can separate a reactive from a neoplastic role in the disease, and where the borderline between transformation and neoplasia occurs. Nevertheless, belief in the immune mechanism remains strong, resting on the overall, rather hazy idea that some features of Hodgkin's disease histology resemble an inflammatory response, that no agent to cause an inflammatory response has been found by methods which have been used to find such agents successfully in other conditions, and that therefore, the only process which could produce this type of histology while masking an infection is an immune one. There is now some more scientific data on which to base an approach to the etiology in immunological terms.

Cell interactions in vitro are the basis for much of the recent information in this field since they allow for study of the interrelationships between individual well-characterized cell types. One of the problems of these methods vis-à-vis Hodgkin's disease is that the cells often form clumps in vitro; this could be highlighting the fact that cell-cell events are the major component of the disease.[62]

To take this further, mitogens are often used such as phytohemagglutinin and pokeweed which activate both T helper and T suppressor cells, and concanavalin A which activates T suppressor cells. Using these methods in Hodgkin's disease, the clumps consist of identifiable T cells around Reed-Sternberg cells.[63]

However, B cells may also be involved in such clumps since spontaneous rosetting can be induced in vitro by mixing lymphoblastoid cell lines and T lymphocytes, and some of the cells in the clumps could be B cells which are transformed. B cells can also clump directly to each other or to macrophages especially when activated by conditioned supernatant from T cells. All these forms of spontaneous rosettes could be represented in one or other form of Hodgkin's disease. The likely postulate is that both in vivo and in vitro the Reed-Sternberg cell acts like the interdigitating cell with regard to the T cell, or the follicular dendritic cell to the B cell.[64]

The importance of this kind of cell-to-cell contact in immune mechanisms cannot be over-emphasized and is less frequently examined than other types of reaction. When it is explored, the results are often surprising. For example, when stimulated T cells are cultivated in modified Marbrook systems over highly purified B cells where only T cell factors have access to the B cell populations, there is little proliferation of B cells, and virtually no conversion to plasma cells. Addition of isogenic purified blood monocytes to the system does not have any effect, but when contact between T and B cells is established then both B cell transformation and conversion to plasma cells occurs even if the T cell concentration is only 2 to 10% of the whole.[65] This illustrates clearly that cell contact and T cell factors are both required for effective interaction.

## A. Epidemiology

Although the cell interaction studies are strongly suggestive of an immune mechanism, the most persuasive evidence for this comes from an interpretation of the epidemiology.

There is a socioeconomic factor which contributes to the disease in the western world. Age-specific incidence has changed significantly in association with development, industrialization, and the institutionalization of health care. From being a disease of childhood and adolescence, Hodgkin's disease is now a disease of young adults. In this age group the patient with Hodgkin's disease belongs to a higher socioeconomic group than controls.[66] There is case clustering and the disease is more frequent in siblings of the same sex as the propositus.[67] A preponderance of Jews compared to Roman Catholics develop the disease.[68] The patient with Hodgkin's disease is more likely to have undergone tonsillectomy[69] and appendectomy[70] although whether this is independent of the higher socioeconomic class is not clear since this group are more likely to consult doctors and hence to undergo elective surgical procedures.[71]

This hypothesis cannot account for all Hodgkin's disease. In less developed countries the disease is also common and here there does not seem to be a class difference.[72] In these countries the more aggressive forms of the disease are more prevalent. The resemblance between the Hodgkin's disease pattern in this population and that of Kaposi's sarcoma is interesting[73] particularly in view of the emerging evidence that an immune mechanism, a viral component, and a social component seem to be important in the pathogenesis of Kaposi's sarcoma in the western world.[74] In immunosuppressed hosts, Hodgkin's disease does occur with a higher risk than in nonimmunosuppressed[75] people; however, Hodgkin's disease is less common in this setting than high grade lymphoma.[76]

An immunological model to cover the epidemiological data suggests that in the western world lower socioeconomic groups are commonly exposed to an agent which results in adequate immunity to the agent. Higher socioeconomic groups are not exposed at an early stage to this agent due to better hygiene. At a later stage they are exposed and at this stage exposure leads to the neoplastic form of the disease. This could be due to aging of the immune system or to idiosyncracy but does not appear to link to any of the known immunogenetic markers, although an intrinsic risk in a target population is a very likely possibility.[76] It is not surprising that there is an association with infectious mononucleosis and with raised titers to EBV[77] since this disease has a similar social and geographic distribution in western countries as well as similar more aggressive variants in less developed countries.[78] Elderly patients with Hodgkin's disease are either those who escaped infection earlier or a recrudescence of a latent infection due to impaired immunity of aging analogous to examples of tuberculosis in a similar population.

## B. Virology

The obvious candidate agent for this type of epidemiology is a virus. There has been an extensive search for such an agent. The suggested framework in which this operates resembles the natural history of poliomyelitis: many are exposed but few contract the disease. Interestingly the immunologic mechanism which presumably determined which patients did develop paralysis and which did not has never been established. The postulate of analogy between poliomyelitis and Hodgkin's disease is that in the case of a Hodgkin's disease, "virus" neoplasia rather than paralysis supervenes.

For a virus to be implicated does not necessarily mean that the virus should persist and be identifiable in the tissues. This has been the type of problem which has bedevilled analysis of all potential viral oncogenic agents.[79] Recently there has been some success in the T cell lymphomas.[80] Interpretation of this kind of data has also been complicated by the observation that there is homology between viral encoded gene sequences and naturally occurring genetic material.[81] Thus even DNA isolation from tumor cells may produce an endogenous product which is not necessarily oncogenic by itself.

The best documented of the numerous attempts at virological analysis in Hodgkin's disease records that both RNA and DNA agents could be isolated from cultured cells but not directly from the tumor.[82] A later series of papers purported to define an antigen in the disease[83] but these data were later shown to be associated with contamination by a monkey virus.[84] The relationship between Hodgkin's disease and EBV has already been mentioned, but there are several other aspects to this question. One is that the titer of antibody to the virus may be raised before the onset of disease when compared to normal controls.[85] Another is that the EBV/Burkitt lymphoma relationship implicates a previous immune onslaught probably due to malaria acting as a kind of cofactor;[86] there may be a requirement for such a nonspecific immune stimulatory role in the etiology of Hodgkin's disease, and EBV would be a candidate for such a role. Whether this is so or not, all the cultures of Hodgkin's cells have been screened for EBV and all have proven negative[87] suggesting that it is not directly implicated as a causative agent.

C. Pathogenesis

The epidemiology and virology combined with the histology add up to considerable evidence that an immune mechanism operates in the disease but combine this with little information as to how this mechanism operates.

The first problem in interpreting Hodgkin's disease in the conventional type model is that since the antigen which acts as an initiator is unknown it is difficult to place the disease into a category of known response. For example; by definition the histology is different from any of the Gell and Coombs hypersensitivity patterns. The only suitable slot suggested is that the features bear some resemblance to a graft vs. host phenomenon.[88] This theory proposes that an antigen (or an acquired oncogenic stimulus) perpetually alters T cells to become nonself cells in such a way that these T cells themselves become presenters to other cytotoxic T cells, despite the absence of residual evidence of the evoking agent. A self-perpetuating mechanism ensues with constant activation of normal T cells which in the end leads to neoplastic transformation of one or another cell type in the node. Another variant of this theme is that an initiating agent could induce the T cell to go into a phase of continual lymphokine production and hence to activate macrophages and related cells; eventually this also leads to a neoplastic rather than a reactive transformation.[89]

Whichever mechanism is operating in the disease, it must incorporate T cell activation either by other T cells or by accessory cells. Thus another point at which an antigen could enter an immune circuit is at the accessory cell level and the neoplastic cell is probably related to this cell compartment.[90] The antigen (such as a virus) could persist in these cells in an occult form and only be reisolated in recognizable form in the culture step[91] but remain active in a T cell stimulatory capacity. This type of mechanism would in turn be dependent on a viral tropism mechanism which is itself unexplained: why are B cells so responsive to EBV, T cells so responsive to retroviruses, and accessory cells so responsive to a possible Hodgkin's disease agent? Part of the explanation may lie in the specific interaction between the Reed-Sternberg cell, and its variants on one hand and the T lymphocytes on the other since this interaction seems to be unlike conventional cytotoxic cell/accessory cell mechanisms and may require a unique receptor on one or another of the cells which is unlike those defined by conventional methods.[92]

Other putative nonviral antigens are also implicated in work on the pathogenesis of Hodgkin's disease. One of the antigens was probably ferritin[93] which supports the general contention that there is a central regulatory role for iron-related proteins in lymphoid tissue and in Hodgkin's disease specifically.[94] This "ecotaxopathy" theory relies upon a microenvironmental defect with sequestration of T cells at distinct sites because of local signals. The local mechanism could operate either as a cofactor in the evolution of an immune response or as a blocking factor in impeding a normal cytotoxic immune reaction. The recent identification of transferrin receptors on proliferating cells in a variety of situations[95] has added emphasis to this kind of postulate.

When one considers these postulates in conjunction with the conventional immune model outlined above a general trend emerges which explains the direction of most of the cell biology studies in Hodgkin's disease. The hypothetical area in which this disease seems to lie is that of occult underlying transforming agents, T cell predominance and activation and neoplasia of a nonlymphoid element. However, none of the studies cited can as yet answer central aspects of the pathogenesis. If the neoplastic event has occurred it is not clear whether this cell can continue to perform the immunoregulatory role for which it was designated. Thus a neoplastic dendritic cell may not be able to elicit cytotoxic responses in the normal fashion expected of it.[96] Further, in the neoplastic context we may have to ignore some aspects of the conventional cell lineages since functionally intermediate forms can occur.

D. Conclusions

Sufficient information is now known about Hodgkin's disease epidemiology to support the notion that some extraneous agent is likely to be involved in the disease. This must operate in an indirect fashion without person-to-person spread and without leaving recognizable evidence of its presence. There is evidence that exposure to this agent may not invariably lead to the disease. Cofactors may be involved in a number of ways; among these could be EBV and other viruses and iron-related proteins. There are several unproven hypotheses of which the most widely respected is the virally altered self mechanism with resultant persistent and unusual local T lymphocyte stimulation. All the mechanisms of etiology and pathogenesis have in common the fact that they implicate the T lymphocyte/accessory cell interaction event at some stage in the process and it is this interaction which represents the key site in the disease.

## VI. HODGKIN'S DISEASE TISSUE

When the diagnosis of Hodgkin's disease has been made the differences between this example of lymph node malignancy on the one hand and other forms of lymph node malignancy on the other have been absorbed into the diagnostic interpretation of the section. The epidemiological and immunological background often plays a part in this interpretation. This common denominator has an air of definition about it so it is then surprising to read that Reed-Sternberg cells can occur in a variety of conditions[97] and that a cynical definition of this cell is that of a cell which a pathologist can convince another pathologist is a Reed-Sternberg cell.

However, pending a more precise definition of the earlier phases of the disease, the biopsy sample has to act not only as the diagnostic material but also as our chief source of information about the disease and in particular about the relative role of the lymphocyte and monocyte.

When interpreting older literature in this field it is important to remember that papers written before the 1960s were looking at a disease which was relatively untreatable and which followed either an unrelenting course or could be paradoxically susceptible to radiation control. The histopathology of the lymphomas was also different from current theory and thus what was considered to be Hodgkin's disease might today be called some other type of lymphoma. More recent literature has to take into account

## A. Histology

The relative preponderance of nonneoplastic cells in a Hodgkin's tumor has already been mentioned. In an involved node there may also be areas which are not involved[98] and these areas may contain both normal and reactive lymph node components including germinal centers and expanded T cell zones in particular. Sometimes reactive monocyte-derived cell populations are identified such as prominent tingible body macrophages in the germinal centers and epithelioid granulomata.[99] The lymphocytes and monocytes which are present in these reactive areas as well as the tumor areas may be important in the disease.

The observation that there is a relationship between the total number of lymphocytes in a sample and the prognosis was made nearly 50 years ago.[100] Since then the chief modification to this concept on strict morphological grounds has been to categorize the disease primarily by this method rather than by the features of the tumor cells. Several mechanisms which could account for the presence of these cells have been mentioned. As this is the prognostic index in the disease[33] the lymphoid infiltrate could be said to suggest that Hodgkin's disease really is an example where immune surveillance[101] operates in the classical sense of the term.

The morphological range of the lymphoid cells themselves is considerable and all stages can occur in the Hodgkin's disease infiltrate. Active DNA synthesis takes place in a high proportion of these cells[102] as judged by tritiated thymidine incorporation. Since the growth in bulk of a Hodgkin's disease node is relatively slow, and since monocytic cells do not label in the same way it has been suggested that there must be a high turnover of lymphoid cells in the tumor. This in turn is consistent with a reactive role for the lymphocyte since if they were the neoplastic element then node growth might be expected to be more rapid.

The monocytic cells have a much less well-defined role in Hodgkin's disease tissue. Normal histiocytes have been regarded as a favorable prognostic marker.[103] Nodular lymphocyte predominant disease may incorporate many of this type of monocyte. Reactive histiocytes have been regarded as a poor prognostic index.[104] There are some instances in which epithelioid cells with or without granuloma formation do predominate.[105] This association was said to be linked to a poor prognostic outcome. However, recently these authors have put forward the view that some of these cases were examples of B cell lymphomas with epithelioid cells rather than Hodgkin's disease.[106] In the lymphocyte-depleted forms of the disease, while there are fewer cells overall, there may be a relative excess of monocytic cells compared to lymphoid cells in a given sample.

The relationship between monocytic cells and other nonlymphoid stromal elements is close. In the mixed cellularity form of the disease where other cells are prominent there are generally more monocytic cells than in the lymphocyte predominant and nodular sclerosing forms of the disease. This could either be relative due to fewer lymphoid cells or absolute due to a real increase in the monocytes. Areas of necrosis are associated with increased numbers of monocytes. This relationship is also not simple. Small areas of fibrinoid necrosis may be related to activation of coagulation as seen in association with most inflammatory responses[107] and the monocytes may be playing an active but nonspecific role since they act as a source of complement[108] and of enzymes such as plasminogen activator.[109] Large areas of necrosis with more monocytes which could still be nonspecific are regarded as being part of more aggressive disease. Unusual concentrations of Reed-Sternberg cells can occur in relationship to areas of necrosis irrespective of size; again the significance is not clear.[87]

Using histochemical methods to identify monocytic cells there are nonspecific esterase-positive cells and acid phosphatase cells in the Hodgkin's disease tissue section which are clearly not neoplastic.[98] There has been no careful analysis of the relative proportion of these cells and also it is not clear how many nonlymphoid cells lack these monocyte enzyme patterns. Taking only the esterase-positive cells as a starting point in the Hodgkin's disease tissues, there is no proliferation of monocytes as judged by tritiated thymidine incorporation.[102] The other forms of accessory cell have been examined solely from the vantage point of malignancy,[61] and cell types such as dendritic cells and follicular dendritics do occur in a nonneoplastic form in the Hodgkin's node but there is no recorded analysis of these cell types as being different in appearance or distribution in the disease.

## B. Immunohistology

The predominant role of immunohistology has been to explore the nature of the neoplastic cell in Hodgkin's disease. This question has been discussed above. As a byproduct, considerable evidence has accumulated about the features of the cells which surround a Reed-Sternberg or Hodgkin cell, but most reports place little emphasis on this aspect.

Using the immunoperoxidase method on Hodgkin's disease tumors there is no evidence to suggest a monoclonal population (see above). There are immunoglobulin-producing cells present in the tumor infiltrate and these show a mixed phenotype with both mu and delta heavy chains, and both kappa and lambda light chains.[110] There are also cells which contain cytoplasmic immunoglobulin; this is predominantly IgG but other isotypes can occur. With regard to T lymphocytes, immunostaining procedures have shown that there is a preponderance of cells which lack immunoglobulin on their surface but which have IgMEA receptors.[111] These cells are particularly prevalent surrounding the atypical cell component.

Recently the advent of monoclonal reagents which identify T cell subsets has led to reevaluation of their role in disease in general and there is a burgeoning literature on the role of helper/inducer and suppressor/cytotoxic cells present in different disease sites. Using this type of method T cells predominate around the atypical cells in most examples of the disease.[175] In the nodular sclerosing form of the disease, T cell predominance is particularly marked and the Reed-Sternberg cells are situated peripherally to the B cell areas surrounded by a T cell population. It could be that there are two forms of Reed-Sternberg cell, one related to the follicular dendritic cell found in the lymphocyte predominant form and the other related to the interdigitating dendritic cell present in the nodular sclerosing form. Within the T cell population it has been suggested that there are helper cells more centrally in relation to the Reed-Sternberg cell and suppressor/cytotoxic cells more peripherally, rather like a normal follicular structure.[9] Whether or not this is so, the T cells themselves are more activated than usual as judged by their expression of OKT 10 and HLADR antigens. Confirming that a direct cytotoxicity pattern between the T cells and the Reed-Sternberg cells is unlikely, in this study the predominant cell around the atypical cells expresses OKT 4 and not OKT 8.

One of the difficulties even on immunohistology is to clarify the monocyte and B cell differences. Both cell types share Fc and C3 receptors and express surface DR antigens. They are also both bone-marrow-derived and thus stain with common leukocyte reagents. There are definitely cells in a Hodgkin's disease tumor which contain lysozyme and are not neoplastic[110] and this has been best shown on immunohistochemistry. These cells have not been shown to have a distinctive distribution and the presence of this marker does not account for all possible monocyte derivatives in a given sample. The cells which express the myeloid-specific monoclonals generally correlate with those which express the lysosomal and lysozyme markers and thus from the point of view of the nonneoplastic component they have not been examined in detail. Nearly all samples of Hodgkin's disease tissue will react strongly with peanut lectin resembling germinal center components and representing part of the so-called sessile cell population.[175]

C. In Vitro Analysis

In vitro analysis of cells from Hodgkin's disease represents an interesting challenge which arises inevitably from this discussion. All the reported studies have stressed difficulties in technology. For this reason most of the documented in vitro work in Hodgkin's disease uses peripheral blood cells (see below).

Most tissue studies have used the nodular sclerosing form of the disease since this is the easiest to obtain in the large western treatment centers; this is not necessarily representative of the entire disease spectrum. It is difficult to be sure whether a given piece of tissue from a Hodgkin's disease patient comes from a tumor-involved site or whether it is part of the uninvolved tissue which may be intimately intermingled. Extracting a viable cell population from the sample is difficult. Once this has been obtained then the requirement for suitable normal controls is difficult to satisfy.

Based on in vitro analysis there is sufficient evidence to confirm that there are more T cells in Hodgkin's disease tissue than in normal control samples.[112] This redistribution of T cells occurs even in uninvolved areas and could thus antecede the disease; but it could also represent disease in which the classic marker cell is not present, thus justifying the unjustifiable epithet uninvolved. When one examines the functional potentials resulting from this observation then the relationship becomes even more complicated. On the one hand (unlike in the peripheral blood) there may be greater responsiveness to phytohemagglutinin in Hodgkin's disease tissue compared with controls.[113] On the other hand the fact that many of these cells express IgMEA may mean that their role as regulators of B cell function is impaired even though they are increased in number.[114] Using a different type of isolation procedure based on density gradient analysis, even though there are more T cells present in total it is interesting that the fraction which is normally composed of E rosetting cells predominantly contains instead a high proportion of null cells;[115] likewise the fraction which gives optimal phytohemagglutinin responses does not do so. One study of Hodgkin's disease lymph nodes using careful statistical methods showed a significant increase in the rosette forming cell population.[116] There was no correlation between the proportion of E rosetting cells and the histological subtype of disease. The spleens involved with the disease showed depressed responses to phytohemagglutinin and concanavalin A; this correlated with nodular sclerosing and mixed cellularity disease, and was not found in lymphocyte predominance. In a given individual sample there is an intrinsic problem: uninvolved spleen lymphocytes may be more reactive but cells from involved areas (which are less reactive) may mask the picture if not analyzed separately. Removal of adherent cells and preincubation to eliminate blocking factors did not alter this pattern.

Using the T cells in a different kind of proliferation assay Hodgkin's-disease-derived cells are poor responders either in the autologous or heterologous mixed leukocyte response.[117] This is not due to monocyte suppression since even after careful adherence the defect in responsiveness is still apparent. When these T cells are placed in contact with the neoplastic cell in vitro then their interaction is dependent upon intact surface proteins and divalent cations[118] but not upon conventional surface receptors, thus suggesting that there is a unique type of interaction different from other forms operating in the immune system.

Studies with monoclonal antibodies applied to cell suspensions have yielded new information about the T cell compartment of these suspensions.[112] Using these markers it is possible to compare directly between E rosetting cells and cells bearing a particular surface antigen. In conjunction with pan T cell reagents the relative proportion of each subset can be analyzed and subtle shifts identified. By these methods there are more OKT-3-bearing cells than E rosetting cells in a normal node but in Hodgkin's disease the two populations are essentially equal. In the Hodgkin's disease node this is associated with active disease involvement rather than with uninvolved samples, but the phenotypic difference is not sufficiently clearcut to allow for discrimination by this kind of technique rather than histology. Another monoclonal antibody, OKT 11, inhibits E rosetting specifically and shows the same pattern as is seen with rosetting. The OKT 10 marker (which is not T-cell-specific) also shows a different distribution in Hodgkin's disease when compared with reactive lymph nodes.

Compared with normal controls there are fewer cells which express surface immunoglobulin in the Hodgkin's disease tissue, but whether this is an absolute phenomenon or relative to the quantitative T cell preponderance is not clear. Functional assay systems have produced the same type of complex pattern as for the T cell, with the added factor that each of the B cell abnormalities could be interpreted as due to altered T cell control mechanisms. When immunoglobulin synthesis is used as the measure of B cell function and corrected for the weight of tumor tissue analyzed then moderately involved Hodgkin's disease tissue derived samples produced more antibody than controls.[119] Secondary in vitro antibody responses in this system also showed enhancement when the disease was less extensive but in massive disease the response became undetectable. Conversely, another system using herpes-specific antibody production as an end assay has shown an impairment in the Hodgkin's tissue.[120] As for the T cell changes, also for the B cell changes, although the abnormalities have been identified, none of them is sufficiently prominent to justify the immunologic deficit with which the disease is associated.

When the monocyte and related cells are considered in vitro there are again difficulties in interpretation since the neoplastic cell may well be included in this fraction, and it is not clear how much of a functional role this cell will play. Further, if T-cell-derived lymphokine type regulatory products are important in the disease then the monocytes could be present but functionally ineffective. There are definitely fewer cells which have monocyte enzyme and receptor properties in a given sample of Hodgkin's-disease-derived tissue than there are in normal controls;[61] this also applies when one examines uninvolved tissue from Hodgkin's disease patients, and exists despite the fact that when adjusted for weight of tissue and assessed by glass adherence alone there is no difference from normal tissue. With regard to functional assays the adherent cells from Hodgkin's disease are poor stimulators of a mixed leukocyte response.[117] This may be due to excess release of prostaglandins by the adherent cells.[121] If the murine model for accessory cell heterogeneity is true in humans then the Hodgkin's adherent cells could show a subtle shift between an effector "peritoneal cell-like" functional role with phagocytic but nonpresenting monocyte derivatives predominating, rather than an inducer situation with "dendritic cell-like" functions more apparent.[122]

D. Conclusions

Hodgkin's disease tissue is composed of a mixture of cells of which lymphocytes and monocytes are the most prominent. The nature of the lymphoid infiltrate is the best-characterized prognostic marker in the disease and the T cell predominates in all the analyses, but there are some features of these T cells which are unusual. These include the predominance of suppressor/cytotoxic cells in some forms of the disease; the poor responsiveness of these cells in some proliferative cultures; and the evidence for a sequestration phenomenon linked to an interaction which differs from conventional T/accessory cell systems. B cells are also abnormal in the disease sample: hyporesponsiveness to some antigens and hyperresponsiveness to others is demonstrable in vitro. The B cells are polyclonal with preserved isotype class distribution suggesting that relatively normal functional activity can be achieved. The monocyte compartment is also altered with some variations associated with the epiphenomena of the disease (such as tissue necrosis) but with other features such as decreased receptor and enzyme expression among the glass adherent cells and decreased in vitro stimulatory capacity. These findings suggest a more direct defect in normal monocyte function over and above the linkage of the neoplastic cell to this cell compartment.

## VII. PERIPHERAL BLOOD CELLS IN HODGKIN'S DISEASE

For the Hodgkin's disease tissue lymphocyte and monocyte there is an obvious dearth of data to explain the discrepant findings and hence clarify the nature of the disease. For the peripheral blood cell there is an extensive literature but the interpretation of this data has proven extremely difficult since no comprehensive pattern has emerged to account for all the defects observed. Part of this may be due to variability intrinsic to peripheral blood estimations, with influences as simple as diurnal variation playing a part. Another factor is that there are inherent technical problems in rosetting and cell separation making the results difficult to reproduce from laboratory to laboratory.

In reviewing the literature a major difficulty is that material has often been analyzed considering Hodgkin's disease as a whole rather than including comparable groups identified by like histology and staging. Another problem is that post-treatment analysis has been included with pre-treatment samples and most treatment regimes, by definition, damage the immune system in some way. However, there are advantages in the peripheral blood systems which have led to the extensive analysis: more cells are available and cells can be obtained repeatedly during the course of the individual illness; and the larger numbers of patients from whom these cells can be derived allows for more statistical objective analysis than has been possible in tissue work.

There is a well-documented leukopenia with lymphopenia in Hodgkin's disease.[123] Overall this is seen in between 40 to 50% of patients and is correlated with staging since in disseminated disease more than half the patients show lymphopenia. In the lymphocyte-depleted form of the disease, which is often disseminated, 80% of the patients are lymphopenic.[124]

There are several possible mechanisms for this lymphopenia. There could be either altered migration and/or sequestration of lymphocytes in tissue[94] or there could be decreased survival due to lymphocytotoxins.[125] The distribution of T cell subsets could be altered in the tissues and this may then be reflected in the bloodstream.[112] Linked to the lymphopenia is the decrease in capping with concanavalin A[126] which reflects membrane alterations, which could in turn influence both migration and responsiveness of lymphocytes.

Morphologically although there are fewer cells overall those present often have the features of blast type activated cells, often hypereosinophilic, and resembling those seen in infectious mononucleosis.[127] These cells show increased spontaneous thymidine incorporation. This activated state includes both T and B lymphocytes and is sometimes regarded as an index of disease progression. It is possible that some of these cells have been considered as circulating Reed-Sternberg cells in earlier reports.[128]

### A. T Lymphocytes

It is widely accepted that T lymphocyte counts are decreased in Hodgkin's disease. This does not always correlate with disease severity.[129] In children with the disease a T lymphopenia is also present but is generally less marked.[53] Since B cell counts are also reduced[130] comparative percentage methods are not useful to demonstrate this. To get an overview of the peripheral blood T cell in the disease it is necessary to examine several types of technique specific for T cells, rather than comparative numerical phenomena.

Using the rosetting method to identify T cells there is a decrease in the number of cells which rosette with sheep erythrocytes using the standard assay,[129] but the so-called active rosetting capacity is unimpaired.[131] The defect in rosetting capacity is corrected either by incubating with fetal serum[132] or with levamisole.[133] It has been shown that this levamisole effect is due to a blocking protein on the cell surface, probably apoferritin. Correlating with this, there is an increase in ferritin synthesis and release[134] by peripheral blood cells in Hodgkin's disease, and abnormal forms of ferritin have been proposed as a factor in pathogenesis. An additional serum glycolipid factor has also been identified,[87] and it is possible that this acts by glycosylation of a surface protein which is reversed in the serum/levamisole incubation procedure.

The in vitro functional T cell responses are impaired in Hodgkin's disease peripheral blood cells. The best example of this is the decrease in responsiveness to the T cell mitogen, phytohemagglutinin.[135] This holds true even if correction for the lymphopenia is included in the analysis, and is irrespective of disease stage but not dissemination. The decrease is not linked to capacity to synthesize either protein or DNA, suggesting a T cell function defect rather than a metabolic failure. In the mixed leukocyte reaction, the Hodgkin's disease peripheral blood cell will show decreased proliferative response.[136] This is confirmed further by a decrease in the generation of allocytotoxic T cells. All these assays are dependent upon carefully controlled in vitro conditions, and it has been suggested that to identify Hodgkin's-disease-related defects it is better to examine proliferation after 3 days rather than 4 days, and to use suboptimal antigen doses.

A different kind of T cell function is the capacity to synthesize lymphokines. In general terms, this too is reduced in Hodgkin's disease peripheral blood cells, as judged by a variety of supernatant activities such as production of macrophage migration inhibition factor, leukocyte migration inhibition factor,[137] and macrophage aggregation factor.[138] An observed defect in interferon production in Hodgkin's disease patients who have symptomatic disease[139] has not been analyzed in detail, but may prove an interesting observation if a viral association is eventually demonstrated in the disease.

Although the T cell defect in the disease is generally regarded as a peripheral one involving the disease site and the peripheral blood only, it has also been suggested that thymic processing of T lymphocytes may be impaired. The evidence for this is based on the lack of so-called thymic factor in the disease[136] and on the experiments which showed that fetal thymic tissue can restore peripheral blood lymphocyte functional parameters to normal.[140] This type of restoration experiment is notoriously difficult to control, especially since the immune mechanism defect in the disease is unknown. The thymic tissue may in fact be acting in a nonspecific fashion rather than reflecting a Hodgkin's-disease-specific reaction.

Another aspect of T cell function is the adoptive transfer capacity of peripheral blood lymphocytes. Under normal circumstances the ability of T cells to transfer hypersensitivity responses is well known. If the recipient has Hodgkin's disease then there is no resultant sensitization.[141] This has been attributed to an excess T cell suppression in the disease;[121] this presumably operates at the tissue level rather than at the peripheral blood level. There is also some evidence to suggest that the Hodgkin's disease patients' peripheral blood T cells have excess suppressive activity; these T cells suppress in a genetically restricted fashion.[142] The postulated explanation is that this is seen as part of disseminated disease where there is relative sparing of a particular subset in otherwise deficient T cell populations; histologically these patients have the lymphocyte-depleted form of the disease.

### B. B Lymphocytes

B cell responses are generally quantified by antibody levels rather than by cellular responses. Taking the serum as a reflection of whole body B cells there is no predictable change in immunoglobulin levels in the disease. Hypogammaglobulinemia may occasionally manifest late in the disease,[143] probably due to the severity of the illness rather than to an intrinsic abnormality. Conversely there is sometimes a mild hypergammaglobulinemia[144] in less severe disease. This is generalized and not a monoclonal gammopathy, although a selective enhancement of IgD with lambda chain expression is a common finding in Hodgkin's disease serology. Others suggest that there is an increase in the IgE level in symptomatic nodular sclerosing patient group.[145] In interpreting this type of information it is important to remember that the immunoglobulin levels will reflect past immunological experience rather than fresh events. With regard to new antigens there is some evidence to suggest a failure of response in the disease.[146] In vitro the analysis of B cell function has been examined using lipopolysaccharide as the nonspecific mitogen, and the response was unimpaired.

The generation of immune complexes is a different kind of reflection on B cell function. Using a variety of indirect methods to demonstrate the presence of complexes in the peripheral blood, there are conflicting reports as to whether or not such complexes are present in the disease. A raised complement level has been reported in one system and increased "macromolecular" C3 has been reported in another[148] and there may be an increase in C5, C8, and C9 rather than C3[149] in yet another system. The Raji type assay is also suggestive of an immune complex associated disease.[150] All these studies are hampered by lack of knowledge about the antigen involved in the disease. As the ferritin-related analyses have not identified a tumor-specific antigen and as there is doubt as to the nature and provenance of the putative antigen isolated from the cultured cells,[151] this aspect of peripheral blood investigation is unsatisfactorily resolved.

An alternative to an exogenous antigen as a component of an immune complex is that antibodies against self antigens are important in the disease.[152] Using direct membrane immunofluorescence there is evidence against this, but in vitro peripheral blood lymphocytes show autologous blast transformation with lymph node derived stimulators. Most of these patients had advanced disease at the time of investigation. In related experiments antibody levels were examined by fluorescence, cytotoxicity on autologous lymphocytes, and hemagglutination assays. However, marked fluctuations in antibody level were observed in the individual patient, making such experiments difficult to interpret.

### C. Monocytes

As for the tissue monocyte compared to the tissue lymphocyte, so the peripheral blood monocyte has been less carefully examined than the peripheral blood lymphocyte. Quantitatively in the blood there is no obvious monocytosis but as a percentage, monocytes are said to comprise more of the mononuclear cell fraction than usual.[153] This could be due to a false negative T cell count as has been mentioned above.

Qualitatively the chief role which has been ascribed to the monocyte is one of immunosuppression,[154] manifest in both alloproliferative and antibody synthesis studies. The more advanced the disease the greater the degree of suppression which was observed. This may be due to excess prostaglandin synthesis,[121] and may be more apparent in vitro than in vivo as normal feedback mechanisms do not operate. The peripheral blood monocyte was at one stage believed to be a source of Reed-Sternberg cells directly,[155] but this is no longer considered to be the case except in advanced disease.

The reason for this postulate was that it was suggested that the disease was blood borne primarily and resembled a leukemic process; the anatomical data about sites of disease have refuted that notion.[156]

## D. Conclusions

The peripheral blood findings in Hodgkin's disease confirm that there is a T cell abnormality in the disease. This is manifest in a number of ways. There are fewer circulating T cells, their rosetting and capping pattern is altered, and the proliferative responses are modified. The precise relationship of these findings to the tissue cell is not clear. There is suggestive evidence that (as in the tissues) the monocyte fraction is abnormal, and this could in turn influence the T cell fraction. The dominant pattern as manifest by the peripheral blood cells is one of a degree of immunosuppression. However, this is a T cell and monocyte suppression since B cell responses are relatively normal except in advanced disease. In vivo the T lymphocyte and monocyte responses may be less impaired than they are in vitro.

Examination of the peripheral blood cells has stimulated investigation of other blood components. An abnormal glycolipid, circulatory immune complexes possibly related to endogenous antigen, and an abnormality in ferritin metabolism have all been identified, and there are several theories which try to link these findings into a comprehensive scheme but none of these can explain the whole pattern of the disease.

## VIII. IMMUNOLOGICAL DEFICIENCY IN HODGKIN'S DISEASE

Against the background of such perturbation of immunological function it is not surprising that there is an immunological deficiency in Hodgkin's disease and that this has clinical implications as well as theoretical. Although this immunological deficiency cannot be categorized neatly into lymphocyte- and monocyte-mediated events, both cell types interact to produce the deficiency, or alternatively it is a manifestation of abnormal interaction between them. It is this deficiency as well as the question of neoplasia which has acted as the stimulus to many of the studies which have been cited above.

### A. Histological Aspects

The histology of the Hodgkin's disease lymph node may itself provide important evidence in interpreting this defect. The germinal centers are often absent in involved tissue although aggregates of lymphoid tissue will often remain. These may resemble primary follicles. These aggregates of B cells are phenotypically of lymphocyte corona type bearing surface IgM and IgD as is seen in association with germinal centers which have been activated. In contrast, unaffected nodes (often those upstream from an affected area) often show marked germinal center activity, the so-called progressive transformation of germinal centers.[157] Similarly, in normal spleen the presence of germinal centers in the white pulp is not usual, while in Hodgkin's disease very marked germinal center formation is frequently found. Germinal center formation is essential for generating "immunological memory" and for producing the highly specific secondary phase of T-cell-dependent humoral immune responses; for their formation T cells, antigen retaining follicular dendritic cells, and complement are necessary, and the predominant B cell population in the germinal center will have complement receptors and bind peanut agglutinin. Two interesting possibilities could account for the comparative defect in germinal center formation in Hodgkin's disease tumors, although as should be apparent there are several possible sites at which this could occur. One is that the immune deficit as demonstrated locally is a T cell defect specifically affecting that subset which is normally implicated in germinal center formation. The second is that the defect lies in the follicular dendritic cell (irrespective of whether or not this cell is implicated in the neoplastic process itself). As in the immunohistology, so in the analysis of the immunological defect, the question is raised that the disease may be characterized by a defect in the regulation of germinal center formation which results in increased elimination of this compartment from the tumor tissues, and accompanied by reactive changes in the surrounding area.

## B. Clinical Aspects

There are two broad views about the immune defect in Hodgkin's disease. One is that the primary lesion is an immunodeficiency which is accompanied by disordered development and/or differentiation in cell lineages functionally related to the immune system. Thus the immune defect is syptomatic of the increasing disorganization and destruction of the normally well-integrated immune system. The other view is that the process is neoplastic *ab initio* and the disorder of immune function is a consequence of neoplastic change affecting a key element which is responsible for coordinating a variety of immune responses.

From the clinical vantage point Hodgkin's disease is a chronic disease and to make the diagnosis in a symptomatic patient requires histology precisely because the clinical features are nonspecific and may resemble a variety of chronic processes. Clinical observation also highlights two further aspects of the immunological defect. First that as chronicity is a feature, the disease and the immune defect may antecede diagnosis by a considerable period in some form. Second, the fact that there are no overt infections and that there are asymptomatic as well as symptomatic patients indicates that the patient compensates for the immunological defect in the earlier and less disseminated forms of the disease. In fact, it is probably true that the pretreatment subclinical immunological defect in Hodgkin's disease seems to be more important in pathogenesis than it is in determining prognosis.

Nonetheless, when the Hodgkin's disease patient is investigated at the time of diagnosis there is a clear but ill-defined deficit in the immune response. The classic example of this is the cutaneous anergy which is due to depressed delayed hypersensitivity reactions. Testing with a wide range of common antigens such as tuberculin, mumps, and candida[158] shows that there is a defective delayed hypersensitivity response in the disease, and that this correlates with the presence of active disease in the first instance. At optimum antigen dosage the results are often equivocal, but using suboptimal doses the anergy is clearly manifest. Another way to look at this is to use skin sensitizing agents such as dinitrochlorobenzene. The response to this agent is depressed,[159] and again this correlates with the extent of disease in that the more disseminated the disease, the more likely there is to be unresponsiveness. It is this form of sensitization which cannot be transferred to a Hodgkin's disease patient by means of adoptive transfer.[141] A similar T-lymphocyte-mediated mechanism underlies the delayed homograft rejection which is present in Hodgkin's disease patients.[160]

As the disease progresses, the susceptibility to infectious complications as a manifestation of the immunological deficit becomes more apparent. This association has been known for many years and is most frequently discussed with tuberculosis.[161] Although the disease-related events and the immunosuppressive effects of treatment are interlinked (see below) the range and nature of the infectious agents is more extensive than can be attributed to treatment alone and the recorded instances of unusual infections antecede modern therapeutic regimes. For example, systemic candidiasis due to defective neutrophil killing of the organisms can occur;[162] *Pneumocystis carinii* infestation is more common,[163] and there is an increased frequency of herpes zoster[164] with more likelihood of disseminated zoster and with cutaneous zoster involvement correlating with disease site or with radiation site.

## C. Tumors

Recent literature has highlighted the occurrence of second tumors in Hodgkin's disease, and the role of therapy in the induction of these tumors has been emphasized.[165] However, second tumors were a feature of the disease even before treatment protocols were introduced which might be tumorigenic.[166] The earlier cases could be linked to the immunological deficiency directly; the more recent examples might arise because of the impaired immunity acting as a cofactor with the pharmacological substances used in treatment, but this is difficult to prove.

The overall incidence of second malignancy is between 5 and 10%, and of these a third are lymphomas of various types, which is far more than the expected number.[167] Since this type of preponderance of a type of second malignancy resembles that seen in immunosuppressed patients it seems reasonable to regard these other neoplasms as a consequence of the immune defect rather than a random phenomenon. Subsequent lymphomas are always of B cell rather than T cell type and are often of the lymphoplasmacytoid variety. The phenotypic analysis of these tumors may be extremely difficult, since to demonstrate polyclonality may depend on the relative proportion of lymphoma B cells and reactive Hodgkin's disease B cells in a given sample. To add further complexity, occasionally Hodgkin's disease can arise after a previous diagnosis of another type of lymphoma or a Hodgkin's disease patient can present as a non-Hodgkin's lymphoma.[168]

In analyzing these kinds of events it is interesting that two-thirds of the simultaneous malignancies (arising within a year of the diagnosis of Hodgkin's disease) were lymphomas, and three of five patients with an antecedent malignancy had a lymphoma; but after treatment one in four malignancies were lymphomas. This kind of analysis suggests that perhaps the immune defect is more relevant than the treatment in the generation of the tumors.

## IX. TREATMENT EFFECTS IN HODGKIN'S DISEASE

The role of treatment as a modulator of cell function in the Hodgkin's disease patient has already been mentioned in several contexts. Since treatment is an invariable accompaniment of most Hodgkin's-disease-derived lymphocytes and monocytes available for analysis in a laboratory, the wide variety of changes which may be induced by therapy need to be understood before making interpretations of the data generated.

Clinically, the major impetus in monitoring many of the treatment effects on lymphocyte and monocyte function is to see how the changes can be used to monitor the presence or absence of residual disease. To date none of the methods used can really advance on the observation that relative dissemination and lymphocyte depletion are poor prognostic indicators *ab initio*.

The chief early effect of therapy is to produce a profound lymphocytopenia involving both T and B cell series; this reverts to pretreatment levels with time[169] but the null cell fraction is increased, and relative to normal controls will remain persistently high irrespective of disease activity. Monocyte counts remain unaltered.

With regard to hypersensitivity responses, patients who are in remission may have normal reactions. However, this is not invariable: mumps skin testing may be impaired for many years after radiation and this is not an index of disease activity.[170] The dinitrochlorobenzene response is quite variable: those previously responsive may become anergic, and sometimes remain so, while others who were anergic may become responsive in remission.

The in vitro tests of cellular function are also altered by treatment.[171] There are fewer cells rosetting with both conventional and active methods and this parallels the lymphocytopenia. This is a real decrease rather than a blocking mechanism activation. In the allogeneic response assay, post-treatment cells remain effective stimulators but not responders, which coincides with the relative radioresistance of monocytic cells. Most patients will recover their responder status with time. With the phytohemagglutinin stimulation response the unresponsiveness increments after therapy is sometimes followed by a rebound effect to above pretreatment levels. If disease activity persists then this rebound does not occur, but since the lag period may be up to 3 years it does not constitute a useful index of recovery.

The specific effects of chemotherapy as opposed to radiotherapy have not been explored to any great extent. The reported studies suggest that the phytohemagglutinin and delayed hypersensitivity responses are impaired in a similar fashion to that seen after irradiation.[172] Splenectomy does not have an untoward effect on cellular immunologic function in Hodgkin's disease;[173] there is a decrease in IgM and IgA levels but IgG levels remain stable. The combination of splenectomy, chemotherapy, and radiotherapy may result in a fall in specific antibody levels to particular antigens but this has to be seen in the context of the indication for combined therapy as being more advanced disease in the first instance.

The morphologic diagnosis of Hodgkin's disease on post-treatment tissue is known to be difficult. The criteria for this diagnosis are the same as those for the pretreatment sample but with some reservations. Sclerosis of nodes is inevitably more frequent and does not necessarily indicate nodular sclerosing disease[174] cellular depletion of nodules can reflect differential sensitivity of cell types to a particular agent rather than an actual depletion. Very few of the in vitro analyses have included posttreatment samples, but when these are included, then the monocytic and hence radioresistant compartment is deficient similarly to the deficit seen in untreated tissue.[61]

## X. FUTURE TRENDS IN HODGKIN'S DISEASE RESEARCH

It should be clear from this discussion that Hodgkin's disease represents an area in which detailed analysis of topics superficially as disparate as cell membrane structure, iron metabolism, and viral DNA extraction all may play a part in future research. The role of immunology in this is twofold: direct investigation of the immune mechanism and its dyscrasia in Hodgkin's disease is one facet, while at the same time immunological techniques will be essential in the examination of some of the other aspects of the disease.

There is much evidence that the central event in Hodgkin's disease is happening at a local site in the lymph node and hence that the tissue cell must be the major focus of research rather than the peripheral blood cell. Detailed analysis of the T lymphocyte/accessory cell interaction comparing Hodgkin's disease with normal control tissue requires isolation procedures which include knowledge of surface membrane properties of the individual cell types. Monoclonal antibodies against membrane determinants on lymphocytes and monocytes are probably going to prove the superior method to do this. At the same time the definition of neoplasia as involving a host response as well as a cell transformation event is highlighted in the Hodgkin's disease morphology; the cells isolated need to be examined with this interaction as an equally important consideration.

There is an obvious requirement for lines and clones of cells derived from these types of sample before it will be possible to do any of the kinds of study which have revealed virus-tumor relationships in both lymphomas and epithelial tumors. In turn, for this too, monoclonal reagents against defined surface products, coded for by specific gene sequences, may prove to be the ideal methodology.

As part of future research on Hodgkin's disease immunology, continued evaluation of epidemiological data is still important. Changing trends in social environments may be related to changes in disease pattern. Equally, the identification of case clusters has made it ethically and scientifically reasonable to suggest that prospective studies on patient contacts at the time of the diagnosis of disease could be useful using peripheral blood samples.

## XI. SUMMARY AND CONCLUSIONS

Analysis of the role of the lymphocyte and monocyte in Hodgkin's disease reveals that cells of these two lineages are the framework for the disease, but that the exact model which fits this framework is unclear.

There is good evidence that the diagnostic sample node is different in biology from conventional tumor samples, including other types of lymph node malignancy. Preceding the diagnosis, there must have been at least partial defect in cell-mediated immune function at the level of the T lymphocyte. This in turn is linked to a general immunosuppression, to serum factors, to local shifts in iron-binding proteins, and to atypical T lymphocyte/accessory cell interaction, but there are also compensatory mechanisms which operate in vivo so that overt and serious immunological deficiency is only a feature of advanced disease. The epidemiological evidence favors a linked viral and social component as prerequisites in the pathogenesis of the disease. None of the identified anomalies are suitable for monitoring the disease.

Future research in Hodgkin's disease must combine identification of at-risk populations for study with single cell investigation of Hodgkin's tumors, and with analysis of the genetic control mechanisms which operate in the isolated cells. These must be interpreted against the background of the microenvironmental lymphocyte/monocyte interaction which is an integral part of the disease.

## REFERENCES

1. Cantor, H. and Weissman, I. L., Development and function of subpopulation of thymocytes and T lymphocytes, *Prog. Allerg.*, 20, 1, 1976.
2. Bollum, F. J., Terminal deoxynucleotidyl transferase as a haemopoietic cell marker, *Blood*, 54, 1203, 1979.
3. Reinherz, E. L., Kung, P. C., Goldstein, G., Levey, R. H., and Schlossman, S., Discrete stages of human intrathymic differentiation: analysis of normal thymocytes and leukaemic lymphoblasts of T cell lineage, *Proc. Natl. Acad. Sci. U.S.A.*, 77, 1588, 1980.
4. Gupta, S. and Tan, C., Subpopulations of human T lymphocytes, *Clin. Immunol. Immunopathol.*, 15, 133, 1980.
5. Greaves, M. F., Owen, J. J. T., and Raff, M. C., T and B lymphocytes: origins, properties and roles in immune responses, *Excerpta Med.*, 1973.
6. Gathings, W. E., Lawton, A. R., and Cooper, M. D., Immunofluorescent studies of the development of pre-B cells, B lymphocytes and isotype diversity in humans, *Eur. J. Immunol.*, 7, 804, 1977.
7. Greaves, M. F., Williams, R. C., and Seymour, G. J., Assays for human lymphocytes, in *Current Research in Rheumatoid Arthritis and Allied Diseases*, Dumonde, D. C. and Maini, R. N., Eds., Med. and Tech. Press, London, 1978.
8. Klaus, G. G. B., B cell maturation: its relationship to immune induction and tolerance in B and T cells, in *Immune Recognition*, Loor, F. and Roelants, G. E., Eds., John Wiley & Sons, New York, 1977.
9. Stein, H., Boak, A., Tolksdorf, G., Lennert, K., Rodt, H., and Gerdes, J., Immunohistological analysis of the organisation of normal lymphoid tissue and non-Hodgkin's lymphomas, *J. Histochem. Cytochem.*, 28, 746, 1980.
10. Swerdlow, S. H., Habeshaw, J. A., Murray, L. J., Dhaliwal, H. S., Lister, T. A., and Stansfeld, A. G., Centrocytic lymphoma: a distinct clinicopathological and immunological entity, submitted for publication.

11. Abo, T., Cooper, M. D., and Balch, C. M., Characterisation of HNK 1+ (Leu 7) human lymphocytes: two distinct phenotypes of human NK cells with different cytotoxic capabilities, *J. Immunol.*, 129, 1752, 1982.
12. Ritchie, A. W. S., James, K., and Micklem, H. S., The distribution and possible significance of cells identified in human lymphoid tissue by the monoclonal antibody HNK-1, *Clin. Exp. Immunol.*, 51, 439, 1983.
13. Poppema, S., Bhan, A. K., Reinherz, E. L., McCluskey, R. T., and Schlossman, S. F., Distribution of T cell subsets in human lymph nodes, *J. Exp. Med.*, 153, 30, 1981.
14. Nossal, G. J. V., Abbot, A., and Mitchell, J., Electron microscopic radioautographic studies of antigen capture in the lymph node medulla, *J. Exp. Med.*, 127, 263, 1968.
15. Niewenhuis, P. and Keuning, F. J., Germinal centres and the origin of the B cell system, *Immunology*, 26, 509, 1974.
16. MacLennan, I. C. M., Gray, D., Kumaratne, D. S., and Bazin, H., The lymphocytes of marginal zones: a distinct B cell lineage, *Immunol. Today*, 3, 305, 1982.
17. Swerdlow, S. H., Murray, L. J., Dorreen, M. S., Lister, T. A., Greaves, M. F., Stansfeld, A. G., and Habeshaw, J. A., Frequency and distribution of NK (Leu 7) cells in reactive lymphoid tissues and malignant lymphomas, submitted for publication.
18. Sandberg, A. A., Chromosomal changes in the lymphomas, *Hum. Pathol.*, 12, 531, 1981.
19. Reddy, E. P., Reynolds, R. K., Santos, E., and Barbacid, M., A point mutation is responsible for the acquisition of transforming properties by the $T23_8$ human bladder cancer oncogene, *Nature (London)*, 300, 149, 1982.
20. Simonsen, M., Graft versus host reactions, *Prog. Allergy*, 6, 349, 1962.
21. Solter, D. and Damjanov, I., Teratocarcinomas rarely develop from embryos transplanted into athymic mice, *Nature (London)*, 278, 554, 1979.
22. Stuart, A. E. and Davidson, A. E., The human reticular cell: morphology and cytochemistry, *J. Pathol.*, 103, 41, 1971.
23. Steinman, R. M. and Cohn, Z. A., Identification of a novel cell type in peripheral lymphoid organs in mice, *J. Exp. Med.*, 137, 1142, 1973.
24. Nossal, G. J. V., Abbott, A., Mitchell, J., and Lummus, Z., Antigens in immunity. XV. Ultrastructural features of antigen capture in primary and secondary lymphoid follicles, *J. Exp. Med.*, 151, 1196, 1968.
25. Heusermann, U., Stutte, H. J., and Muller-Hermelink, H. K., Interdigitating cells in the white pulp of human spleen, *Cell Tissue Res.*, 153, 415, 1974.
26. Silberberg-Sinankin, I. and Thorbecke, G. J., The Langerhans cell, in *The Reticulo-Endothelial System*, Vol. 1, Carr, I. and Daems, W. T., Eds., Plenum Press, New York, 1980, 555.
27. Kelly, R. H., Balfour, B. M., Armstrong, J. A., and Griffiths, S., Functional anatomy of lymph nodes. II. Peripheral lymph borne mononuclear cells, *Anat. Rec.*, 190, 5, 1978.
28. Streefkerk, J. G., Streefkerk, J. G., and Veerman, A. J. P., Histochemistry and electron microscopy of follicle linings. Reticular cells in the rat spleen, *Z. Zellforsch Mikroskop Anat.*, 115, 524, 1971.
29. Dorfman, R. F., Classification of non-Hodgkin's lymphomas, *Lancet*, 1, 1295, 1974.
30. Bennett, M. H., Farrer-Brown, G., Henry, K., and Jelliffe, A. M., Classification of non-Hodgkin's lymphomas, *Lancet*, 2, 405, 1974.
31. Gerard-Marchant, R., Hamlin, I., Lennert, K., Rilke, E., Stansfeld, A. G., van Unnik, J. A. M., Classification of non-Hodgkin's lymphomas, *Lancet*, 2, 406, 1974.
32. Lukes, R. J. and Collins, R. D., Immunological characterisation of human malignant lymphomas, *Cancer*, 14, 1488, 1974.
33. Lukes, R. J., Craver, L., Hall, T. C., Rappaport, H., and Ruben, P., Report of the nomenclature committee, *Cancer Res.*, 26, 1311, 1966.
34. Jackson, J., Jr., and Parker, F., Jr., *Hodgkin's Disease and Allied Disorders*, Oxford University Press, New York, 1947, 177.
35. Azar, H. A., Significance of the Reed-Sternberg cell, *Hum. Pathol.*, 6, 479, 1975.
36. Anagnostou, D., Parker, J. W., Taylor, C. R., Tindle, B. H., and Lukes, R. J., Lacunar cells of nodular sclerosing Hodgkin's disease, *Cancer*, 39, 1032, 1977.
37. Taylor, C. R., An immunohistological study of follicular lymphoma, reticulum cell sarcoma and Hodgkin's disease, *Eur. J. Cancer*, 12, 61, 1976.
38. Aisenberg, A. C., Cell surface markers in lymphoproliferative disease, *N. Engl. J. Med.*, 304, 331, 1981.
39. Levy, R., Warnke, R., Dorfman, R. F., and Haimovich, J., The monoclonality of human B cell lymphomas, *J. Exp. Med.*, 145, 1014, 1977.
40. Ramot, B., Levanon, M., Hahn, Y., Lahat, N., and Moroz, C., The mutual clonal origin of the lymphoplasmacytic and lymphoma cell in alpha chain disease, *Clin. Exp. Immunol.*, 27, 440, 1977.

41. Bloomfield, C. D., Kersey, J. H., Brunning, R. D., and Gajl-Pacjalska, K. J., Prognostic significance of lymphocyte surface markers in adult non-Hodgkin's malignant lymphomas, *Lancet*, 2, 1330, 1976.
42. Mann, R. B., Jaffe, E. S., and Berard, C. W., Malignant lymphomas — a conceptual understanding of morphological diversity, *Am. J. Pathol.*, 94, 104, 1979.
43. Leech, J. H., Glick, A. D., and Waldron, J. A., Malignant lymphomas of follicular center cell origin in man. I. Immunologic studies, *J. Natl. Cancer Inst.*, 54, 11, 1975.
44. Ziegler, J. L., Burkitt's lymphoma, *N. Engl. J. Med.*, 305, 735, 1981.
45. Dorfman, R. F., Enzyme histochemistry of the cells in Hodgkin's disease and related disorders, *Nature (London)*, 190, 25, 1961.
46. Kadin, M. E., Stiles, D. P., Levy, R., and Warnke, R., Exogenous immunoglobulin and macrophage origin of Reed-Sternberg cells in Hodgkin's disease, *N. Engl. J. Med.*, 299, 1208, 1978.
47. Poppema, S., Elema, J. D., and Halie, M. R., The localisation of Hodgkin's disease in lymph nodes. A study with immunohistological enzyme histochemical and rosetting techniques on frozen sections, *Int. J. Cancer*, 24, 532, 1979.
48. Papadimitriou, C. S., Stein, H., and Lennert, K., The complexity of immunohistochemical staining patterns of Hodgkin and Reed-Sternberg cells — demonstration of immunoglobulin, albumin, alpha-1-antichymotrypsin and lysozyme, *Int. J. Cancer*, 21, 531, 1978.
49. Boyd, A. W. and Schrader, J. W., Derivation of macrophage-like lines from the pre-B lymphocyte ABLS81 using 5-azacytidine, *Nature (London)*, 297, 691, 1982.
50. Schwab, U., Stein, H., Gerdes, J., Lemke, H., Kirchner, H., Schandt, M., and Diehl, V., Production of a monoclonal antibody specific for Hodgkin and Sternberg-Reed cells of Hodgkin's disease and a subset of normal lymphoid cells, *Nature (London)*, 299, 65, 1982.
51. Habeshaw, J. A., Bailey, D., Stansfeld, A. G., and Greaves, M. F., The cellular content of non-Hodgkins lymphomas: an evaluation of monoclonal antibodies, *Br. J. Cancer*, p. 46, 1983.
52. Halper, J. P., Knowles, D. M., and Wang, C. Y., Ia antigen expression by human malignant lymphomas: correlation with conventional lymphoid markers, *Blood*, 55, 373, 1980.
53. Tan, C. T. C., De Sousa, M., and Good, R. A., Distinguishing features of the immunology of Hodgkin's disease in children, *Cancer Treat. Rep.*, 66, 969, 1982.
54. Fialkow, P. J., Klein, E., Klein, G., Clifford, P., and Singh, S., Immunoglobulin and glucose 6 phosphate dehydrogenase as markers of cellular origin in Burkitt lymphoma, *J. Exp. Med.*, 138, 89, 1973.
55. Epstein, A. L., Herman, M. M., Kim, H., Dorfman, R. F., and Kaplan, H. S., Biology of the human malignant lymphomas, *Cancer*, 37, 2158, 1976.
56. Nilsson, K., Giovanella, B. C., Stehlin, J. S., and Klein, G., Tumourigenicity of haemopoietic cell lines in athymic nude mice, *Int. J. Cancer*, 19, 337, 1977.
57. Kaplan, H. S., Hodgkin's disease: biology, treatment and progress, *Blood*, 57, 813, 1981.
58. Fogh, J., *Human Tumour Cells In Vitro*, Plenum Press, New York, 1975.
59. Purtilo, D. T., Cassel, C. K., Yang, J. P. S., Harper, R., X-linked recessive progressive combined variable immunodeficiency (Duncan's disease), *Lancet*, 1, 935, 1975.
60. Purtilo, D. T., Epstein-Barr-virus-induced oncogenesis in immune deficient individuals, *Lancet*, 1, 300, 1980.
61. Katz, D. R., The macrophage in Hodgkin's disease, *J. Pathol.*, 133, 145, 1981.
62. Payne, S. V., Newell, D. G., Jones, D. B., and Wright, D. H., The Reed-Sternberg cell/lymphocyte interaction, *Am. J. Pathol.*, 100, 7, 1980.
63. Stuart, A. E., The pathogenesis of Hodgkin's disease, *J. Pathol.*, 126, 239, 1978.
64. Feldmann, M., Katz, D. R., and Sunshine, G. H., *RES-Leucocyte Interactions in Reticulo-Endothelial System Treatise*, Vol. 4, Reichert, S., Ed., in press.
65. Delves, P., M.Sci. thesis, Brunel University, 1980.
66. Gutensohn, N. and Cole, P., Epidemiology of Hodgkin's disease, *Semin. Oncol.*, 7, 92, 1980.
67. Gutensohn, N. and Cole, P., Epidemiology of Hodgkin's disease in the young, *Int. J. Cancer*, 19, 595, 1977.
68. Gutensohn, N. and Cole, P., Childhood social environment and Hodgkin's disease, *N. Engl. J. Med.*, 304, 135, 1980.
69. Vianna, N. T., Lawrence, C. E., Davies, J. N. P., Arbuckle, J., Harris, S., Marani, W., and Wilkinson, J., Tonsillectomy and childhood Hodgkin's disease, *Lancet*, 2, 338, 1980.
70. Ruuskanen, O., Vanha-Perttula, T., and Kouvalainen, K., Tonsillectomy, appendectomy and Hodgkin's disease, *Lancet*, 1, 1127, 1979.
71. Cartwright, A. and O'Brien, X., Social class variation in health care, in *Sociology of the N.H.S.*, Stacey, M., Ed., Kiel University Press, Kiel, 1976.
72. Burn, C., Davies, J. N. P., Dodge, O. G., and Nias, B. C., Hodgkin's disease in English and African children, *J. Natl. Cancer Inst.*, 46, 37, 1971.

73. Taylor, J. F., Templeton, A. C., Vogel, C. L., Ziegler, J. L., and Kyalwazl, S. K., Kaposi's sarcoma in Uganda: a clinico-pathological study, *Int. J. Cancer,* 8, 122, 1971.
74. Centre for Disease Control, Epidemiological aspects of the current outbreak of Kaposi's sarcoma and opportunistic infections, *N. Engl. J. Med.,* 306, 248, 1982.
75. Cerilli, J., Rynasiewicz, J. J., and Rothermel, W. S., Hodgkin's disease and human renal transplantation, *Am. J. Surg.,* 133, 182, 1977.
76. Bjorkholm, M., Holm, G., Mellstedt, H., Johansson, B., Killander, D., Sundblad, R., and Soderberg, G., Prognostic factors in Hodgkin's disease, *Scand. J. Haematol.,* 20, 306, 1978.
77. Evans, A. S. and Comstock, G. W., Presence of elevated antibody titres to Epstein-Barr virus before Hodgkin's disease, *Lancet,* 1, 1183, 1981.
78. Epstein, M. A. and Achong, B. G., Various forms of Epstein-Barr virus infection in man: established facts and a general concept, *Lancet,* 2, 836, 1973.
79. Schwartz, R. S., Epstein-Barr virus — Oncogen or Mitogen?, *N. Engl. J. Med.,* 302, 1307, 1980.
80. Poiesz, B. J., Ruscetti, F. W., Reitz, M. S., Kalyanaraman, V. S., and Gallo, R. C., Isolation of a new type C retrovirus (HTLV) in primary uncultured cells of a patient with Sezary-T cell leukaemia, *Nature (London),* 294, 268, 1981.
81. Prodha, L. E., Tobin, C. J., Shih, C., and Weinberg, R. A., Human EJ bladder carcinoma oncogene is homologue of Harvey sarcoma virus rat gene, *Nature (London),* 297, 474, 1982.
82. Eisinger, M., Fox, S. M., DeHarven, E., Biedler, J. L., and Sanders, F. K., Virus-like agents from patients with Hodgkin's disease, *Nature (London),* 233, 104, 1971.
83. Long, J. C., Aisenberg, A. C., Zamecnik, M. V., and Zamecnik, P. C., A tumour antigen in tissue cultures derived from patients with Hodgkin's disease, *Proc. Natl. Acad. Sci. U.S.A.,* 70, 1540, 1973.
84. Harris, N., Gang, D. L., Quay, S. C., Poppema, S., Zamecnik, P. C., Nelson-Rees, W. A., and O'Brien, S. J., Contamination of Hodgkin's disease cell cultures, *Nature (London),* 289, 228, 1981.
85. Evans, A. S., and Comstock, G. W., Presence of elevated antibody titres to Epstein-Barr virus before Hodgkin's disease, *Lancet,* 1, 1183, 1981.
86. Burkitt, D. P., Etiology of Burkitt's lymphoma — an alternative hypothesis to a vectoral virus, *J.* 42, 19, 1969.
87. Kaplan, H. S., *Hodgkin's Disease,* Harvard University Press, Cambridge, 1979, 598.
88. Kaplan, H. S. and Smithers, D. W., Autoimmunity in man and homologous disease in mice in relation to the malignant lymphomas, *Lancet,* 2, 1, 1959.
89. Order, S. E. and Hellman, S., Pathogenesis of Hodgkin's disease, *Lancet,* 1, 571, 1972.
90. Kaplan, H. S. and Gartner, S. Sternberg-Reed giant cells of Hodgkin's disease — cultivation in vitro, heterotransplantation and characterisation as neoplastic macrophages, *Int. J. Cancer,* 19, 511, 1977.
91. Reitz, M. S., Poiesz, B. J., Ruscetti, F. W., and Gallo, R. C., Characterisation and distribution of nucleic acid sequences of a novel type C retrovirus isolated from neoplastic human T lymphocytes, *Proc. Natl. Acad. Sci. U.S.A.,* in press.
92. Payne, S. V., Jones, D. B., and Wright, D. H., Reed-Sternberg cell/lymphocyte interaction, *Lancet,* 2, 768, 1977.
93. Moroz, C., Giler, S., Kupfer, B., and Urca, I., Lymphocytes bearing surface ferritin in patients with Hodgkin's disease and breast cancer, *N. Engl. J. Med.,* 296, 1172, 1977.
94. DeSousa, M., Yang, M., Lopes-Corrales, E., Tan, C., Hansen, J. A., Dupont, B., and Good, R. A., Ecotaxis: the principle and its application to the study of Hodgkin's disease, *Clin. Exp. Immunol.,* 27, 143, 1977.
95. Trowbridge, I. S., Omary, M. B., Human cell surface glycoprotein related to cell proliferation is the receptor for transferrin, *Proc. Natl. Acad. Sci. U.S.A.,* 78, 4515, 1981.
96. Czitrom, A. A., Katz, D. R., and Sunshine, G. H., Alloreactive cytotoxic T lymphocyte responses to H-2 products on purified accessory cells, *Immunology,* 134, 117, 1982.
97. Tindle, B. H., Parker, J. W., and Lukes, R. J., Reed-Sternberg cells in infectious mononucleosis, *Am. J. Clin. Pathol.,* 58, 607, 1972.
98. Curran, R. C. and Jones, E. L., Hodgkin's disease: an immunohistochemical and histological study, *J. Pathol.,* 115, 45, 1979.
99. Kadin, M. E., Donaldson, S. S., and Dorfman, R. F., Isolated granulomas in Hodgkin's disease, *N. Engl. J. Med.,* 283, 858, 1978.
100. Rosenthal, S. R., Significance of tissue lymphocytes in the prognosis of lymphogranulomatosis, *Arch. Pathol.,* 21, 628, 1936.
101. Thomas, L., *Immune surveillance in Cellular and Humoral Aspects of the Hypersensitivity States,* Lawrence, H. S., Ed., Cassell, 1959, 529.
102. Peckham, M. J., Quantitative cytology and cytochemistry of Hodgkin's disease tissue labelled in vitro with tritiated thymidine, *Br. J. Cancer,* 28, 332, 1973.
103. Lukes, R. J. and Butler, J. J., The pathology and nomenclature of Hodgkin's disease, *Cancer Res.,* 26, 1063, 1966.

104. Lohmann, H., Prognostic significance of histopathology in Hodgkin's granuloma, *Acta Pathol. Microbiol. Scand.*, 64, 16, 1965.
105. Lennert, K. and Mestdagh, J., Lymphogranulomatosen mit konstant hohen Epithelioidzellgehalt, *Virchows Arch. A*, 34, 41, 1968.
106. The Lennert lymphoma, *Lancet*, ii, 507, 1976.
107. Colvin, R. B., Johnson, R. A., Mihm, M. C., and Dvorak, H. F., Role of the clotting system in cell-mediated hypersensitivity. I. Fibrin deposition in delayed skin reactions in man, *J. Exp. Med.*, 138, 686, 1973.
108. Wyatt, C., Kessler, D., and Burkholder, P. M., Production of the second (C2) and fourth (C4) components of guinea pig complement by single peritoneal cells: evidence that one cell may produce both components, *J. Immunol.*, 108, 1609, 1972.
109. Unkeless, J. C., Gordon, S., and Reich, E., Secretion of plasminogen activator by stimulated macrophages, *J. Exp. Med.*, 139, 834, 1974.
110. Landaas, T. O., Godal, T., and Halvorsen, T. B., Characterisation of immunoglobulins in Hodgkin cells, *Int. J. Cancer*, 20, 717, 1977.
111. Stuart, A. E., Williams, A. R., and Habeshaw, J. A., Rosetting and other reactions of the Reed-Sternberg cell, *J. Pathol.*, 122, 81, 1977.
112. Dorreen, M. S., Habeshaw, J. A., Wrigley, P. J. M., and Lister, T. A., Distribution of T lymphocyte subsets in Hodgkin's disease characterised by monoclonal antibodies, *Br. J. Cancer*, 45, 491, 1982.
113. Twomey, J. J., Laughter, A. H., Lazar, S., and Douglass, C. C., Reactivity of lymphocytes from primary neoplasms of lymphoid tissue, *Cancer*, 38, 740, 1976.
114. Hunter, C. P., Pinkus, G., Woodward, L., Moloney, W. C., and Churchill, W. H., Increased T lymphocytes and IgMEA receptors bearing lymphocytes in Hodgkin's disease spleens, *Cell Immunol.*, 31, 193, 1977.
115. Rocha, B., Ferreira, A. A., Mann, G., de Sousa, M., and Freitas, A. A., Spleen lymphocyte populations in patients with Hodgkin's disease — properties of cells with different densities, *Clin. Exp. Immunol.*, 48, 300, 1982.
116. Baroni, O. D., Ruco, L., Occini, S., Foschi, A., Occhionero, M., and Marcorelli, E., Tissue T lymphocytes in untreated Hodgkin's disease, *Cancer*, 50, 259, 1967.
117. Hillinger, S. M. and Herzig, G. P., Impaired cell-mediated immunity in Hodgkin's disease mediated by suppressor lymphocytes and monocytes, *J. Clin. Invest.*, 61, 1620, 1978.
118. Payne, S. V., Newall, D. G., Jones, D. B., and Wright, D. H., The Reed-Sternberg cell/lymphocyte interaction, *Am. J. Pathol.*, 100, 7, 1980.
119. Longmire, R. L., Macmillan, R., Yelenosky, R., Armstrong, S., Long, J. E., and Craddock, C. A., In vitro splenic IgG synthesis in Hodgkin's disease, *N. Engl. J. Med.*, 289, 763, 1973.
120. Aisenberg, A. C., Immunologic status of Hodgkin's disease, *Cancer*, 19, 385, 1966.
121. Goodwin, J. S., Messner, R. P., Bankhurst, A. D., Peake, G. T., Saiki, J. H., and Williams, R. C., Prostaglandin producing suppressor cells in Hodgkin's disease, *N. Engl. J. Med.*, 297, 963, 1977.
122. Katz, D. R., Czitrom, A. A., Feldmann, M., and Sunshine, G. H., Ia and macrophages in alloproliferation and allocytotoxicity, in *Macrophages and Nk Cells*, Normann, S. J. and Sorkin, E., Eds., Plenum Press, New York, 1982, 601.
123. Aisenberg, A. C., Lymphocytopenia in Hodgkin's disease, *Blood*, 25, 1037, 1965.
124. Neiman, R. S., Rosen, P. J., and Lukes, R. J., Lymphocyte depletion Hodgkin's disease: a clinicopathological entity, *N. Engl. J. Med.*, 288, 751, 1973.
125. Longmire, R. L., Ryan, S., MacMillan, R., Lightsey, A., and Heath, V., Antibody dependent lymphocytotoxicity induced by immunoglobulin G from Hodgkin's disease splenic lymphocytes, *Science*, 199, 71, 1978.
126. Ben Bassat, H. and Goldblum, N., Con A receptors on the surface membrane of lymphocytes from patients with Hodgkin's disease and other malignant lymphomas, *Proc. Natl. Acad. Sci. U.S.A.*, 72, 1046, 1973.
127. Crowther, D., Fairley, G. H. and Sewell, R. L., DNA synthesis in lymphocytes of patients with malignant disease, *Eur. J. Cancer*, 3, 417, 1967.
128. Schiffer, C. A., Levi, J. A., and Wiernik, P. H., The significance of abnormal circulating cells in patients with Hodgkin's disease, *Br. J. Haematol.*, 31, 177, 1975.
129. Bobrove, A. M., Fuks, Z., Strober, S., and Kaplan, H. S., Quantitation of T and B lymphocytes and cellular immune function in Hodgkin's disease, *Cancer*, 36, 169, 1975.
130. Case, D. C., Hansen, J. A., Corrales, E., Young, C. W., du Pont, B., Pinsky, C. M., and Good, R. A., Depressed in vitro responses to phytohaemagglutinin in patients with Hodgkin's disease in continuous long remissions, *Blood*, 49, 5, 1977.
131. Lang, J. M., Bigel, P., Oberling, F., and Mayer, S., Normal active rosette forming cells in untreated patients with Hodgkin's disease, *Biomedicine*, 27, 322, 1977.

132. Fuks, Z., Strober, S., King, D. P., and Kaplan, H. S., Reversal of cell surface abnormalities of T lymphocytes in Hodgkin's disease after in vitro incubation in foetal calf sera, *J. Immunol.*, 117, 1331, 1976.
133. Moroz, C., Lahat, M., Biniaminov, M., and Ramot, B., Ferritin on the surface of lymphocytes in Hodgkin's disease patients. A possible blocking substance removed by levamisole, *Clin. Exp. Immunol.*, 29, 30, 1977.
134. Bieber, C. P. and Bieber, M. M., Detection of ferritin as a circulating tumour associated antigen in Hodgkin's disease, *Natl. Cancer Inst. Monogr.*, 36, 147, 1973.
135. Levy, R. A. and Kaplan, H. S., Impaired lymphocyte function in untreated Hodgkin's disease, *N. Engl. J. Med.*, 290, 181, 1974.
136. Twomey, J. J. and Rice, L., Impact of Hodgkin's disease upon the immune system, *Semin. Oncol.*, 7, 114, 1980.
137. Churchill, W. H., Rocklin, R. R., and Maloney, W. C., In vitro evidence of normal lymphocyte function in some patients with Hodgkin's disease and negative delayed cutaneous hypersensitivity, *Natl. Cancer Inst. Monogr.*, 36, 99, 1973.
138. Gorski, A. J., du Pont, B., Hansen, J. A., and Good, R. A., Leucocyte migration inhibition factor induced by Concanavalin A. Standardised microassay for production in vitro, *Proc. Natl. Acad. Sci. U.S.A.*, 72, 3197, 1975.
139. Rassiga-Pidot, A. L. and MacIntyre, O. R., In vitro leucocyte interferon production in patients with Hodgkin's disease, *Cancer Res.*, 34, 2995, 1974.
140. Marcolongo, R. and diPaolo, N., Foetal thymic transplantation in patients with Hodgkin's disease, *Blood*, 41, 625, 1973.
141. Good, R. A., Kelly, W. D., Rotsten, J., and Varco, R. L., Hodgkin's disease and other lymphomas, *Prog. Allerg.*, 6, 275, 1962.
142. Engleman, E. G., Hoppe, R., Kaplan, H. S., Comminskey, J., and McDevitt, H. O., Suppressor cells of the mixed leucocyte response in healthy subjects and patients with Hodgkin's disease and sarcoidosis, *Clin. Res.*, 26, 513, 1978.
143. Aisenberg, A. C. and Leskowitz, S., Antibody formation in Hodgkin's disease, *N. Engl. J. Med.*, 268, 1269, 1963.
144. Stuart, A. E., The pathogenesis of Hodgkin's disease, *J. Pathol.*, 26, 239, 1978.
145. Amlot, P. C., and Green, L. A., Atopy and IgE concentrations in Hodgkin's disease and other lymphomas, *Br. Med. J.*, 1, 327, 1978.
146. Barr, M. and Fairley, G. H., Circulating antibodies in reticuloses, *Lancet*, 1, 1305, 1961.
147. Rottino, A. and Levy, A. C., Behaviour of total serum complement in Hodgkin's disease and other malignant lymphomas, *Blood*, 14, 246, 1959.
148. Amlot, P. C., Slaney, J. M., and Williams, B. D., Circulating immune complexes and symptoms in Hodgkin's disease, *Lancet*, 1, 449, 1976.
149. Lichtenfeld, J. L., Wiernik, P. H., Mardiney, M. R., and Zarco, R. M., Abnormalities of complement and its components in patients with acute leukaemia Hodgkin's disease and sarcoma, *Cancer Res.*, 36, 3678, 1976.
150. Brown, C. A., Hall, C. L., Long, J. C., Carey, K., Weitzman, S. A., and Aisenberg, A. C., Circulating immune complexes in Hodgkin's disease, *Am. J. Med.*, 64, 289, 1978.
151. Eshhar, Z., Order, S. E., and Katz, D. H., Ferritin, a Hodgkin's disease associated antigen, *Proc. Natl. Acad. Sci. U.S.A.*, 71, 3956, 1974.
152. Grifoni, V., Recent immunological findings in Hodgkin's disease, *Tumori*, 59, 363, 1973.
153. Schecter, G. P. and Soehlen, F., Monocyte mediated inhibition of lymphocyte mitogenesis in Hodgkin's disease, *Blood*, 52, 261, 1978.
154. Twomey, J. J., Laughter, A. H., Farrow, S., and Douglass, C. C., Hodgkin's disease. An immunodepleting and immunosuppressive disorder, *J. Clin. Invest.*, 56, 467, 1975.
155. Halie, M. R., Huiges, W., and Nieweg, H. O., Abnormal cells in the peripheral blood of patients with Hodgkin's disease. Observations with light microscopy, *Br. J. Haematol.*, 28, 317, 1974.
156. Kaplan, H. S. and Rosenberg, S. A., The management of Hodgkin's disease, *Cancer*, 36, 796, 1975.
157. Lennert, K., *Malignant Lymphomas Other Than Hodgkin's Disease*, Springer Verlag, Basel, 1978, 38.
158. Ziegler, J. B., Hansen, P., and Penny, R., Intrinsic lymphocyte defect in Hodgkin's disease — analysis of the phytohaemagglutinin dose response, *Cell Immunol. Immunopathol.*, 3, 451, 1975.
159. Aisenberg, A. C., Studies on delayed type hypersensitivity in Hodgkin's disease, *J. Clin. Invest.*, 41, 1964, 1962.
160. Kelly, W. D., Good, R. A., Varco, R. L., and Levitt, M., The altered response to skin homografts and to delayed allergens in Hodgkin's disease, *Surg. Forum*, 9, 785, 1958.
161. Ewing, J., *Neoplastic Diseases*, W. B. Saunders, Philadelphia, 1928.
162. Louria, D. B., Stiff, D. P., and Bennett, B., Disseminated moniliasis in the adult, 41, 307, 1962.

163. Gordell, B., Jacobs, J. B., Powell, R. D., and de Vita, V. T., Pneumocystis carinii — the spectrum of diffuse interstitial pneumonias in patients with neoplastic disease, *Ann. Int. Med.*, 72, 337, 1970.
164. Goffinel, D. R., Goldstein, M. D., and Kaplan, H. S., Herpes zoster infections in lymphoma patients, *Natl. Cancer Inst. Monogr.*, 36, 463, 1973.
165. Arsenau, J. C., Canellos, G. P., Johnson, R., and de Vita, V. T., Risk of new cancers in patients with Hodgkin's disease, *Cancer*, 40, 1912, 1977.
166. Warthin, A. S., The genetic neoplastic relationships of Hodgkin's disease aleukaemic and leukaemic lymphoblastoma and mycosis fungoides, *Ann. Surg.*, 93, 153, 1931.
167. Pedersen-Bjergaard, J. and Larsen, S. O., Incidence of acute nonlymphocytic leukaemia, preleukaemia and acute myeloproliferative syndrome up to 10 years after treatment of Hodgkin's disease, *N. Engl. J. Med.*, 307, 965, 1982.
168. Wolter, J., Hammann, W., and Ostendorf, P., Ein Fall von grosfollikularen Lymphoblastom mit finalem lymphoma maligneum Hodgkin, *Med. Welt*, 21, 1778, 1970.
169. Bjorkholm, M., Hohn, G., and Mellstedt, H., Persisting lymphocyte deficiencies during remission in Hodgkin's disease, *Clin. Exp. Immunol.*, 28, 389, 1977.
170. Check, J. H., Damsker, J. I., Brady, L. W., and O'Neill, E. A., Effect of radiation treatment on mumps delayed type hypersensitivity reactions in lymphoma and carcinoma patients, *Cancer*, 32, 580, 1973.
171. Fuks, Z., Strober, S., Bobrove, A. M., Sasazuki, T., MacMichael, A., and Kaplan, H. S., Long term effects of radiation on T and B lymphocytes in peripheral blood of patients with Hodgkin's disease, *J. Clin. Invest.*, 58, 803, 1976.
172. Weitzmann, S. A., Aisenberg, A. C., Siber, G. R., and Smith, D. H., Impaired humoral immunity in treated Hodgkin's disease, *N. Engl. J. Med.*, 297, 245, 1977.
173. Wagener, D. J. T., Geestman, E., Borgonjen, A., and Haanen, C., The influence of splenectomy on cellular immunologic parameters in Hodgkin's disease, *Cancer*, 12, 683, 1976.
174. Sutcliffe, S. B., Katz, D. R., Stansfeld, A. G., Wrigley, P. J. M., Shand, W. S., and Malpas, J. S., Post treatment laparotomy in the management of Hodgkin's disease, *Lancet*, 2, 57, 1978.
175. Dorreen, M. S. and Habeshaw, J. A., unpublished observations.

Chapter 3

# NON-HODGKIN'S LYMPHOMA CONCEPTS OF CLASSIFICATION

John R. Krause

## TABLE OF CONTENTS

| | | |
|---|---|---|
| I. | Introduction | 66 |
| II. | Historical Perspectives | 66 |
| III. | Current Concepts | 67 |
| | A. Rappaport Classification | 67 |
| IV. | Immunological Concepts | 67 |
| | A. Lukes and Collins Classification | 67 |
| V. | Kiel Classification | 69 |
| VI. | British Classification | 69 |
| VII. | Dorfman Classification | 71 |
| VIII. | World Health Organization (WHO) Classification | 72 |
| IX. | NCI Working Formulation of Non-Hodgkin's Lymphomas | 73 |
| X. | Summary | 73 |
| References | | 77 |

## I. INTRODUCTION

The non-Hodgkin's lymphomas (NHL) are a group of neoplastic disorders that have undergone considerable reexamination and evaluation in the last few years. The significance and concepts of the changes that have occurred can perhaps be better appreciated if a brief review of the milestones in the history of the lymphomas is presented.

## II. HISTORICAL PERSPECTIVES

The first clinical account of a primary lymph node disorder was described in the now classic paper by Thomas Hodgkin in 1832.[1] His contribution was significant in that he emphasized that a disease process could involve the lymph nodes and spleen as a syndrome at a time when the functions and interrelation between these organs were unrecognized. Virchow next conceived of and defined leukemia (1845),[2] and introduced the concepts of lymphosarcoma and lymphoma (1863) for nonleukemic conditions.[3] However, he included under the name lymphosarcoma, not only sarcomas of lymphoid tissues, but also Hodgkin's disease and a number of other conditions. Cohnheim (1865) proposed the term pseudoleukemia, a condition in which the histologic features of leukemia were present but without an accompanying leukocytosis.[4] Samuel Wilks (1865) published a second series of cases similar to those described by Hodgkin and he introduced the eponym Hodgkin's disease for this disorder.[5] Kundrat later (1893) proposed that the term lymphosarcoma should not be used in the broad sense as Virchow described, but be restricted to a sarcomatous tumor involving only lymphoid cells.[6] At the turn of the century Sternberg (1898)[7] and Reed (1902)[8] both described and illustrated the characteristic giant cell of Hodgkin's disease that accords them eponymic recognition.

Although the concept of the reticuloendothelial system had been slowly evolving, it was Aschoff (1924) that first presented a comprehensive account of the system.[9] Maximow[10] followed with the idea of the pleuripotentiality of the undifferentiated mesenchyme cell (1927). Meanwhile, Ewing's histologic description (1928)[11] of lymphosarcoma received general acceptance. He described two types of lymphosarcoma; the malignant lymphosarcoma containing small cells and the large round cell lymphosarcoma or reticulum cell sarcoma.

In America another course was emerging. In 1925 Brill, Bauer, and Rosenthal described follicular lymphomas as a distinct clinicopathological entity.[12] Two years later Symmers[13] independently made the same observations and this type of lymphoma has since been termed giant follicle hyperplasia, follicular lymphoblastoma, or Brill-Symmers disease. Gall and Mallory (1942)[14] reported a series of over 600 cases of lymphoma which they classified as lymphocytic, lymphoblastic, stem cell, clasmatocytic, Hodgkin's lymphoma, and Hodgkin's sarcoma. It was Gall and Mallory in this review who proposed the use of the term reticulum cell sarcoma to describe poorly differentiated malignant neoplasms, either of stem cell or histiocytic origin. Far more influential was the publication of Jackson and Parker (1947)[15] of *Hodgkin's Disease and Allied Disorders*. They gave a clinical-pathological review of approximately 800 cases of primary lymph node disorders, over a third of which were Hodgkin's disease. The main interest of their work was their approach to Hodgkin's disease, which on histological grounds they divided into three types; paragranuloma, granuloma, and sarcoma; they also showed that each had a different natural history and prognosis. However they included the clinical and pathological features of giant follicle lymphoma, myeloma, leukemia, and reticulosarcoma and their review had a valuable influence as they emphasized the distinct clinical-pathological features of the various lymphadenopathies.

Table 1
RAPPAPORT
CLASSIFICATION OF NON-
HODGKINS' LYMPHOMA

Nodular          Diffuse

Lymphocytic, well differentiated
Lymphocytic, poorly differentiated
Mixed cell (lymphocytic and histiocytic)
Histiocytic
Undifferentiated

*Note:* All types may occur in a nodular or diffuse form.

The final entrant to date into the lymphoma family was not reported until Burkitt (1958),[16] and O'Connor and Davies (1960)[17] described a unique lymphoma in African children that now goes by the eponymic name of Burkitt's lymphoma. This lymphoma has a predilection for the bones of the jaw, orbit, and for the gonads. This tumor has received intense interest because of its epidemiologic behavior and its relationship to infections caused by the Epstein-Barr virus.

## III. CURRENT CONCEPTS

### A. Rappaport Classification

In 1956 Rappaport, Winter, and Hicks[18] studied a group of cases of lymphoma from the Armed Forces Institute of Pathology and proposed a new system to classify malignant lymphomas based on morphological criteria. Rappaport's initial classification is presented in Table 1 but was later revised in 1966.[19] In the original report, Rappaport and colleagues described five cytologic categories and emphasized that within each cytologic class, lymphomas with a nodular architecture tend to have a better prognosis than those with a diffuse pattern, and that those patients with well and poorly differentiated lymphocytic lymphoma had a longer survival than patients with mixed cell and histiocytic lymphomas. This classification gained little attention or acceptance until the studies of Jones et al.[20] demonstrated that this classification is applicable to clinicopathologic investigations and provides information that is prognostically significant. Other studies[21-24] confirmed these conclusions. This consensus allowed clinicians from many medical institutions to compare the results of treatment trials, and Rappaports classification was accepted and adopted by the Lymphoma Pathology Panel for Clinical Trial Studies,[25] which serves cancer chemotherapy groups throughout the United States and in a number of other countries. However, the Rappaport classification was proposed prior to the implementation of immunologic tests to determine more precisely the origin of the abnormal cells in non-Hodgkin's lymphomas and is not biologically correct. In particular, strong criticism has been directed toward Rappaport's category of histiocytic lymphomas which actually includes a number of immunologically and morphologically different categories, most of them being of lymphoid rather than of histiocytic origin. This has led to a number of other classifications.

## IV. IMMUNOLOGICAL CONCEPTS

### A. Lukes and Collins Classification

Two lymphocytic systems are generally accepted to exist in man. They are the T cell or thymic-dependent system and the B cell or bursal equivalent (thymic-independent)

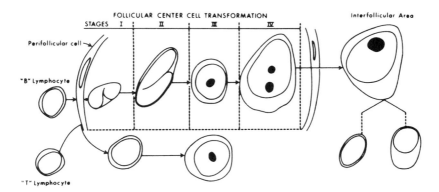

FIGURE 1. Schematic representation of normal transformation of follicular center cells (FCC) in comparison with transformation of T cells. (I) Small cleaved cell; (II) large cleaved cell; (III) small noncleaved transformed cell; (IV) large noncleaved transformed cell, gives rise to a B immunoblast, which may revert to a small lymphocyte or become a plasma cell. T immunoblast results from T lymphocyte transformation. Lymphomas appear to develop from either a "block" in or a "switch-on" of this lymphocyte transformation in vivo. (From Lukes, R. J., et al., *Semin. Hematol.*, 15, 322, 1978. With permission.)

system. A group of lymphocytes without membrane markers is also recognized; the so-called null cells. The T and B cells are distributed in a consistent manner. The T cells are found in the paracortical area of lymph nodes, perivascular region of the spleen, and small foci in the lamina propria of the gastrointestinal tract. The B cells concentrate in the follicular centers of lymph nodes, spleen, the lamina propria of the gastrointestinal tract, and wherever follicles occur. B lymphocytes are also found interspersed in the marrow.

Lukes and Collins and Lennert have been the main proponents of new approaches to the classification of non-Hodgkin's lymphomas. Lukes and Collins have proposed a classification of non-Hodgkin's lymphomas based upon the T and B cell system and the concept of lymphocyte transformation (Figure 1).[26,27] These authors included the knowledge that the follicular center is the site of B cell transformation and that with rare exceptions the histiocytic lymphomas of Rappaport are really lymphomas of transformed lymphocytes. Their classification is listed in Table 2. The different cell types in the sequence of B and T cell transformation form the basis of their classification in that lymphomas possibly develop through a block or a "switch-on" at various stages of B or T cell transformation,[26] and that the morphologic features are predictive of the specific type. Lukes and Collins' classification contains two additional cell types; the U cell (undefined) and the true histiocyte. Lukes and Collins have emphasized that lymphomas with cleaved nuclei originate in lymphoid follicles and thus can be recognized as follicular center cell (FCC) lymphomas even when a nodular pattern is not evident. The authors imply that the prognosis of lymphomas of follicular center cell origin is dependent on the specific cell type and not on the architectural pattern. In the Lukes and Collins classification the individuals with cleaved cell lymphomas have a better survival than those having noncleaved cell lymphomas or lymphomas with convoluted lymphocytes. Furthermore, within the cleaved group the trend seems to indicate that those with small cell types survive longer than those with large cell types. The category of mixed cell lymphomas has been eliminated and this has made it difficult for many pathologists to classify lymphomas in which small and large cells are present without preponderance of either type. The terminology in this classification is somewhat unwieldy and clinicians as well as pathologists have had difficulty with its use and the appropriate clinical-pathological correlations.

Table 2
LUKES AND COLLINS'
FUNCTIONAL CLASSIFICATION OF
MALIGNANT LYMPHOMA

U cell (undefined cell) type
T cell types
    Mycosis fungoides and Sezary's syndrome
    Convoluted lymphocyte
    Immunoblastic sarcoma of T cells
B cell types
    Small lymphocyte (CLL)
    Plasmacytoid lymphocyte
    Follicular center cell (FCC) types (follicular,
        diffuse, follicular and diffuse, and sclerotic)
    Small cleaved
    Large cleaved
    Small noncleaved
    Large noncleaved
    Immunoblastic sarcoma of B cells
Histiocytic type
Unclassifiable

## V. KIEL CLASSIFICATION

This classification was proposed by Lennert from the University of Kiel and is appropriately termed the Kiel classification. The classification is based primarily on cytologic features and like the Lukes and Collins classification it ascribes no conceptual or prognostic relevance to pattern (follicular or diffuse). Unlike the other classifications, the Kiel classification uses the terms low and high grade malignancy to indicate two major prognostically different subgroups. The classification was initially published for the European Lymphoma Club in 1974.[28] A revised classification appears in Table 3.[29] The suggestion that all lymphomas with a nodular pattern are of germinal center (follicular center) origin, a view which is now universally accepted, was first proposed by Lennert.[30-32] He designated cells within the germinal centers of three types: small centrocytes, large centrocytes, and centroblasts in contrast to Lukes and Collins who classified the follicular center cells into four types: small cleaved, large cleaved, small noncleaved, and large noncleaved. The authors of the Kiel classification also stress that the cytologic type of a lymphoma is of much greater importance for the prognosis than the architectural pattern. The Kiel classification has not caught on in America as the terminology is unfamiliar.

## VI. BRITISH CLASSIFICATION

The classification of NHL proposed by Bennett, Farrer-Brown, and Henry is often referred to as the British classification. This was first presented at a meeting in Chicago in 1973 and was published in 1974 (Table 4).[33] This classification was later expanded[34] and is referred to as the British National Lymphoma Investigation Classification. As in the Rappaport classification, the NHL are subdivided on the basis of pattern into follicular and diffuse forms (all lymphomas with a follicular pattern are considered to be low grade malignant tumors). There have been objections to this classification. The British classification uses the terms well differentiated and poorly differentiated with reference to the lymphocytic lymphomas and objections have been raised since the concept of differentiation as applied to the lymphocyte may not be true. The term poorly differentiated lymphocytic (lymphoblastic) in this classification includes a heterogeneous group of lymphomas; (1) the non-Burkitt's type; (2) the Burkitt's lympho-

## Table 3
## MODIFICATION OF THE KIEL CLASSIFICATION OF NON-HODGKIN'S LYMPHOMA

Low grade malignancy
  ML lymphocytic
    Chronic lymphocytic leukemia, B cell type
    Chronic lymphocytic leukemia, T cell type
    Hairy-cell leukemia (?)
    Mycosis fungoides and Sezary's syndrome
    T-zone lymphoma
  ML lymphoplasmacytic/lymphoplasmacytoid (lymphoplasmacytoid immunocytoma)
  ML plasmacytic (plasmacytoma[a])
  ML centrocytic
  ML centroblastic/centrocytic
    Follicular
    Follicular and diffuse
    Diffuse with or without sclerosis
High grade malignancy
  ML centroblastic
    Primary
    Secondary
  ML lymphoblastic
    B lymphoblastic, Burkitt type, and others
    T lymphoblastic, convoluted cell type, and others
    Unclassified
  ML immunoblastic
    With plasmablastic/plasmacytic differentiation (B)
    Without plasmablastic/plasmacytic differentiation (B or T)

*Note:* ML = malignant lymphoma.

[a] Only extramedullary plasmacytoma.

From Gerard-Marchant, R., et al., *Lancet,* 2, 406, 1974. With permission.

## Table 4
## BRITISH NATIONAL LYMPHOMA INVESTIGATION CLASSIFICATION

Follicular lymphoma
  Follicle cells, predominantly small
  Follicle cells, mixed small and large
  Follicle cells, predominantly large
Diffuse lymphoma
  Lymphocytic, well differentiated (small round lymphocyte)
  Lymphocytic, intermediately differentiated (small follicle lymphocyte)
  Lymphocytic, poorly differentiated (lymphoblast)
    Non-Burkitt
    Burkitt's tumors
    Convoluted cell mediastinal lymphoma
  Lymphocytic/mixed small lymphoid and large cell (mixed follicle cells)
  Undifferentiated large cell (large lymphoid cell)
  Histiocytic cell (mononuclear phagocytic cell)
  Plasma cell (extramedullary plasma cell)
  Malignant lymphoma, unclassified
  Plasmacytoid differentiation
  Sclerosis, banded
  Sclerosis, fine

Table 5
DORFMAN CLASSIFICATION OF NON-HODGKIN'S LYMPHOMAS

Follicular lymphomas[a]

(Follicular or follicular and diffuse)
    Small lymphoid
    Mixed small and large lymphoid
    Large lymphoid

Diffuse lymphomas[a]

    Small lymphocytic[b]
    Atypical small lymphoid
    Lymphoblastic
        Convoluted
        Nonconvoluted
    Large lymphoid
    Mixed small and large lymphoid
    Histiocytic
    Burkitt's lymphoma
    Mycosis fungoides
    Undefined

[a] Composite lymphomas, comprising two well defined and apparently different types of lymphoma within the same tissue; lymphomas associated with sclerosis.
[b] Lymphomas showing plasmacytoid differentiation; and those diffuse lymphomas associated with epithelioid cells are suitably designated.

From Dorfman, R. F., *Lancet*, 1, 1295, 1974. Modified 1976. With permission.

mas; and (3) the convoluted cell mediastinal lymphoma. No reason is given for including the Burkitt's lymphoma and the convoluted cell mediastinal lymphoma as lymphoblastic lymphomas. These lymphomas are quite different from each other and have recognizably dissimilar morphologic features as well as very different natural histories and responses to therapy. This classification also fails to include a category for the mycosis fungoides-Sezary (T cell) lymphomas.

## VII. DORFMAN CLASSIFICATION

In 1974 Dorfman published a "working classification" for the non-Hodgkin's lymphomas.[35,36] This classification (Table 5) was introduced as a compromise between that of Rappaport and Lukes, and the classification proposed by Farrer-Brown, et al. (Table 5). It relates to Rappaport's classification in that a major prognostic feature is whether the neoplastic proliferation is follicular or diffuse, with a follicular pattern having a favorable prognosis. Dorfman implied a fundamental division between low grade and high grade malignant lymphomas being implicit in the terminology. The low grade lesions comprise the group of follicular lymphomas and in the diffuse category, the small lymphocytic lymphoma which corresponds to Rappaport's well differentiated

Table 6
WHO CLASSIFICATION OF
MALIGNANT LYMPHOMAS

    Lymphosarcomas
        Nodular lymphosarcoma
            Prolymphocytic
            Prolymphocytic, lymphoblastic
        Diffuse lymphosarcoma
            Lymphocytic
            Lymphoplasmacytic
            Prolymphocytic
            Lymphoblastic
            Immunoblastic
            Burkitt's tumor
    Mycosis fungoides
    Plasmacytoma
    Reticulosarcoma
    Unclassified malignant lymphomas

lymphocytic type. Rappaport's five diffuse categories were increased by Dorfman to nine and there was provision for a composite lymphoma and whether or not there was accompanying sclerosis. This classification also employs descriptive terminology, and many of the discredited histogenetic names are replaced by terms that indicate the size of the malignant cells which therefore becomes another major criterion for classification. Again, this classification while having merits has not found general acceptance and usage.

## VIII. WORLD HEALTH ORGANIZATION (WHO) CLASSIFICATION

The WHO classification of neoplastic diseases of hematopoietic and lymphoid tissues appeared in 1976.[37] It includes a far broader group of conditions than is ordinarily included under non-Hodgkin's lymphoma although the demarcation line of this group is not clear. In the original WHO list the primary division is between systemic diseases which includes the leukemias and related diseases, and tumors which includes Hodgkin's disease. The classification of the NHL portion is listed in Table 6. This classification has not received a wide or warm reception. While it has incorporated some of the new terms such as immunoblastic, it includes the retrogressive term lymphosarcoma which has engendered much confusion in the past as to its meaning. The term prolymphocytic is also used which may be clear on examination of Romanovsky-stained smears but not to those working with histologic sections. Likewise, Galton[38] has recently described an entity called prolymphocytic leukemia which differs from the phase of the nodular (follicular) lymphomas of lymphocyte type.[39] The WHO monograph is well illustrated with colored photographs and there is a short description of each of the conditions. However, the cytological account of each of the individual cell types is somewhat lacking.

The six most prevalent classification systems for the non-Hodgkin's lymphomas have been presented. Some of these new classification systems have not been based upon extensive clinical correlations and they have been subject to modifications as new entities have been recognized. Obviously no consensus exists as to which system is most satisfactory with regard to clinical relevance, scientific accuracy and reproducibility, or really whether any is more valuable than the modified and revised Rappaport system. This has resulted in much confusion and controversy and prominent investigators in this field have attempted to discuss and resolve their differences at numerous international conferences including London, England (1973), Florence, Italy (1974), and Airlie House, Warrenton, Virginia (1975). These efforts were unsuccessful largely because inadequate clinical data were available to resolve the controversial issues and because a common base data was not available for the many proposed classifications.

## IX. NCI WORKING FORMULATION OF NON-HODGKIN'S LYMPHOMAS

In the spring of 1976 the National Cancer Institute (NCI) agreed to organize a retrospective review of biopsies from over a thousand cases of NHL that had an adequate follow-up period. It was the hope that the analysis of results from such an undertaking might create the basis for a new classification that would prove as satisfactory as was Rappaport's classification for almost 20 years. The reviews were completed in the latter part of 1978 and conferences were held in Stanford, California in June 1979 and January 1980. The results of this study have recently been published.[29]

The NCI study has been based primarily on clinical correlations, particularly survival curves, age, sex, and presenting sites and stage of disease. No immunologic methods were employed. This classification is listed in Table 7. Some interesting findings resulted from this study. In each of the six classifications that have been discussed, within the same cytologic subtypes, those patients with follicular or nodular patterns had a more favorable survival experience than those with diffuse patterns. The presence of a follicular or nodular pattern, therefore, is an important favorable prognostic indicator. This is true whether there was a totally follicular or nodular pattern or a partially follicular pattern with areas of diffuse proliferation in the same specimen. However, the cell type (size and shape) is also of great importance and the lymphomas were grouped based upon survival into low grade, intermediate grade, and high grade malignancies. A provision was made for the inclusion of additional morphological observations as subtypes under each major grouping, e.g., plasmacytoid differentiation, diffuse areas, sclerosis, and epithelial cell components. While these features may have clinical importance, none could be shown to have statistically significant correlations with survival or any other tested clinical parameters.

The participants of this study emphasize that this formulation is not devised to replace any of the currently utilized classifications. It is hoped that by using the related terms, pathologists and clinicians may continue to employ those systems with which they feel most comfortable. A comparison of the NCI classification with Rappaport's, Lukes-Collins', and Lennert's classifications is presented in Table 8. Unquestionably, the NCI formulation is an important contribution and step forward in alleviating the controversy that exists by encouraging translations of the various classifications. Most likely, the final word(s) on the classification system for the non-Hodgkin's lymphomas has not been written.

## X. SUMMARY

During the past decade the classification of the non-Hodgkin's lymphomas has been one of the most hotly debated topics in the medical literature. The profusion of nomenclatures and classifications has led to confusion and uncertainty among clinicians and pathologists alike. The general acceptance of the Rappaport classification, even with its recognized deficiencies, has been very useful for therapeutic selection and for the evaluation of results.

Perhaps the most important development in the last few years in the search of the pathogenesis of the non-Hodgkin's lymphomas has been the application and utilization of immunological techniques. This has been directed primarily to the study of surface

## Table 7
## NCI WORKING FORMULATION OF NON-HODGKIN'S LYMPHOMAS

### Low grade

A. Malignant lymphoma
   Small lymphocytic
      Consistent with CLL
      Plasmacytoid
B. Malignant lymphoma, follicular
      Predominantly small cleaved cell
      Diffuse areas
      Sclerosis
C. Malignant lymphoma, follicular
      Mixed, small cleaved and large cell
      Diffuse areas
      Sclerosis

### Intermediate grade

D. Malignant lymphoma, follicular
      Predominantly large cell
      Diffuse areas
      Sclerosis
E. Malignant lymphoma, diffuse
      Small cleaved cell
      Sclerosis
F. Malignant lymphoma, diffuse
      Mixed, small and large cell
      Sclerosis
      Epithelioid cell component
G. Malignant lymphoma, diffuse
      Large cell
         Cleaved cell
         Noncleaved cell
      Sclerosis

### High grade

H. Malignant lymphoma
      Large cell, immunoblastic
         Plasmacytoid
         Clear cell
         Polymorphous
         Epithelioid cell component
I. Malignant lymphoma
      Lymphoblastic
         Convoluted
         Nonconvoluted cell
J. Malignant lymphoma
      Small noncleaved cell
         Burkitt's
         Follicular areas

### Miscellaneous

Composite
Mycosis fungoides
Histiocytic
Extramedullary plasmacytoma
Unclassifiable
Other

## Table 8
## COMPARISON OF NON-HODGKIN'S LYMPHOMA CLASSIFICATIONS

| NCI Formulation | Rappaport | Lukes-Collins | Kiel |
|---|---|---|---|
| **Low grade** | | | |
| A. ML, small lymphocytic Consistent with CLL Plasmacytoid | Well-differentiated lymphocytic | Small lymphocyte (B cell) Plasmacytoid lymphocytic (B cell) | ML, lymphocytic, CLL ML, lymphoplasmacytic/lymphoplasmacytoid |
| B. ML, follicular Predominantly small cleaved cell | Nodular, poorly differentiated lymphocytic | Small cleaved FCC, follicular (B cell) | |
|   Diffuse areas   Sclerosis | | | ML, centroblastic-centrocytic, follicular, ± diffuse |
| C. ML, follicular Mixed small cleaved and large cell   Sclerosis | Nodular mixed lymphocytic and histiocytic | | |
| **Intermediate grade** | | | |
| D. ML, follicular Predominantly large cells | Nodular, histiocytic | Large cleaved FCC, follicular Large noncleaved FCC, follicular | ML, centroblastic-centrocytic, follicular, ± diffuse |
|   Diffuse areas   Sclerosis | | | |
| E. ML, diffuse Small cleaved cell   Sclerosis | Diffuse, poorly differentiated lymphocytic | Diffuse small cleaved FCC With sclerosis | ML, centrocytic, small |
| F. ML, diffuse Mixed, small and large cell   Sclerosis | Diffuse, mixed | | ML, centroblastic-centrocytic (small), diffuse ML, lymphoplasmacytic/cytoid, polymorphic |
|   Epitheloid cell   Component | Lymphoepitheloid cell | | |

Table 8 (continued)
## COMPARISON OF NON-HODGKIN'S LYMPHOMA CLASSIFICATIONS

| NCI Formulation | Rappaport | Lukes-Collins | Kiel |
|---|---|---|---|
| G. ML, diffuse, large cell | Diffuse, histiocytic | Large cleaved FCC, diffuse | ML, centroblastic-centrocytic (large), diffuse |
| Cleaved cell | | | ML, centrocytic, large |
| Noncleaved cell | | Large noncleaved FCC, diffuse | ML, centroblastic |
| Sclerosis | | | |
| High grade | | | |
| H. ML, large, immunoblastic | Diffuse histiocytic | Immunoblastic sarcoma | ML, immunoblastic |
| Plasmacytoid | | B cell type | |
| Clear cell | | T cell type | T zone lymphoma |
| Polymorphous | | | |
| Epithelioid cell component | | Lymphoepithelioid cell (T cell) | Lymphoepithelioid cell lymphoma |
| I. ML, lymphoblastic | Lymphoblastic | Convoluted T cell | ML, lymphoblastic convoluted cell type |
| Convoluted cell | | | ML, lymphoblastic unclassified |
| Nonconvoluted cell | | | |
| J. ML, small noncleaved cell | Diffuse, undifferentiated | Small noncleaved FCC, diffuse (B cell) | ML, lymphoblastic, Burkitt type and other B lymphoblastic |
| Burkitt's | | Burkitt's variant (B cell) | |
| Follicular areas | | | |
| K. Miscellaneous | | | |
| Composite | | | |
| Mycosis fungoides | | Cerebriform T cells | Mycosis fungoides |
| Histiocytic | | Histiocytic (true) | |
| Extramedullary plasmacytoma | | | ML, plasmacytic |
| Unclassifiable | | | |
| Other | | | |

*Note:* ML = malignant lymphoma; CLL = chronic lymphocytic leukemia; FCC = follicular center cell.

membrane markers and to a lesser degree of intracytoplasmic markers. Indeed it is now possible to identify the lymphocytic type, and in some cases subtype, of the majority of the non-Hodgkin's lymphomas. Several studies based upon immunologic identification of lymphomas have demonstrated that 75 to 80% are B cell, 8 to 20% are T cell, 5 to 10% are undefined, and <1% are true histiocytic lymphomas.[40,41] Lukes and Collins, and Karl Lennert and co-workers introduced the concept of the follicular center cell (FCC) lymphoma. Their suggestion that all lymphomas with a nodular pattern are of follicular or germinal center origin is now universally accepted. The recognition of specific cell types within a diffuse lymphoma, however, can also identify the lymphoma as being of follicular center cell (FCC) origin (Table 2). From comparisons of morphologic observations with immunologic techniques, the lymphomas formerly regarded as reticulum cell sarcoma or histiocytic lymphoma of Rappaport are really lymphomas of transformed lymphocytes, with rare exceptions. The true histiocytic lymphoma is not very common.[42-48] The T cell group of lymphomas includes cytologic types with prominent nuclear configurations; the convoluted T cell lymphoblastic lymphoma and the cerebriform cell of Sezary syndrome and mycosis fungoides. Whereas immunologic studies of the non-Hodgkin's lymphomas have contributed greatly in the study and pathogenesis of these tumors, the techniques are costly and require expertise to perform and hence are not yet widely used in routine hospital practice. Likewise, data remains to be correlated whether immunologic typing of the lymphomas will contribute significantly more than careful morphologic classification of these tumors for clinicopathologic correlation.

From the NCI study (no immunologic studies included) certain features are apparent. A follicular or nodular architectural pattern implies a more favorable prognosis no matter what classification is used or whether the lesion is totally follicular or only partially follicular with areas of diffuse proliferation in the same specimen. Likewise, the lymphomas may be classified into low, intermediate, or high grade malignancies (Table 7), depending on the morphologic cell type. Over the next years we will most likely see a further definition of the subtypes of the T and B cell non-Hodgkin's lymphomas. A great therapeutic challenge remains with the non-Hodgkin's lymphoma and perhaps the combined use of chemotherapeutic agents with innovative immunologic therapy such as specific anti-idiotypic antisera might lead to an improved prognosis and survival in these lesions.

## REFERENCES

1. Hodgkin, T., On some morbid appearances of the absorbent glands and spleen, *Med. Chir. Trans.*, 17, 56, 1865.
2. Virchow, R., Weiss Blut, Neue Notizen aus dem Gebeit der Natur - und Heilkunde, *Froriep's neue Notizen*, 36, 151, 1845.
3. Virchow, R., Die krankhaften Geschwulste, Dreissig Vorlesungen, gehalten wahrend des Wintersemesters, 1862-1863, an der Universitat zu Berlin, Vol. 2, Berlin, A. Hirschweld, 1864-65.
4. Cohnheim, J., Ein Fall von Pseudoleukamie, *Virchows Arch. A,* 33, 451, 1865.
5. Wilks, S., Cases of enlargement of the lymphatic glands and spleen (or, Hodgkin's disease) with remarks, *Guys Hosp. Rep. (Series 3),* 11, 56, 1865.
6. Kundrat, H., Uber Lympho-Sarkomatosis, *Wien Klin. Wochenschr.,* 6, (211) 234, 1893.
7. Sternberg, C., Uber eine eigenartige unter dem Bilde der Pseudoleukamie verlaufende Tuberculose des lymphatischen Apparates, *Z. Heilk,* 19, 21, 1898.
8. Reed, D. M., On the pathological changes in Hodgkin's disease with special reference to its relation to tuberculosis, *Johns Hopkins Hosp. Rep.,* 10, 133, 1902.
9. Aschoff, L., *Ergeb. Inn. Med. Kinderheilkd.,* 26, 1, 1924.
10. Maximow, A. A., *Handbuch der Mikrosp Anat des Menschen,* Von Mullendorf, W., Ed., Springer II, Berlin, 1, 1927, 359.

11. Ewing, J., Neoplastic diseases, in *A Treatise on Tumors,* 3rd ed., W. B. Saunders, Philadelphia, 1928, 368.
12. Brill, N. E., Bauer, G., and Rosenthal, N., Generalized lymph follicle hyperplasia of lymph nodes and spleen. A hitherto undescribed type, *JAMA,* 84, 668, 1925.
13. Symmers, D., Follicular lymphadenopathy with splenomegaly, *Arch. Pathol. Lab. Med.,* 3, 816, 1927.
14. Gall, E. A. and Mallory, T. B., Malignant lymphoma — a clinico-pathologic survey of 618 cases, *Am. J. Pathol.,* 18, 381, 1942.
15. Jackson, H., Jr. and Parker, F., Jr.,*Hodgkin's Disease and Allied Disorders,* Oxford University Press, New York, 1947.
16. Burkitt, D. P., A sarcoma involving the jaws in African children, *Br. J. Surg.,* 46, 218, 1958.
17. O'Connor, G. T. and Davies, J. N. P., Malignant tumors in African children, with special reference to malignant lymphoma, *J. Pediatr.,* 56, 526, 1960.
18. Rappaport, H., Winter, W. J., and Hicks, E. B., Follicular lymphoma: a re-evaluation of its position in the scheme of malignant lymphoma based on a survey of 253 cases, *Cancer,* 9, 729, 1956.
19. Rappaport, H., Tumors of the hematopoietic system, in *Atlas of Tumor Pathology, Section 3,* Fascicle 8, U.S. Armed Forces Institute of Pathology, Washington, D.C., 1966.
20. Jones, S. E., Fuks, Z., Bull, M., et al., Non-Hodgkin's lymphomas. IV. Clinico-pathologic correlation in 405 cases, *Cancer,* 31, 806, 1973.
21. Bonadonna, Q., DeLena, M., Lattuada, A., et al., Combination chemotherapy and radiotherapy in non-Hodgkin's lymphomata, *Br. J. Cancer,* 31, (Suppl. 2), 481, 1975.
22. Brown, T. C., Peters, M. V., Bergsagel, D. E., et al., A retrospective analysis of the clinical results in relation to the Rappaport histological classification, *Br. J. Cancer,* Suppl. 2, 174, 1975.
23. Canellos, G. P., DeVita, V. T., Young, R. C., et al., Therapy of advanced lymphocytic lymphoma — a preliminary report of a randomized trial between combination chemotherapy (CVP) and intensive radiotherapy, *Br. J. Cancer,* 31, (Suppl. 2), 474, 1975.
24. Johnson, R. E., DeVita, V. T., Kun Le, et al., Patterns of involvement with malignant lymphoma and implications for treatment decision making, *Br. J. Cancer,* 31, (Suppl. 2), 237, 1975.
25. DeVita, V. T., Rappaport, H., and Frea, E., Announcement of formation of the Lymphoma Task Force and Pathology Reference Center, *Cancer,* 22, 1087, 1968.
26. Collins, R. D. and Lukes, R. J., Studies on possible derivation of some malignant lymphomas from follicular center cells, *Am. J. Pathol.,* 62, 63a, 1971.
27. Lukes, R. J. and Collins, R. D., New observations on follicular lymphoma, in *Malignant Diseases of the Hematopoietic System,* GANN Monogr. Cancer Res., No. 15, Akazaki, K., Rappaport, H., and Borard, C. W., Eds., University of Tokyo Press, Japan, 1973, 209.
28. Gerard-Marchant, R., Hamlin, J., and Lennert, K., et al., Classification of non-Hodgkin's lymphomas, *Lancet,* 2, 406, 1974.
29. Rosenberg, S. A., et al., National Cancer Institute sponsored study of classification of non-Hodgkin's Lymphomas, summary and description of a working formula for clinical usage, *Cancer,* 49, 2112, 1982.
30. Lennert, K., Classification on malignant lymphomas (European concept), in *Progress in Lymphology,* Ruttimann, A., Ed., Thieme, Stuttgart, 1967, 103.
31. Lennert, K., Follicular lymphoma; a special entity of malignant lymphomas, in *Plenary Session Papers J.,* Meeting Europ. Div. of Int. Soc. of Haemat., Milano, 1971, Milano, Arti Grafiche, Fratelli Ferrari, 1971, 109.
32. Lennert, K., Follicular lymphoma — a tumor of the germinal centers, in *Malignant Diseases of the Hematopoietic System,* GANN Monogr. on Cancer Res., Vol. 15, Akazaki, K., Rappaport, H., and Berard, C. W., Eds., University of Tokyo Press, Japan, 1973, 217.
33. Bennett, M. H., Farrer-Brown, G., Henry, K., et al., Classification of non-Hodgkin's lymphomas, *Lancet,* 2, 405, 1974.
34. Henry, K., Bennett, M. H., and Farrer-Brown, G., Morphological classification of non-Hodgkin's lymphomas, *Recent Results Cancer Res.,* 64, 38, 1978.
35. Dorfman, R. F., Classification of non-Hodgkin's lymphoma, *Lancet,* 1, 1295, 1974.
36. Dorfman, R. F., The non-Hodgkin's lymphomas, in *The Reticuloendothelial System,* Int. Acad. Pathol. Monogr., No. 16, Williams & Wilkins Co., Baltimore, 1975, 262.
37. Mathe, G., Rappaport, H., O'Conner, G. T., et al., Histological and cytological typing of neoplastic diseases of hematopoietic and lymphoid tissues in *WHO International Histological Classification of Tumors,* No. 14, World Health Organization, Geneva, 1976.
38. Galton, D. A. G., Goldman, E. W., Catovsky, D., et al., Prolymphocytic leukemia, *Br. J. Haematol.,* 27, 7, 1974.
39. Schnitzer, B., Loesel, L. S., and Reed, R. E., Lymphosarcoma cell leukemia, *Cancer,* 26, 1082, 1970.

40. Lukes, R. J., Parker, J. W., Taylor, C. R., et al., Immunologic approach to non-Hodgkin's lymphomas and related leukemias, analysis of the results of multiparameter studies of 425 cases, *Semin. Hematol.*, 15, 322, 1978.
41. Lukes, R. J., The immunologic approach to the pathology of malignant lymphomas, *Am. J. Clin. Pathol.*, 72, 657, 1979.
42. Lennert, K., Mohri, N., Stein, H., and Kaiserling, E., The histopathology of malignant lymphoma, *Br. J. Haematol.*, Suppl. 31, 193, 1975.
43. Aisenberg, A. C. and Long, J. C., Lymphocytic surface characteristics in malignant lymphoma, *Am. J. Med.*, 58, 300, 1975.
44. Bloomfield, C. D., Kersey, J. H., Brunning, R. D., and Gajl-Peczalska, K. J., Prognostic significance of lymphocytic surface markers in adult non-Hodgkin's malignant lymphoma, *Lancet*, 1, 1330, 1976.
45. Brouet, J. C., Labaume, S., and Seligmann, M., Evaluation of T and B lymphocyte membrane markers in human non-Hodgkin's malignant lymphomata, *Br. J. Cancer*, Suppl. 22, 121, 1975.
46. Jaffe, E. S., Braylan, R. C., Nanba, K., et al., The cellular origin of histiocytic lymphomas (HL), *Am. Soc. Hematol.*, Abstract 239, 1976.
47. Leech, J. H., Glick, A. D., Waldron, J. A., et al., Malignant lymphomas of follicular center cell origin in man. I. Immunologic studies, *J. Natl. Cancer Inst.*, 54, 11, 1975.
48. Morris, M. W. and Davey, F. R., Immunologic and cytochemical properties of histiocytic and mixed lymphocytic lymphomas, *Am. J. Clin. Pathol.*, 63, 403, 1975.

Chapter 4

# IMMUNE DYSFUNCTION IN NON-HODGKIN'S LYMPHOMA

### H. S. Dhaliwal and T. A. Lister

## TABLE OF CONTENTS

| | | |
|---|---|---|
| I. | Introduction | 82 |
| | A. Histopathological Classifications of Non-Hodgkin's Lymphoma | 82 |
| | B. Tests of Immune Function | 83 |
| II. | Immune Function in Non-Hodgkin's Lymphoma | 85 |
| | A. Cellular Immunity | 85 |
| |     1. Lymphocyte Count | 85 |
| |     2. Delayed Hypersensitivity | 86 |
| |     3. Lymphocyte Response to Mitogens and Allogeneic Lymphocytes | 88 |
| | B. Humoral Immune Function | 88 |
| |     1. Serum Immunoglobulins | 88 |
| |     2. Primary and Secondary Antibody Responses | 94 |
| III. | Nonimmune Host Defense Mechanisms | 94 |
| IV. | Chronic Lymphocytic Leukemia | 95 |
| | A. Cellular Immunity | 96 |
| |     1. Delayed Hypersensitivity | 96 |
| |     2. Response of CLL Lymphocytes to Mitogens or Allogeneic Lymphocytes | 96 |
| | B. Humoral Immunity | 96 |
| |     1. Serum Immunoglobulins | 96 |
| V. | Summary of Immune Defects | 97 |
| VI. | Etiology and Significance of Immune Dysfunction | 97 |
| VII. | Concluding Remarks | 99 |
| VIII. | Abbreviations | 100 |
| Acknowledgments | | 100 |
| References | | 100 |

## I. INTRODUCTION

Non-Hodgkin's lymphomas (NHL) are malignant disorders of the lymphoreticular system.[1] The immune system is intimately involved in the etiology, pathogenesis, and clinical presentation of these disorders. Not only may the host immune response be profoundly affected by the proliferation and accumulation of a particular clone of cells but in turn these cells may be subject to normal biological immunoregulatory mechanisms.[2] Furthermore, the cytotoxic drugs used for therapy have immediate effects on the host defense mechanisms and in particular the immune system.[3-6] The observed frequency of immune dysfunction[7-13] and the predilection of NHL patients to develop infections[14-17] must evidently relate to the interaction of the above factors. In spite of advances in supportive care, infection is the most frequent cause of death in NHL patients.[15,17]

Early studies of immunocompetence in lymphoproliferative disorders (LPD) focused on patients with Hodgkin's disease (HD),[18-20] chronic lymphocytic leukemia (CLL),[21-23] and multiple myeloma (MM);[24,25] each of these disorders is characterized by a unique pattern of immune dysfunction. Although many of the early studies also included patients with NHL, the interpretation of the results is complicated by the heterogeneity of the patient population studied, particularly with regard to the histological subgroups included and the treatment status of patients.

Remarkable progress in our understanding of lymphocyte biology over the past decade has led to new concepts of the immunopathology of the lymphoma[1] and new insights into the immunological disorders accompanying lymphomas. This review will focus on the immunological abnormalities associated with NHL. The tests of immune function that are useful clinically shall be briefly discussed and the early and more recent studies of the immune function of NHL patients shall be evaluated in the light of recent progress in the field of immunobiology. Immunological abnormalities of immunodeficient or immunosuppressed patients who develop lymphomas will not be discussed in detail (see Reference 26). Data regarding the correlation of delayed hypersensitivity (102 patients) and serum immunoglobulins (444 patients) to clinicopathological factors in previously untreated patients managed at St. Bartholomew's Hospital over the past decade will be presented. The significance of immune defects noted in NHL patients will be considered and finally strategies for future evaluation of NHL patients will be suggested.

Although myeloma and Waldenström's macroglobulinemia (WM) are clearly B cell disorders,[25,27] the immune defects associated with these diseases will only be considered in order to demonstrate that the mechanisms of immune dysfunction that have been elucidated in some detail in these disorders are of general relevance.

### A. Histopathological Classifications of Non-Hodgkin's Lymphoma

NHL encompasses a diverse group of disorders. Excluding CLL, the majority of adult NHL patients in the Western World have tumors of germinal center cell (GCC) origin.[1] Many histopathological classifications have been proposed of which the most frequently used are the Rappaport, Lukes and Collins, and Kiel classifications. The latter two incorporate recent concepts of lymphocyte heterogeneity and differentiation. More recently, some consensus of opinion has been reached by an international working committee, culminating in the publication of an "International Working Formulation" (Working Formulation Committee[28]). The reader is referred to this review for the equivalent terms of other classifications for the Kiel classification used currently at St. Bartholomew's Hospital.

All classifications recognize two broad categories of NHL; the low grade, "good prognosis" or "favorable" variety, and the high grade, "bad prognosis" or "unfa-

Table 1
TESTS OF IMMUNE FUNCTION

General Tests
  Lymphocyte count
  T and B cell count
  Serum immunoglobulins
Cellular Immunity
    In vivo
        Delayed Hypersensitivity — skin tests
           1°: Response to DNCB, KLH
           2°: Response to recall antigens, e.g., Candida, mumps, and PPD
    In vitro
        Subsets of T cells
        T cell response to: mitogens, e.g., PHA, Con A; alloantigens, e.g., MLR assay
        Interaction of T and B cells, e.g., PWM-induced B cell differentiation; suppression in MLR assay
        Production of lymphokines: MIF, LIF, IL, IFN
        Cell-mediated cytotoxicity: ADCC, NK cell activity
Humoral Immunity
    In vivo antibody response to antigens
        1°: KLH, bacteriophage 174
        2°: Bacterial antigens (tetanus or diphtheria toxoids), viral antigens (influenza, polio)
    In vitro
        Subsets of B cells
        B cell response to: polyclonal mitogens: PWN, LPS, SpA, PPD, and EBV
        B cell stimulatory capacity in MLR

*Note:* See text for abbreviations.

vorable" group. The indolent nature of the low grade NHL, particularly the follicular lymphomas, is reflected in the prolonged natural survival (median survival greater than 6 years) while the latter frequently cause death within a short time (median survival of untreated patients being less than 6 months).

The nodular or follicular lymphomas and the well differentiated lymphocytic lymphomas (Rappaport classification) are virtually always due to proliferation of B cells. Most diffuse lymphomas, in which the lymph node architecture is completely effaced by malignant cells, are also B-cell-derived, but may involve T or null cells (see References 29 to 32). The existence of the null cell[33] or its neoplastic[10] counterpart has been questioned.[32] T and B cell surface marker characteristics may be of prognostic importance, particularly in the high grade lymphomas[34,35] and may correlate with the frequency of immune dysfunction,[12] but this needs to be confirmed.

The monoclonal origin of most non-Hodgkin's lymphomas is well established[36-40] but considerable heterogeneity may exist within a given clone;[41] this has important biological and therapeutic implications. The phenotypic characteristics of the predominant cells in any given lymphoma may reflect the developmental potential of the progenitor cells or may be related to the "block" in differentiation of that particular clone of cells.[41,42]

## B. Tests of Immune Function

Clinically useful tests employed most frequently for the assessment of immune status of NHL patients are listed in Table 1. The majority of the tests cannot be used routinely and require careful standardization to achieve reproducible results. Of the general tests, lymphocyte count and serum immunoglobulin (Ig) estimation have proven to be remarkably reliable. Although regulation of lymphopoiesis is not well understood,[43] the lymphocyte count reflects T cell numbers most closely since the majority of the human blood lymphocytes are T cells. Serum immunoglobulins can be measured with considerable accuracy but the concentration of any Ig class depends on many factors including synthesis, distribution in body fluids, catabolism, and excretion as well as age, sex, and race.[44-46]

Human T cells are commonly identified by their capacity to form rosettes with sheep erythrocytes.[29] With the use of monoclonal antibodies many functionally distinct subsets of T cells can be defined (also see References 47 and 48). So far, helper/inducer ($T_H$) and suppressor or cytotoxic ($T_S$) subpopulations have been analyzed, primarily of CLL[49-51] and MM patients.[27]

Expression of immunoglobulin on the cell membrane (SmIg) or in the cytoplasm (cIg) is the most reliable marker of B lymphocytes. Direct immunofluorescence (DIF), the most commonly used assay for detection of B cells, is subject to many artifacts[52-54] and may seriously underestimate the proportion of B cells,[33] particularly if SmIg expression is weak as on CLL lymphocytes.[55] Many subsets may be defined by the presence of other surface markers such as receptors for complement components (C3b and C3d), immunoglobulin Fc component (FcIgG, FcIgM), and mouse erythrocytes as well as antigens defined by monoclonal antibodies[56-59] (see also References 29, 59, and 60). However, functionally distinct B cell subpopulations are not well defined.[59]

The in vivo tests used to assess the primary and secondary, cellular or antibody responses depend on complex interactions of cells and antigens. Both afferent and efferent arms of the immune response must be intact and it is often impossible to pinpoint the defect precisely. Nevertheless, defective reponses have been noted with considerable consistency in NHL patients *(vide infra)*. It is worth stressing that antibodies are elaborated by cells and the antibody response to any antigen involves not only a particular clone of B cells but a whole series of cell to cell interactions. On the other hand the presence of antibodies may affect the delayed hypersensitivity reactions. Therefore, strict division of immune function into cell mediated immunity (CMI) and humoral immunity is artificial.

Delayed type hypersensitivity (DTH) is assessed by intradermal injections of either antigens to which the individual is likely to have been exposed previously (secondary response) or antigens such as dinitrophenolchlorobenzene (DNCB) or keyhole limpet hemocyanin (KLH) which test the patient's ability to mount an immune response *de novo*. Similarly, KLH and bacteriophage 0174 are used to elicit a primary antibody response, while antigens like tetanus or diphtheria toxoids are used to assess the secondary antibody response of sensitized individuals.

Stimulation of T or B cells by specific antigens and measurement of the antibody response in vitro have not proven very useful. Lack of specific antigens has also restricted the use of biological assays of lymphokine production in NHL patients. These assays are difficult to standardize[61] but the use of specific antisera for direct quantification of lymphokines[62] may overcome these problems in the near future.

Response to nonspecific mitogenic agents is the most widely used in vitro parameter of T or B cell function, but only the overall response of the lymphocytes is evaluated in these assays.[63] While phytohemagglutinin (PHA) and concanavalin A (Con A) are relatively T-cell-specific and bacterial lipopolysaccharide (LPS), purified protein derivative (PPD), and protein A (SpA) or formalin-fixed Cowan strain staphylococci are relatively B-cell-specific. Other mitogens, for example pokeweed mitogen (PWM), may affect both B and T cells, even though differentiation of only B cells is induced. Since the PWM-induced B cell differentiation is T-cell-dependent, this system has been exploited extensively to dissect functional activities of T cells or B cells.[63] Recent evidence suggests PWM may stimulate only the "mature" B cell subset expressing sIgG,[64] while the subset bearing receptors for mouse erythrocytes responds poorly.[65] In contrast Epstein-Barr virus (EBV) activates most B cells and the activation is T-cell independent.[66]

Activation and differentiation may be measured by a variety of methods (see Reference 63). In the mixed lymphocyte reaction (MLR), T cells are the responder cells and B cells the stimulator cells. The presence of other cells may modify the reaction.[67] Generation of cytotoxic cells in the MLR or the activity of preactivated T cells can also be measured in this assay.

Antibody-dependent cell-mediated cytotoxicity (ADCC) or the natural, spontaneous cytotoxic activity (NK cell activity) are often used as indicators of in vivo sensitization to tumors. The former is mediated primarily by the null or "third population" cells,[68] while a subset of these cells, the large granular lymphocytes (LGL) account for most of the NK cell activity in some assays.[69,70]

## II. IMMUNE FUNCTION IN NON-HODGKIN'S LYMPHOMA

### A. Cellular Immunity

Relatively few studies have assessed comprehensively the cellular immune function of NHL patients. Studies of DTH as assessed by skin reaction to antigens are difficult to compare because of the variable composition of the antigens used, geographic variations in exposure to the antigens, and the subjective nature of assessing skin reactions.

The response of lymphocytes to mitogens has been the most common in vitro test of CMI but is difficult to standardize, and normal individuals show wide day-to-day variations.

*1. Lymphocyte Count*

Although the absolute lymphocyte count embraces changes in T and B cells, it reflects more closely the integrity of cellular immunity. Lymphopenia in lymphoma has been observed for nearly 50 years[71] but not systematically investigated or related to histology and stage until recently. Jones et al.[9] found severe lymphopenia (absolute lymphocyte count $<1.0 \times 10^9/\ell$) in 32% of patients with diffuse histiocytic NHL. The mean lymphocyte count ($1.14 \times 10^9/\ell$) of these patients was significantly lower than those with nodular or diffuse nodular, poorly differentiated lymphocytic lymphomas (PDLL) or the control population. The lymphopenia was correlated with B symptoms, advanced disease, skin anergy, and depression of immunoglobulin levels. The latest study by the same group, of 186 patients confirmed these findings,[13] and documented depression of both T and B cell numbers. However, correlation with the stage of disease or immunoglobulin levels was not confirmed, although a positive correlation with IgA levels and an inverse relationship to bulk of disease was demonstrated. Opat et al.[72] also noted T lymphopenia in six patients with advanced lymphoma and 16 patients in remission of lymphoma, but in this study patients with Hodgkin's disease and NHL were grouped together.

Of the 444 previously untreated NHL patients managed at Barts (see Table 2 for clinicopathological details) during the past decade severe lymphopenia was found in 40% of patients with high grade NHL and 14% of patients with low grade NHL. The mean lymphocyte count values were 1.53 and $5.75 \times 10^9/\ell$, respectively (Table 3). If patients with overt leukemia (CLL, lymphoplasmacytoid, and some centrocytic NHL patients) are excluded from the low grade NHL group the mean lymphocyte count is nearly halved, but remains significantly higher than that of high grade NHL patients. Most of the patients in the latter group with severe lymphopenia had advanced disease (Table 3). Patients with small cell centrocytic NHL (excluding leukemic patients) had lymphopenia frequently (56%), which was severe in 23%. Lymphopenia was associated in the high grade NHL patients with skin anergy to recall antigens and depression of serum immunoglobulins, response to treatment and survival, but the correlation was not independent of stage, bulk of disease, and the presence of systemic symptoms.

Table 2
GENERAL CLINICOPATHOLOGICAL FEATURES OF 444
PREVIOUSLY UNTREATED PATIENTS WITH NHL[a]

| | Histological Subtype[b] | | | | | | | | |
|---|---|---|---|---|---|---|---|---|---|
| | | | | | Cc | | | | |
| Stage | Ib | Cb | Lb | HGu | Cb/Cc | Sc | Lc | Ly | Lpc | LGu |
| I, I$_E$, II | 18 | 8 | 4 | 6 | 24 | 1 | 6 | 0 | 5 | 1 |
| III, IV | 46 | 17 | 22 | 14 | 95 | 30 | 4 | 102 | 32 | 13 |
| Total | 64 | 25 | 26 | 20 | 119 | 31 | 10 | 102 | 37 | 14 |

Note: Kiel Classification — Ib, immunoblastic; Cb, centrocytic; Lb, lymphoblastic (includes subgroups B or T, Burkitt's and unclassified); HGu, high grade unclassified; Cb/Cc, centroblastic/centrocytic (includes subgroup Cb/Cc-diffuse), Cc, centrocytic (Sc, small cell; Lc, large cell); Ly, lymphocytic; Lpc, lymphoplasmacytoid; LGu, low grade unclassified.

[a] Mean age (range) = 55.0 years (17 to 87); Male: female ratio = 1.6:1; Survival — median (months) = 50; % survival, 5 years = 42%.
[b] Patients with malignant histiocytosis, angioimmunoblastic lymphadenopathy, and subgroups with <10 patients are excluded.

Table 3
RELATIONSHIP OF LYMPHOCYTE COUNT TO
STAGE AND HISTOLOGICAL SUBGROUP OF
NON-HODGKIN'S LYMPHOMA

| Lymphocyte count | High grade[a] stage | | Low grade[b] stage | |
|---|---|---|---|---|
| | I & II[c] | III & IV[d] | I & II[e] | III & IV[f] |
| <1.0 × 10⁹/ℓ | 4 | 47 | 7 | 35 |
| >1.0 × 10⁹/ℓ | 22 | 54 | 17 | 235 |

Note: Lymphopenia (count <1.0 × 10⁹/ℓ) frequency: a V b, $p < 0.01$; c V d, $p < 0.003$; e V f, $p < 0.001$; d V f, $p < 0.000$.

In a detailed immunological analysis of blood lymphocytes of 186 consecutive patients, Cader et al.[73] found severe lymphopenia of both B and T cells in 63% of high grade NHL patients and approximately one-third of all low grade NHL patients. Overall, 53% of 47 patients with B lymphopenia also had reduced T cell numbers and selective T lymphopenia was found in only 4 out of 111 nonleukemic NHL patients. Thus patients with nonleukemic NHL frequently have lymphopenia that can be severe in those with high grade NHL.

*2. Delayed Hypersensitivity*

In contrast to the well-established depression of DTH in Hodgkin's disease, the frequency of skin anergy in NHL patients is controversial.[7-11,13,74] Most early studies noted marked anergy in symptomatic patients with extensive disease and relative preservation of skin reactivity in patients with local disease who were well.[7,8,74] The heterogeneity of the patients studied is probably the major variable when older studies are compared, for example the disease spectrum of patients included in the lymphosarcoma group may extend from CLL to acute lymphoblastic leukemia (ALL).

Table 4
SKIN TEST REACTIVITY OF NON-HODGKIN'S
LYMPHOMA PATIENTS TO RECALL ANTIGENS

| Number of antigens<br>Histological subtype[a] | No. | 2 or more<br>+ve reaction | 1<br>(% of patients) | 0 |
|---|---|---|---|---|
| High grade | 17 | 12[b] | 47 | 41 |
| Ib | 7 | 0 | 71 | 29 |
| Low grade | 71 | 31[c] | 30 | 36 |
| Cb/Cc-f | 37 | 32 | 24 | 43 |
| Lymphocytic | 19 | 32 | 53 | 15 |
| Lpc | 7 | 29 | 14 | 57 |

[a] Subgroups within each subtype with <5 patients not included.
[b] V c, p value <0.05; others not statistically significant.

Table 5
FREQUENCY OF ANERGY TO FOUR
RECALL ANTIGENS

| | NHL subgroup | | | |
|---|---|---|---|---|
| | High grade | | Low grade | |
| Anergy to | No | % | No | % |
| 1-2 antigens | 1 | 6 | 20 | 29 |
| 3-4 antigens | 15 | 94[a] | 49 | 71[b] |

*Note:* a V b, *p* value <0.01.

The most detailed study of DTH in NHL patients is that of Jones et al.[9] It was extended recently to 186 untreated patients.[13] The mean induration diameter of response at 48 hr to six recall antigens was quantificated and some degree of impairment demonstrated in most patients. However, the results varied from almost no abnormality in patients with diffuse well differentiated lymphoma to marked anergy in those with diffuse histiocytic lymphoma (DHL). The response was related to stage; for example positive reactions were obtained to four of six antigens in localized DHL and only one out of six antigens in advanced (stages III and IV) DHL. In contrast, most follicular lymphoma patients reacted to at least four antigens. Response to SK-SD antigens was the most discriminatory test.

Similarly Advani et al.[11] noted relative preservation of response to recall antigens in well differentiated lymphoma and localized DHL. In contrast, only 18% of patients with generalized DHL showed any response. Response to the primary antigen DNCB was negative, while a diminished response was found in other lymphomas. Lapes et al.[10] noted anergy to KLH, but in contrast to above and in agreement with earlier studies, found anergy to recall antigens only in patients with stage IV disease.

The results of the Barts study of 102 patients tested for recall reaction to four antigens (candida, mumps, PPD, and SK-SD) were similar to those reported by Anderson et al.[13] Of the 89 patients tested with all four antigens, only 2 of 17 patients with high grade NHL (14 of whom had stage IV disease) responded to at least two antigens (Table 4), while about 30% of low grade NHL responded to two or more antigens. The relationship of anergy to histological subgroup is shown in Table 5. The response was related to stage of low grade NHL but could not be related to stage in the high grade

NHL patients because of insufficient numbers with localized disease. No relationship between skin reactivity and lymphocyte count, serum immunoglobulin levels, bone marrow dysfunction, systemic symptoms, response to treatment, or survival (minimum follow-up 6 years), could be demonstrated.

### 3. Lymphocyte Response to Mitogens and Allogeneic Lymphocytes

The response of blood lymphocytes of patients with NHL to mitogens and allogeneic lymphocytes has been studied frequently with inconsistent results.[13,21,75-78] The degree of lymphopenia, leukemic spill-over of nodal disease, and drugs, modify the proportions of responder cells and contribute to the variability of the reported results. Most studies have demonstrated diminished responses. Anderson et al.[13] observed correlation of the response to PHA or PWM response with T lymphocyte count and diffuse histology.

Whisler et al.[78] investigated in detail the response of blood lymphocytes of 18 NHL patients to Con A and suggested that a variety of mechanisms may be responsible for the observed hyporesponsiveness. Significant improvement in response occurred upon culturing lymphocytes for 3 days in media alone. Further the recultured cells augmented but did not normalize the response of freshly isolated lymphocytes in mixing experiments. Suppressor activity of adherent cells partly accounted for the hyporesponsiveness of lymphocytes. An intrinsic cell defect was postulated but seems unlikely since this would involve both T and B cells. Alteration of the proportion of circulating mitogen reactive cells would be a more plausible explanation for the depressed responses.[79]

In mixed lymphocyte culture experiments, response (T cell function) has been reported to be normal[13,21] or depressed[77] but the stimulatory capacity was normal.[77]

## B. Humoral Immune Function

The overall frequency of immunoglobulin abnormalities depends on the histological spectrum of the NHL patients tested; thus some studies do and others do not include CLL with NHL patients. Hypogammaglobulinemia occurs in at least 50% of CLL patients and hence can affect the overall frequency of Ig abnormalities.

### 1. Serum Immunoglobulins

Hypogammaglobulinemia was noted frequently in the earlier studies which often included patients with lymphosarcoma-cell leukemia, in whom low gammaglobulin levels had been found in up to 50% of patients.[80] Profound hypogammaglobulinemia occurs in probably 10% of the patients.[1] The presence of a monoclonal paraprotein has also been described but its frequency among various forms of lymphomas depends on the histological classification in use. Thus in the Kiel classification, although the lymphoplasmacytoid lymphomas in which an M band is found frequently (20% in the series reported by Lennert and Mohri[1]) are classified as a distinct subgroup, unlike other classifications, WM is included in this group.

In the series of 444 previously untreated non-Hodgkin's lymphoma patients managed at Barts since 1972, in whom immunoglobulin levels were measured the overall incidence of hypogammaglobulinemia was 23%. The clinicopathological features of these patients are shown in Table 2 and the frequency of serum immunoglobulin abnormalities according to histological subtype are shown in Table 6, while Table 7 shows the frequency of depressed levels in relation to the immunoglobulin class.

Analysis of Ig levels in this series revealed that normal immunoglobulin levels were found in less than 65% of the patients. Abnormalities were equally frequent in high grade and low grade NHL subtypes (37% vs. 40%). However, in the former group depressed Ig levels were much less common (8% vs. 31%, Table 6). The most fre-

Table 6
FREQUENCY OF SERUM IMMUNOGLOBULIN
ABNORMALITIES ACCORDING TO HISTOLOGICAL
SUBTYPE

| Kiel histology subtype | No. | Ig concentration | | |
|---|---|---|---|---|
| | | Normal | Decreased[a] | Elevated[b] |
| High Grade NHL | | | | |
| Immunoblastic | 64 | 69[b] | 6 | 25 |
| Centroblastic | 22 | 77 | 14 | 9 |
| Centrocytic large cell | 9 | 56 | 0 | 44 |
| Lymphoblastic | 26 | 69 | 12 | 19 |
| High grade unclassified | 20 | 80 | 5 | 15 |
| Low Grade NHL | | | | |
| Lymphocytic | 102 | 39 | 50 | 11 |
| Lymphoplasmacytoid | 37 | 24 | 24 | 51 |
| Centroblastic/centrocytic | 119 | 71 | 18 | 12 |
| Centrocytic small cell | 31 | 45 | 23 | 32 |
| Low grade unclassified | 14 | 64 | 36 | 0 |
| Total | 444 | | | |

[a]  Values below the 5th percentile of normal range.
[b]  Values above the 95th percentile of normal range.
[c]  Figures represent percent of patients.

Table 7
FREQUENCY OF SERUM Ig
ABNORMALITIES ACCORDING TO Ig
ISOTYPE

| Ig Level | High grade | | | Low grade | | |
|---|---|---|---|---|---|---|
| | IgG | IgA | IgM | IgG | IgA | IgM |
| Normal | 86[a] | 91 | 85 | 73 | 72 | 73 |
| Elevated | 7 | 7 | 14 | 8 | 5 | 14 |
| Depressed | 7 | 2 | 1 | 19 | 23 | 12 |

[a]  Figures represent percent of patients.

quently depressed Ig class was IgA in low grade NHL and IgG in high grade NHL. The presence of a monoclonal Ig peak was detectable by serum electrophoresis in 2% of patients with high grade NHL and 10% of low grade NHL patients.

Elevated Ig levels were equally frequent in both major subgroups but were most frequently attributed to IgM in low grade NHL, reflecting the inclusion of patients with lymphoplasmacytoid NHL, some of whom had WM. The cause of the elevated Ig levels in patients with high grade NHL is not clear since only 2% were noted to have a monoclonal peak. Elevated levels may reflect the minimal secretory capacity of the neoplastic B cell clone since the subgroup of patients with immunoblastic NHL frequently had hypergammaglobulinemia. However, electrophoretic analysis suggested a polyclonal increase. Alternatively, raised Ig levels may be related to inclusion of patients with T cell NHL since neoplastic T cells can induce polyclonal B cell differentiation. However, elevated levels were not confined to this group as noted by Lichtenstein and Taylor.[12] Polyclonal hypergammaglobulinemia was also observed in centroblastic NHL and most frequently of all in centrocytic (large or small cell type) NHL (Table

Table 8
CLINICOPATHOLOGICAL CHARACTERISTICS OF
PATIENTS WITH HIGH GRADE NON-HODGKIN'S
LYMPHOMA

| | Relationship to Ig Levels | | | | | |
|---|---|---|---|---|---|---|
| | Normal | | Depressed | | Elevated | |
| Characteristic | No. | % | No. | % | No. | % |
| No. patients | 101 | 100 | 11 | 100 | 30 | 100 |
| Mean age (years) | 56.2 | | 53.4 | | 52.5 | |
| Sex ratio, M:F | 2.3 | | 0.8 | | 1.3 | |
| Stage | | | | | | |
| I/II | 29 | 29 | 1 | 9 | 8 | 27 |
| III | 17 | 17 | 1 | 9 | 3 | 10 |
| IV | 55 | 55 | 9 | 81[b] | 19 | 63 |
| B symptoms | 37 | 37 | 10 | 90[c] | 15 | 50 |
| BM involvement | 17 | 17 | 3 | 27 | 2 | 7 |
| Lymphocyte count ($<1.0 \times 10^9/\ell$) | 14 | 14 | 5 | 46[c] | 11 | 36 |
| Response to Rx[a] | | | | | | |
| CR/GPR | 42 | 47 | 3 | 30 | 16 | 58 |
| PPR/F | 45 | 53 | 7 | 70[b] | 11 | 42 |
| Median survival (months) | 20 | | 9[b] | | 25 | |

Note: CR = complete remission; GPR, PPR = good or partial remission; F = failure to respond.

[a] Only evaluable patients included (10% not evaluable in each group).
[b] $p$ value = 0.05 compared to patients with normal Ig level.
[c] $p$ value < 0.01 compared to patients with normal Ig level.

6). A recent study showed that blood T lymphocytes of NHL patients exhibited increased helper activity.[81]

Preliminary analysis by isoelectric focusing has demonstrated a more restricted pattern of increase in that multiple discrete bands with high pI values were apparent in some patients.[151] The nature and significance of these bands is currently under investigation.

Considering each histological subtype separately it was apparent (Table 8) that high grade NHL patients who had depressed Ig levels were more likely to be female with symptomatic stage IV disease. BM involvement and severe lymphopenia were significantly more frequent in these patients. Thus 46% of patients with depressed Ig had severe lymphopenia compared with 14% of those with normal Ig levels. Although survival of patients with depressed Ig levels was significantly poorer than those with normal or elevated levels, hypogammaglobulinemia was not an independent prognostic factor.

Among patients with low grade NHL the majority of the abnormalities in Ig levels occurred in patients with non-GCC lymphomas. Within the GCC group, in agreement with the previous observations[9,12,13] hypogammaglobulinemia was less common in follicular lymphoma. Of the few patients with follicular lymphoma (Cb/Cc-f) who had depressed Ig levels, male predominance and increased frequency of BM involvement were noted (Table 9). Although the overall survival of patients with or without normal Ig levels was similar, response rates were significantly higher in those with normal Ig levels (Table 9).

Table 9
CLINICOPATHOLOGICAL CHARACTERISTICS OF PATIENTS WITH CENTROBLASTIC/CENTROCYTIC NON-HODGKIN'S LYMPHOMA (STAGE III TO IV)

| Characteristic | Relationship to Ig Levels | | | | | |
|---|---|---|---|---|---|---|
| | Normal | | | Depressed | | |
| | No. | % | | No. | % | |
| No. patients[a] | 71 | 100 | | 15 | 100 | |
| Mean age (years) | 54 | | | 53 | | |
| Sex ratio, M:F | 0.9 | | | 2.0 | | |
| Stage | | | | | | |
| III | 22 | 30 | | 0 | | |
| IV | 49 | 70 | | 15 | 100 | |
| BM involvement | 33[b] | 48 | $p<0.05$ | 12 | 75 | |
| Response to Rx | | | | | | |
| CR/GPR | 44[c] | 70 | $p<0.05$ | 5[d] | 35 | |
| PPR/F | 21 | 30 | $p<0.01$ | 9 | 63 | |

[a] Patients with elevated level (only nine) excluded.
[b] Involvement not assessed in two patients.
[c] Six patients not evaluable.
[d] One patient not evaluable.

Table 10
CLINICOPATHOLOGICAL CHARACTERISTICS OF PATIENTS WITH LYMPHOCYTIC NON-HODGKIN'S LYMPHOMA

| Characteristic | Relationship to Ig Levels | | | | | |
|---|---|---|---|---|---|---|
| | Normal | | | Depressed | | |
| | No. | % | | No. | % | |
| No. patients | 40 | 100 | | 51 | 100 | |
| Mean age (years) | 58 | | | 58 | | |
| Sex ratio, M:F | 1:8 | | | 1:5 | | |
| Stage IV | 38 | 98 | | 50 | 99 | |
| Splenomegaly | 5 | 13 | $p<0.01$ | 27 | 54 | |
| Hb <10 g/dℓ or P1 <100 × 10⁹/ℓ | 5 | 13 | $p<0.01$ | 26 | 51 | |
| Lymphocyte count | | | | | | |
| (×10⁹/ℓ mean + SD) | 18.5 + 18.4 | | $p=$ N.S. | 72 + 107.8 | | |
| Median survival | not reached | | $p=$ N.S. | 4.5 years | | |

The lymphocytic lymphoma group in the Kiel classification includes patients who would otherwise be classified as CLL. However, nearly 15% of patients in this group had absolute lymphocyte counts within the normal range. Patients with depressed Ig levels were noted to have splenomegaly and bone marrow dysfunction (hemaglobin < 10.0 g/dℓ and/or platelet count < $100 \times 10^9/\ell$) more frequently (Table 10). This may reflect the greater tumor load since the lymphocyte count exceeded $15 \times 10^9/\ell$ in 72% of patients with depressed Ig compared with 40% of those with normal Ig levels, even

Table 11
COMPARISON OF CLINICOPATHOLOGICAL DATA OF PATIENTS WITH MONOCLONAL Ig PROTEIN AND THOSE WITH DEPRESSION OF ALL THREE Ig CLASSES

| Characteristic | M band No. | M band % | All three Ig Depressed No. | All three Ig Depressed % |
|---|---|---|---|---|
| No. patients | 34 | 100 | 20 | 100 |
| Histology |  |  |  |  |
|   HG | 3 | 9 | 0 |  |
|   LG  — Ly | 8 | 24 | 14 | 70 |
|       — Lpc | 18 | 54 | 1 | 5 |
|       — Cc (Sc) | 1 | 3 | 3 | 15 |
|       — Cb/Cc | 0 | 0 | 2 | 10 |
|       — Unclass | 3 | 9 |  |  |
| Stage |  |  |  |  |
|   — I/Ie | 4 | 12 | 0 | 0 |
|   — IV | 31 | 88 | 20 | 100 |
| Lymphocyte count (×10s/ℓ) |  |  |  |  |
|   — <1.0 | 4 | 12 | 1 | 5 |
|   — 1.1-2.0 | 21 | 63 | 2 | 10 |
|   — >2.0 | 9 | 25 | 17 | 85 |

though the mean lymphocyte counts did not differ significantly (Table 10). All other characteristics examined, including age, stage, bone marrow involvement, response to treatment, and survival, did not correlate with Ig level at presentation.

Table 11 shows that lymphocytic NHL accounted for the majority of patients (14 out of 20) who had panhypogammaglobulinemia viz., depression of all three Ig classes measured. All of these patients had BM involvement. No patient with high grade NHL had panhypogammaglobulinemia. The majority (15 of 20) also had splenomegaly and 50% had bone marrow dysfunction. Fourteen of these patients (70%) failed first line therapy (CB ± prednisolone) compared with an expected *response* rate of more than 60% in patients with lymphocytic NHL. The survival was significantly worse in this group comared with the whole group.

Serum immunoglobulin levels in patients with lymphoplasmacytoid NHL did not correlate with clinicopathological features. It is worth stressing that only 18 of the 34 patients (54%) with a monoclonal M band had lymphoplasmacytoid NHL, while three patients had high grade NHL, eight had lymphocytic NHL, three had low grade unclassified NHL and there was one each with centrocytic and follicular NHL (Table 11). The bone marrow was not involved in 63% of the patients and 75% had a normal lymphocyte count. Thus the majority of these patients did not have typical WM. Mean concentration of M band paraprotein in those patients in whom it was quantifiable was 9 g/dℓ. In contrast, the majority of patients with multiple myeloma have a paraprotein

Table 12
RECENT STUDIES OF SERUM
IMMUNOGLOBULINS OF NON-HODGKIN'S
LYMPHOMA PATIENTS

| First author (year) | No. of patients | Ig level (% patients) | | |
|---|---|---|---|---|
| | | Normal | Elevated | Decreased |
| Jones[a] (1977) | 71 | IgG decreased in diffuse NHL IgA decreased in diffuse histiocytic NHL and in nodular NHL | | |
| Lapes (1977) | 27 | ? | ? | 33 |
| Rosett (1978) | 57 | 48 | 37 | 16 |
| Leonard (1979) | 101-105 | IgG, IgA and Ig decreased in 17%, 29%, and 32%, respectively | | |
| Amlot[c] (1979) | 64 | 14% had IgA/IgM/IgG < mean − 2 SD  12% male NHL had IgM > mean + 2 SD  4% had IgG/IgA > mean + 2 SD | | |
| Lichtenstein (1980) | 120 | 82 | 14 | 4 |
| Advani (1980) | 62 | IgM elevated in most subtypes of NHL  IgM decreased in 13% of PDLL | | |
| Anderson[b] (1981) | 172 | Nodular NHL, IgG and IgA decreased  Diffuse histiocytic NHL IgA decreased | | |
| Dhaliwal (1983) | 444[d] | 57 | 23 | 23 |
| | 407[e] | 60 | 18 | 23 |

[a] See footnote c.
[b] Values calculated from Figure 1 of reference no. 86.
[c] Includes patients reported in a.
[d] Some patients had one Ig class elevated and others depressed.
[e] Excluding patients with paraprotein bands.

band in excess of 15 g/dℓ. Alexanian[82] in a review of 1649 patients with NHL found a mean M band level of only 2 g/dℓ but in this study patients with WM were excluded.

Comparison with other recent studies (Table 12) demonstrates that the results reported here are broadly comparable but important differences also emerge. Thus Jones et al.[9] and Leonard et al.[83] did not report hypergammaglobulinemia, although the latter study noted paraproteins in a number of patients. In contrast, at least immunoglobulin was elevated in 37% of NHL patients studied by Rosset et al.[84] Advani et al.[11] reported hypergammaglobulinemia in all patients but in this study a quantitative hemagglutination-inhibition method was used for measuring Ig levels which may be far more sensitive than immunoplates used in other studies. Also the patients were of Asian origin, in whom frequent antigen stimulation may account for the hypergammaglobulinemia which was noted in many apparently healthy subjects. Lichtenstein and Taylor[12] found hypergammaglobulinemia in 14% of 120 patients, the incidence being higher (38%) in those with diffuse type of NHL and the highest values were noted in patients with T cell NHL.

Of the 171 to 189 NHL patients (excluding CLL) reported by Galton and MacLennan,[85] in whom IgG, IgA, and IgM levels were measured, low levels in each class were noted in 0 to 32%, 0 to 37%, and 0 to 38% of the patients, respectively, depending on the NHL subgroup. Thus patients with centroblastic NHL had normal Ig levels (only five patients studied) while about 15% of patients with immunoblastic NHL had low Ig levels and a slightly high incidence (about 20%) in patients with low grade GCC NHL. Approximately a third of the patients with lymphoplasmacytoid or lymphocytic lymphoma had hypogammaglobulinemia. In this study, a paraprotein was detected least frequently (<5%) in low grade GCC lymphoma and in the majority of patients with lymphoplasmacytoid NHL. In contrast with other studies, a paraprotein was also found in 43% of patients with immunoblastic NHL. Whether this high incidence is related to the sensitivity of the technique used is not clear.

Anderson et al.[13] noted depressed mean concentrations of IgG and IgA in nodular lymphoma and IgA only in DHL but did not relate the *frequency* of Ig abnormalities to histological subtype. The mean values may mask the frequency of Ig abnormalities. Thus 14% of patients studied by Amlot and Green[86] had low Ig levels but significant depression of mean Ig levels was apparent only of IgA of patients with diffuse PDLL.

Hypogammaglobulinemia was found in 16% of patients with B cell NHL and none of the T cell NHL patients studied by Lichtenstein and Taylor.[12] IgG and IgA levels were significantly depressed in nodular lymphoma like the other major study,[13] but mean Ig levels were normal in diffuse histiocytic or PDLL, although 13% of DHL patients had at least one subnormal Ig level. The incidence of hypogammaglobulinemia in nodular GCC lymphoma (18%) and the overall frequency of Ig abnormalities (40%) found is remarkably similar to the Barts study. Other studies[10,84] had insufficient numbers of patients in each histological subgroup.

In summary, marked depression of Ig levels occurs infrequently in high grade NHL except in symptomatic patients with extensive or bulky disease. Most patients with low grade lymphomas of germinal or follicular center cell origin also have normal Ig levels. In contrast, hypogammaglobulinemia affecting any Ig class or panhypogammaglobulinemia is found frequently in lymphocytic and lymphoplasmacytoid NHL, even in the absence of a paraprotein. The not-uncommon occurrence of a paraprotein in lymphocytic NHL suggests that this may be a tumor of functionally mature B cells. Secretion of Ig leading to a detectable serum paraprotein is uncommon in high grade NHL. However an unusually high incidence was noted by Galton and MacLennan.[85] Polyclonal hypergammaglobulinemia is often observed, particularly in NHL of immunoblastic or centrocytic type, or NHL of T cell origin. The etiology of Ig abnormalities is discussed later.

*2. Primary and Secondary Antibody Responses*

There is marked paucity of recent data regarding the antibody responses to antigens in NHL patients. Lapes et al.[10] found near-normal response to KLH in a small number of patients including those with advanced disease. However, impaired antibody response has been noted in patients in long-term remission following chemotherapy.

## III. NONIMMUNE HOST DEFENSE MECHANISMS

Although neutrophil and monocyte dysfunction may contribute to the increased frequency of infections in patients with lymphoma, the function of these cells has been measured in surprisingly few studies. Sbarra et al.[87] found phagocytic capacity in 24 out of 37 patients with lymphoreticular disorders, but many had hypogammaglobulinemia (mostly patients with lymphosarcoma and CLL-like disorders), and some were treated with steroids. Normal serum reversed the minor defects noted, suggesting hypogammaglobulinemia as the major factor responsible for the defects. Phagocytosis was reported to be normal or increased in lymphoma patients[88] in another study.

McCormack et al.[4] studied migratory function, phagocytic capacity, and chemiluminescence in 17 untreated NHL patients (histology not recorded) and found neutrophil function to be normal. Further, eight patients were tested before and after chemotherapy; only neutrophil migration was impaired during therapy and returned rapidly to normal after cessation of therapy.

Cutaneous inflammatory response as revealed by skin window exudates showed reduced cellularity of the exudates and significant differences (compared with controls) in macrophage surface morphology.[89] This study suggested that maturation or activation of monocytes may be impaired.

## IV. CHRONIC LYMPHOCYTIC LEUKEMIA

Chronic lymphocytic leukemia deserves special consideration for several reasons. First, unlike most other NHL, circulating leukemic lymphocytes are readily available and have been studied extensively; bone marrow is always involved. Second, some but not all previous studies of NHL patients have excluded CLL. Third, according to the Kiel classification used in the Barts study, CLL can be diagnosed on histology alone and the presence of blood lymphocytosis (lymphocyte count $> 5.0 \times 10^9/\ell$) is not essential. Other classifications also recognize that the histological picture of CLL may be identical to that seen in lymphocytic NHL (WDLL-D) without lymphocytosis. Thus most of the studies of lymphoma patients discussed so far include some patients with the Kiel equivalent of B-CLL. On the other hand, most studies of CLL include some patients with a paraprotein band and histological features that are recognized to comprise a distinct group of NHL viz., lymphoplasmacytoid NHL. Fourth, the relatively well characterized immunological abnormalities found in B-CLL can provide a basis for understanding similar defects in other lymphomas.

In the majority of patients with CLL the leukemic lymphocytes have the properties of a single clone of B cells which, it has been postulated, have become "frozen" at a certain stage of differentiation.[42] The SmIg molecules expressed are of single light chain type indicating the monoclonal nature of the disorder. Convincing evidence of monoclonality has been obtained by demonstrating the antigen specificity of SmIg or the presence of idiotypic determinants.[90-92]

Most commonly, the heavy chain classes expressed on the cell surface are of IgM and IgD type with IgG occurring in a few cases as a single isotype. More recently, the presence of IgG in addition to IgM and IgD has been demonstrated in some cases by more sensitive techniques of SmIg detection, but the presence of multiple heavy chain isotypes does not argue against monoclonality since the SmIg has been shown to be of single light chain type.[73,93,94]

The leukemic B cells are said to be incapable of normal immune function which led Dameshek[95] to describe CLL as an accumulative disorder of immunoincompetent lymphocytes. This view was based primarily on the poor blastogenic response to mitogens and allogeneic lymphocytes, as well as poor secretion of immunoglobulin following mitogen stimulation (see References 23 and 96). However, most studies have compared the monoclonal CLL lymphocytes with normal blood lymphocytes that are composed not only of T cells but a heterogeneous population of polyclonal B cells consisting of many subsets, some of which may also respond poorly to mitogens.[64,65] The more recent studies[51,92,97] suggest that this functional deficiency may reflect abnormalities in the T cell population as well as T and B cell interactions. With improved culture conditions, CLL B cells can be stimulated by PHA, PWM mitogen, or EB virus particles.[96,98]

## A. Cellular Immunity

### 1. Delayed Hypersensitivity

Skin reaction to a number of recall antigens (PPD, candida, mumps, SK-SD) have been reported to have been normal[8,99,100] except in patients with advanced disease. Recently, Rai and Sawitsky[23] reported that 17% of 43 patients were unable to respond to SK-SD and all these patients had Rai stage III and IV disease, while all patients with stages 0 to 1 responded. Impairment of primary sensitization to DNFB was found in 6/7 patients who responded to recall antigens, but Block et al.[100] had noted only minimal depression of response to a similar hapten DNCB.

### 2. Response of CLL Cells to Mitogens or Allogeneic Lymphocytes

In the past, the majority of studies reported marked depression of lymphocyte response to mitogens. With the realization that PHA-responsive T cells may be diluted by CLL B lymphocytes,[101] considerable controversy was generated regarding the responsiveness of the residual T cells (see References 92 and 102). The consensus of current opinion suggests that T cell subpopulations in B-CLL are not normal, in that both helper and suppressor T cell abnormalities as well as unusual T cell phenotypes have been noted.[49,51,92,102,103] T cell abnormalities may be more frequent in advanced disease.[94] The abnormal T cell populations may also account for the poor blastogenic response in MLC of lymphocytes of CLL patients[104,105] but the stimulatory capacity in one-way MLC reactions has been reported to be normal.[77,106] Others maintain that CLL B lymphocytes are poor stimulators in MLC reactions and suggest that this is related to the reduced expression of Ia antigens.[107] However, Halper et al.[108] found normal or increased expression of Ia antigens on CLL B cells which nevertheless proved to be poor stimulators in MLC response. However, intrinsic B cell abnormalities may be responsible for the poor stimulatory capacity.

## B. Humoral Immunity

Poor antibody response to antigens in CLL patients has been observed since 1914 (Moreschi, Rotsky, quoted by Howell[109]) and confirmed in more recent studies.[110,111] Primary antibody response (immunization with bacteriophage 0174) was markedly depressed, while secondary response was weak and delayed.[112]

### 1. Serum Immunoglobulins

With the advent of paper electrophoresis, marked and frequent depression of gammaglobulins was soon documented[113] and confirmed.[99] Hypogammaglobulinemia is frequently present in untreated patients and can occur in up to 90% of patients.[113-117] Fiddes et al.[115] tested 54 patients and not one had all three normal immunoglobulin levels (IgG, IgA, IgM). Association of the hypogammaglobulinemia with lymphocyte count, duration of disease, lymphadenopathy, duration of treatment, particularly continuous Chlorambucil therapy, and frequency of infections was noted. Correlation with increased frequency of infections[118,119] had been noted previously but Hansen[120] in a detailed study of a large number of patients failed to confirm this as did Ben-Bassat et al.[121]

Jayaswal et al.[122] noted that all patients with null cell CLL had depressed Ig levels but 70% of these also had extensive extramedullary disease. This relationship to SmIg levels may be due to underdetection of SmIg isotypes since with the use of a more sensitive technique very few patients (<2%) were found to have null cell CLL[117] and no relationship of Ig level to any surface marker was apparent.

Foa et al.[116] also found depression of at least one serum Ig in 87% of patients (48 patients tested) but no relationship to SmIg type was noted. Normal values were found in 18.5% of Rai stage I and II patients compared with only 5% of patients with stage III to IV disease. Only 17% of the patients had normal IgG levels.

Analysis of immunoglobulin levels of patients managed at Barts is shown in Table 10. The only significant features associated with depressed Ig levels were splenomegaly and bone marrow dysfunction.

Generally the hypogammaglobulinemia is associated with extensive disease of long duration. The depression in immunoglobulin levels persists even if clinical remission is achieved following treatment. It has been suggested that this should be one of the factors used for documenting complete remission following treatment with experimental intensive chemotherapy or radiotherapy regimens.[123]

## V. SUMMARY OF IMMUNE DEFECTS

Patients with NHL often have abnormalities of both cellular and humoral immune function which become more pronounced with progression of the disease. The pattern of immunological abnormalities is related to the histological subtype of NHL.

Patients with high grade NHL have relative preservation of humoral immunity but impairment of cellular immunity is found frequently in advanced lymphoma. This is reflected in the marked lymphopenia, skin anergy to recall antigens, and the depressed lymphocyte response to mitogens that are observed frequently. Polyclonal hypergammaglobulinemia is not uncommon particularly in immunoblastic NHL but a monoclonal paraprotein is found only infrequently.

Of the low grade or good prognosis NHL group, patients with nodular or follicular lymphomas rarely have marked immune dysfunction compared with those with diffuse lymphoma, even though most patients have advanced disease at presentation. In contrast, humoral dysfunction as evidenced by B and T cell lymphopenia, hypogammaglobulinemia, depressed primary and secondary antibody responses, as well as development of autoantibodies, is found early and frequently in CLL and lymphocytic lymphoma. Although abnormalities of T cells may be frequent, CMI is generally intact except in advanced disease. A similar pattern of immune dysfunction but with more marked depression of B cell function occurs in MM or WM patients.

## VI. ETIOLOGY AND SIGNIFICANCE OF IMMUNE DYSFUNCTION

The non-Hodgkin's lymphomas are not a single disease entity. The heterogeneity of NHL patients studied is likely to be an important determinant of the variation of reported frequency and severity of immune dysfunction. Other factors which affect immunocompetence that have to be frequently taken into account include the effect of age,[46] nutritional status and drugs,[3,5,6,124,125] and the previous history of immune disorder.[26] Nevertheless, the pattern of immunological abnormalities and their relationship to specific histological subtypes cannot be explained on the basis of these factors alone, and indicates a more intimate relationship of the host's immune system to the development and evolution of the lymphoma.

The defects of humoral immunity that occur more commonly in patients with lymphocytic or lymphoplasmacytoid and some GCC tumors are similar to the better studied abnormalities found in CLL and MM. The latter, therefore, provide useful models for this pattern of immune dysfunction.

In CLL, hypogammaglobulinemia is a prominent feature of the disease and appears to be irreversible. Although more frequent in advanced disease, the hypogammaglobulinemia is common even in patients with Rai stage I disease which suggests that the proliferation of monoclonal B cells affects the overall function of normal B cells. How often hypogammaglobulinemia precedes clinical disease is not known but it can be present when monoclonal lymphocytosis is the only evidence of disease.[117]

CLL lymphocytes differ from normal B cells in many respects: poor response to mitogens and antigens, defective MLC stimulatory capacity, defective production of lymphokines, impaired activity of cAMP enzymes, and reduced density of many cell surface receptors such as SmIg, C3, Fc, and catchecholamine receptors. CLL cells are less motile, demonstrate defective capping, and have an immature cell phenotype (References 23 and 126). Also, T cell abnormalities may be intrinsic to the disease.[127] Taken together, these suggest the oncogenic event(s) leading to emergence of the malignant clone result in marked cellular dysfunction.

The long life of CLL cells and perhaps the lack of response to regulatory influences may lead to progressive infiltration of the reticuloendothelial system. This replacement may interfere with cell migration and cell-cell interactions which are critical determinants of a normal immune response.[128,129] Thus the bulk of disease, which is difficult to measure in NHL, may be important in the association of advanced disease with defective immunity. However, the bulk of disease or the infiltration of vital sites of B cell development like the bone marrow cannot entirely explain the impairment of humoral immunity. Alterations in "regulatory cells" also do not provide an adequate explanation even though abnormalities of T cell subpopulations have been documented frequently in CLL. The hypogammaglobulinemia is likely to be multifactorial in origin and related to the intrinsic B and T cell defect, progressive replacement of lymphoid tissues, and the defective B cell generation and development.

In myeloma a variety of mechanisms have also been proposed for the pathogenesis of the marked and frequent depression of normal immunoglobulin levels (see Reference 25 for full discussion). The presence of suppressor macrophages/monocytes has been consistently observed[25,130] but other important mechanisms include defective proliferation of antigen responsive cells and the presence of cytotoxic lymphocytes.[131-133] In the murine model of human prolymphocytic leukemia ($BCL_1$ tumor), immunosuppression mediated by phagocytic cells has also been demonstrated but similar cells in CLL or other lymphomas have not been defined.

The aforementioned studies of CLL and MM patients need to be extended to NHL patients. So far the inaccessibility of malignant B cells of nonleukemic NHL has led to lack of functional studies. This difficulty is compounded by the frequency of lymphopenia particularly in high grade NHL patients. However, with improved techniques and the increasing acceptance of bone marrow and lymph node biopsy as essential investigations in NHL patients, the study of blood, BM and nodal lymphocytes should be feasible and rewarding.

In mice the development of B cells in the marrow is a carefully regulated process.[134,135] The BM may also be the most important site of Ig production, and its importance may increase with age (reviewed by Benner et al.[136]). Thus the lymphopenia and the hypogammaglobulinemia of NHL patients may be reflections of the disordered regulatory mechanisms controlling lymphopoiesis and the replacement of bone marrow. It would be important to study not only the function of malignant T and B cells but also the production and function of normal B cells. The importance of functional studies is stressed by the recent studies of patients with hypogammaglobulinemia[137] and NHL patients.[81] In the latter study increased T helper activity was found in spite of normal T cell subpopulations. Could this account for the polyclonal hypergammaglobulinemia observed in many NHL patients? T cell colony assays[138,139] suggest that T cell abnormalities may be present in most NHL patients.

Further studies to evaluate the primary and secondary antibody responses in vivo and in vitro particularly in untreated patients are required and serial studies may be necessary. Some immunological abnormalities may persist for years after the end of treatment as has been shown in ALL patients.[140] In this context, it is interesting that Ballester et al.[141] recently found impaired antibody responses in 6/8 NHL patients in long-term remission.

The relative preservation of humoral and cellular immunity even in advanced follicular lymphoma is intriguing. It has been suggested that follicular lymphomas may be benign rather than malignant tumors of the immune system.[142] The indolent nature of the disease, nondestructive development of follicules confined to B cell areas, absence of cellular atypia, lack of involvement of CNS and other privileged sites have been cited as evidence favoring this hypothesis. Akin to this is the hypothesis proposed by Habeshaw[143] which suggests that follicular lymphomas represent aberrant immune responses to unidentified antigens. Results of immune function of NHL patients reviewed herein would be consistent with this view.

Recent studies of immunocompetence of HD patients[144,145] and ALL patients[146] suggest that immunocompetence is a powerful independent discriminant risk factor. Similar multiparameter studies in histologically well-defined subgroups of NHL patients need to be undertaken. Such studies are likely to provide further insights into the biology of NHL and may even define subgroups of patients at particular risk of developing infections. Vaccination against bacterial antigens may be worthwhile for these patients although similar procedures have yielded disappointing results in myeloma patients.[147]

## VII. CONCLUDING REMARKS

In conclusion, a variety of defects of cellular and humoral immunity occur in non-Hodgkin's lymphomas. These defects are related to the histological subtype and extent of disease but their pathogenesis remains obscure. In some disorders, like CLL, multiple factors seem to be responsible for the humoral dysfunction that may be an intrinsic component of the disease. The hypogammaglobulinemia and defective humoral immune responses may explain the propensity of NHL patients to succumb to bacterial infections. Cellular immunity is affected less often and the impairment noted particularly in advanced high grade lymphoma, in contrast with Hodgkin's disease, is not associated with increased tendency to develop viral infections.

Although the immunological abnormalities do not have a dominant effect on prognosis, response to treatment, or survival, elucidation of the underlying mechanisms has already yielded considerable insight into the biology of some immunoproliferative disorders. Increasing experimental and clinical evidence suggests that tumors of the lymphoid system are subject to immunoregulatory influences and can be exploited as models to define biochemical mechanisms underlying such regulation. Regulatory mechanisms are likely to be important, particularly in low grade NHL which differ markedly from high grade NHL. Hopefully, it may be possible to manipulate the immune system like the endocrine system.

Monoclonal antibodies, anti-idiotypic antibodies, and allogeneic or autologous bone marrow transplantation are increasingly being considered as alternative therapeutic strategies for the treatment of NHL patients.[91,148,149] In the near future, monoclonal antibodies conjugated to toxins or cytotoxics may prove useful.[150] Modulation of the immune response with highly active synthetic peptides may also be possible. Therefore, knowledge of the immunological abnormalities and their pathogenesis is likely to assume greater importance for the successful application of these techniques in the management of NHL patients.

## VIII. ABBREVIATIONS

| | |
|---|---|
| NHL — | Non-Hodgkin's Lymphoma |
| LPD — | Lymphoproliferative Disorders |
| HD — | Hodgkin's disease |
| CLL — | Chronic Lymphocytic Leukemia |
| MM — | Multiple Myeloma |
| WM — | Waldenström's Macroglobulinemia |
| GCC — | Germinal Center Cell |
| DIF — | Direct Immunofluorescence |
| CMI — | Cell-Mediated Immunity |
| DTH — | Delayed Type Hypersensitivity |
| DNCB — | Dinitrophenolchlorobenzene |
| KLH — | Keyhole Limpet Hemocyamin |
| PHA — | Phytohemagglutinin |
| Con A — | Concanavalin A |
| LPS — | Lipopolysaccharide |
| MIF — | Macrophage Inhibitory Factor |
| LIF — | Lymphocyte Inhibitory Factor |
| IL — | Interleukin |
| IFN — | Interferon |
| PPD — | Purified Protein Derivative |
| SpA — | Staphylococcal Protein A |
| PWM — | Pokeweed Mitogen |
| EBV — | Epstein-Barr Virus |
| MLR — | Mixed Lymphocyte Reaction |
| ADCC — | Antibody-Dependent Cell Cytotoxicity |
| NK — | Natural Killer |
| LGL — | Large Granular Lymphocytes |
| PDLL — | Poorly Differentiated Lymphocytic Lymphomas |
| DHL — | Diffuse Histiocytic Lymphoma |
| BM — | Bone Marrow |

## ACKNOWLEDGMENTS

We are grateful to Lisa White for typing the manuscript, Katy Ash for compilation and retrieval of data, and Walter Gregory for his assistance with statistical calculations.

## REFERENCES

1. Lennert, K. and Mohri, N., Histopathology and diagnosis of non-Hodgkin's lymphomas, in *Malignant Lymphomas Other Than Hodgkin's Disease,* 1st ed., Lennert, K., Mohri, N., Stein, H., Kaiserling, E., and Muller-Hermelink, H. K., Eds., Springer-Verlag, Berlin, 1978, 111.
2. Abbas, A. K., Immunologic regulation of lymphoid tumor cells: model systems for lymphocyte function, *Adv. Immunol.,* 32, 301, 1982.
3. Hersh, E. M. and Freireich, E. J., Host defense mechanisms and their modification by cancer chemotherapy, in *Methods of Cancer Research,* Vol. 4, Academic Press, New York, 1968, 355.
4. McCormack, R. T., Nelson, R. D., Bloomfield, C. D., Quie, P. G., and Brunning, R. D., Neutrophil function in lymphoreticular malignancy, *Cancer,* 44, 920, 1979.

5. Cupps, T. R. and Fauci, A. S., Corticosteroid-mediated immunoregulation in man, *Immunol. Rev.,* 65, 133, 1982.
6. Turk, J. L. and Parker, D., Effect of cyclophosphamide on immunological control mechanisms, *Immunol. Rev.,* 65, 99, 1982.
7. Sokal, J. E. and Primikirios, N., The delayed skin test response in Hodgkin's disease and lymphosarcoma. Effect of disease activity, *Cancer,* 14, 597, 1961.
8. Miller, D. G., Patterns of immunological deficiency in lymphomas and leukaemia, *Ann. Intern. Med.,* 57, 703, 1962.
9. Jones, S. E., Griffith, K., Dombrowski, P., and Gaines, J. A., Immunodeficiency in patients with non-Hodgkin's lymphomas, *Blood,* 49, 335, 1977.
10. Lapes, M., Rosenzweig, M., Barbieri, B., Joseph, R. A., and Smalley, R. V., Cellular and humoral immunity in non-Hodgkin's lymphoma, *Am. J. Clin. Pathol.,* 67, 347, 1977.
11. Advani, S. H., Dinshaw, K. A., Nair, C. N., Gopal, R., Talwalkar, G. V., Iyyer, Y. S., Bhatia, H. M., and Desai, P. B., Immune dysfunction in non-Hodgkin's lymphoma, *Cancer,* 45, 2843, 1980.
12. Lichtenstein, A. and Taylor, C. R., Serum immunoglobulin levels in patients with non-Hodgkin's lymphoma, *Am. J. Clin. Pathol.,* 74, 12, 1980.
13. Anderson, T. C., Jones, S. E., Soehnlen, B. J., Moon, T. E., Griffith, K., and Stanley, P., Immunocompetence and malignant lymphoma: immunologic status before therapy, *Cancer,* 48, 2702, 1981.
14. Casazza, A. R., Duvall, C. P., and Carbone, P. P., Infection in lymphoma. Histology, treatment, and duration in relation to incidence and survival, *JAMA,* 197, 710, 1966.
15. Feld, R. and Bodey, G. P., Infections in patients with malignant lymphoma treated with combination chemotherapy, *Cancer,* 39, 1018, 1977.
16. Valdivieso, M., Bacterial infection in haematological diseases, *Clin. Haematol.,* 5, 229, 1976.
17. Ostrow, S., Diggs, C. H., Sutherland, J., and Weirnik, P. H., Causes of death in patients with non-Hodgkin's lymphoma, *Cancer,* 48, 779, 1981.
18. Twomey, J. J., Good, R. A., and Case, D. C., Immunological changes with Hodgkin's disease, in *The Immunopathology of Lymphoreticular Neoplasms,* Twomey, J. J. and Good, R. A., Eds., Plenum, New York, 1978, 585.
19. Gupta, S., Immunodeficiencies in Hodgkin's disease. I. Cell-mediated immunity, *Clin. Bull.* 11, 10, 1981.
20. Gupta, S., Immunodeficiencies in Hodgkin's disease. II. B cell immunity, complement systems and phagocytic cell systems, *Clin. Bull.* 11, 58, 1981.
21. Hansen, J. A., Bloomfield, C. D., Dupont, B., Gajl-Peczalska, K., Kiszkiss, D., and Good, R. A., Lymphocyte subpopulations and immunodeficiency in lymphoproliferative malignancies, in *Proc. 8th Leukocyte Culture Conf.,* Lindahl-Kiessling, K. and Osoba, D., Eds., Academic Press, New York, 1973, 119.
22. Gupta, S. and Good, R. A., Immunodeficiencies associated with chronic lymphocytic leukaemia and non-Hodgkin's lymphomas, in *The Immunopathology of Lymphoreticular Neoplasms,* Twomey, J. J. and Good, R. A., Eds., Plenum, New York, 1978, 565.
23. Rai, K. R. and Sawitsky, A., Studies in clinical staging, lymphocyte function and markers as an approach to the treatment of chronic lymphocytic leukaemia, in *Contemporary Hematology/Oncology,* Vol. 2, Silber, R., Gordon, A. S., LoBue, J., and Muggia, F. M., Eds., Plenum, New York, 1981, 227.
24. Pruzanski, W., Gidon, M. S., and Roy, A., Suppression of polyclonal immunoglobulins in multiple myeloma: relationship to the staging and other manifestations at diagnosis, *Clin. Immunol. Immunopathol.,* 17, 280, 1980.
25. Ullrich, S. and Zolla-Pazner, S., Immunoregulatory circuits in myeloma, *Clin. Haematol.,* 11, 87, 1982.
26. Louie, S., Daoust, P. R., and Schwartz, R. S., Immunodeficiency and the pathogenesis of non-Hodgkin's lymphoma, *Semin. Oncol.,* 7, 267, 1980.
27. Mellstedt, H., Holm, G., Pettersson, D., and Peest, D., Idiotype-bearing lymphoid cells in plasma cell neoplasia, *Clin. Haematol.,* 11, 65, 1982.
28. National Cancer Institute, The non-Hodgkin's lymphoma pathologic classification project National Cancer Institute sponsored study of classifications of non-Hodgkin's lymphomas, *Cancer,* 49, 211, 1982.
29. Siegal, F. P. and Good, R. A., Human lymphocyte differentiation markers and their application to immune deficiency and lymphoproliferative disease, *Clin. Haematol.,* 6, 355, 1977.
30. Stein, H., Gerdes, J., and Mason, D. Y., The normal and malignant germinal centre, *Clin. Haematol.,* 11, 531, 1982.
31. Aisenberg, A. C., Cell surface markers in lymphoproliferative disease, *N. Engl. J. Med.,* 304, 331, 1981.

32. Gajl-Peczalska, K. J., Bloomfield, C. D., Frizzera, G., Kersey, J. H., and LeBein, T. W., Diversity of phenotypes of non-Hodgkin's malignant lymphoma, in B and T Cell Tumors, U.C.L.A. Symp. Mol. Cell. Biol., Vol. 24, Vitetta, E. S., Eds., Academic Press, New York, 1982, 63.
33. Haegert, D. G. and Coombs, R. R. A., Do human B and "null" lymphocytes form a single immunoglobulin-bearing population? Lancet, 2, 1051, 1979.
34. Bloomfield, C. D., Gajl-Peczalska, K. J., and Frizzera, G., Clinical utility of lymphocyte surface markers combined with the Lukes-Collins histologic classification in adult lymphoma, N. Engl. J. Med., 301, 512, 1979.
35. Warnke, R., Miller, R., and Grogan, T., Immunologic phenotype in 30 patients with diffuse large-cell lymphoma, N. Engl. J. Med., 303, 293, 1980.
36. Jaffe, E. S., Braylan, R. C., and Brunning, R. D., et al., Functional markers: a new perspective on malignant lymphomas, Cancer Treat. Rep., 94, 218, 1977.
37. Levy, R., Warnke, R., Dorfman, R. F., and Haimovich, J., The monoclonality of human B cell lymphomas, J. Exp. Med., 145, 1014, 1977.
38. Stein, H., Bonk, A., Tolksdorf, G., Lennert, K., and Geroes, J., Immunohistologic analysis of the organization of normal lymphoid tissue and non-Hodgkin's lymphomas, J. Histochem. Cytochem., 28, 746, 1980.
39. Failkow, P. J., Najfeld, V., Reddy, A. L., Singer, J., and Steinmann, L., Chronic lymphocytic leukaemia: clonal origin in a committed B lymphocyte progenitor, Lancet, 2, 444, 1978.
40. Janossy, G., Thomas, J. A., Pizzolo, G., Granger, S. M., McLaughlin, J., Habeshaw, J. A., Stansfeld, A. G., and Sloane, J., Immuno-histological diagnosis of lymphoproliferative diseases by selected combinations of antisera and monoclonal antibodies, Br. J. Cancer, 42, 224, 1980.
41. Godal, T. and Funderud, S., Human B cell neoplasms in relation to normal B cell differentiation and maturation processes, Adv. Cancer Res., 36, 221, 1982.
42. Salmon, S. E. and Seligman, M., B cell neoplasia in man, Lancet, 2, 1230, 1974.
43. Micklem, H. S., B lymphocytes, T lymphocytes and lymphopoiesis, Clin. Haematol., 8, 395, 1979.
44. Waldman, T. A. and Strober, W., Metabolism of immunoglobulins, Clin. Immunobiol., 3, 71, 1976.
45. Solomon, A., Current developments in immunoglobulins, in Contemporary Hematology/Oncology, Vol. 2, Silber, R., Gordon, A. S., LoBue, J., and Muggia, F. M., Eds., Plenum, New York, 1981, 399.
46. Buckley, C. E. and Dorsey, F. C., The effect of aging on human serum immunoglobulin concentrations, J. Immunol., 105, 964, 1970.
47. Hansen, J. A., and Martin, P. L., Human T cell differentiation antigens, in Mitchell, M. S. and Oettgen H. F., Eds., Raven Press, New York, 1982, 75.
48. Janossy, G. and Prentice, H. G., T cell subpopulations, monoclonal antibodies and their therapeutic applications, Clin. Haematol., 11, 631, 1982.
49. Matutes, E., Wechsler, A., Gomez, R., Cherchi, M., and Catovsky, D., Unusual T cell phenotype in advanced B chronic lymphocytic leukaemia, Br. J. Haematol., 49, 635, 1981.
50. Mills, K. H. G., Worman, C. P., and Cawley, J. C., T cell subsets in B chronic lymphocytic leukaemia (CLL), Br. J. Haematol., 50, 710, 1982.
51. Herrmann, F., Lochner, A., Philippen, H., Jauer, B., and Ruhl, H., Imbalance of T cell subpopulations in patients with chronic lymphocytic leukaemia of the B cell type, Clin. Exp. Immunol., 49, 157, 1982.
52. Kumagai, K., Abo, T., Sekizawa, T., and Sasaki, M., Studies of surface immunoglobulins on human B lymphocytes. I. Dissociation of cell-bound immunoglobulins with acid pH or at 37°C, J. Immunol., 115, 982, 1975.
53. Winchester, R. J. and Fu, S. M., Lymphocyte surface membrane immunoglobulin, Scand. J. Immunol., 5 (Suppl. 5), 77, 1976.
54. Pettersson, D., Mellstedt, H., and Holm, G., IgG on human blood lymphocytes studied by immunofluorescence, Scand. J. Immunol., 8, 535, 1978.
55. Dighiero, G., Bodega, E., Mayzner, R., and Binet, J. L., Two new applications of the immunoperoxidase method: cell-by-cell quantitation of surface immunoglobulins and automated recognition of B-lymphocytes, Blood Cells, 6, 371, 1980.
56. Ross, G. D. and Polley, M. J., Specificity of human lymphocyte complement receptors, J. Exp. Med., 141, 1163, 1975.
57. Dickler, H. B., Studies of human lymphocyte receptor for heat-aggregated or antigen complexed immunoglobulin, J. Exp. Med., 140, 508, 1974.
58. Forbes, I. J., Zalewski, P. D., Valente, L., and Gee, D., Two maturation-associated mouse erythrocyte receptors of human B cells. I. Identification of four human B-cell subsets, Clin. Exp. Immunol., 47, 396, 1982.
59. McKenzie, I. F. C. and Zola, H., Monoclonal antibodies to B cells, Immunol. Today, 4, 10, 1983.
60. Ling, N. R. and MacLennan, I. C. M., Analysis of lymphocytes in blood and tissues, in Techniques in Clinical Immunology, 2nd ed., Thompson, R. A., Ed., Blackwell Scientific, Oxford, 1981, 222.

61. Hamblin, A. S. and Maini, R. N., An evaluation of lymphokine measurement in man, *Recent Adv. Clin. Immunol.*, 2, 243, 1980.
62. Altman, A. and Katz, D. H., The biology of monoclonal lymphokines secreted by T cell lines and hybridomas, *Adv. Immunol.*, 33, 73, 1982.
63. Waldman, T. A. and Broder, S., Polyclonal B cell activators in the study of the regulation of immunoglobulin synthesis in the human system, *Adv. Immunol.*, 32, 1, 1982.
64. Ault, K. A. and Towle, M., Human B lymphocyte subsets. I. IgG-bearing B cell responses to pokeweed mitogen, *J. Exp. Med.*, 153, 339, 1981.
65. Lucivero, G., Lawton, R. A., and Cooper, M. D., Rosette formation with mouse erythrocytes defines a population of human B lymphocytes unresponsive to pokeweed mitogen, *Clin. Exp. Immunol.*, 45, 185, 1981.
66. Bird, A. G. and Britton, S., A new approach to the study of human B lymphocyte function using an indirect plaque assay and a direct B cell activator, *Immunol. Rev.*, 45, 41, 1979.
67. DuPont, B., Hansen, J. A., and Yunis, E. J., Human mixed-lymphocyte culture reaction: genetics, specificity and biological implications, *Adv. Immunol.*, 23, 108, 1976.
68. Revillard, J. P., Samarut, C., Cordier, G., and Brochier, J., Characterization of human lymphocytes bearing Fc receptors with special reference to cytotoxic (K) cells, in *Inserm Symposium I*, Seligman, M., Preud'homme, J-L., and Kourilsky, F. M., Eds., American-Elsevier, New York, 1975, 171.
69. Herberman, R. B., Djeu, J. Y., Kay, H. D., Ortaldo, J. R., Riccardi, G. D., Bonnard, H. T., Fagnani, R., Santoni, A., and Puccetti, P., Natural killer cells: characteristics and regulation of activity, *Immunol. Rev.*, 44, 43, 1979.
70. Roder, J. C. and Pross, H. F., The biology of the human natural killer cell, *J. Clin. Immunol.*, 2, 249, 1982.
71. Wiseman, B. K., The blood pictures in the primary disease of the lymphatic system, *JAMA*, 107, 2016, 1936.
72. Opat, R., Kolar, V., Lauerova, L., Pintera, J., and Zemanova, D., Humoral and cellular immunity in long-term surviving patients with malignant lymphoma, *Neoplasma*, 27, 301, 1980.
73. Cader, A., Richardson, P., Walsh, L., Ling, N. R., MacLennan, I. C. M., Jones, E. L., and Leyland, M., The incidence of B cell leukaemia and lymphopenia in B cell neoplasia in adults, in press.
74. Lamb, D., Pilney, F., Kelly, W. D., and Good, R. A., A comparative study of the incidence of anergy in patients with carcinoma, leukaemia, Hodgkin's disease and other lymphomas, *J. Immunol.*, 89, 555, 1962.
75. Hersh, E. M., Curtis, J. E., Harris, J. E., McBride, C., Alexanian, R., and Rossen, R., Host defense mechanisms in lymphoma and leukaemia, in *Leukaemia-Lymphoma*, Year Book Medical Publishers, Chicago, 1970, 149.
76. Catovsky, D., Holt, P. J. L., and Galton, D. A. G., Lymphocyte transformation in immunoproliferative disorders, *Br. J. Cancer*, 26, 154, 1972.
77. Ruhl, H., Vogt, W., Bochert, G., Schmidt, S., Moelle, R., and Schaqua, H., Mixed lymphocyte culture stimulatory and responding capacity of lymphocytes with lymphoproliferative diseases, *Clin. Exp. Immunol.*, 19, 55, 1976.
78. Whisler, R. L., Balcerzak, S. P., and Murray, J. L., Heterogeneous mechanisms of impaired lymphocyte responses in non-Hodgkin's lymphoma, *Blood*, 57, 1081, 1981.
79. Farrant, J. and Knight, S. C., Help and suppression by lymphoid cells as a function of cellular concentration, *Proc. Natl. Acad. Sci. U.S.A.*, 76, 3507, 1979.
80. Aisenberg, A. C. and Long, J. C., Lymphocyte surface characteristics in malignant lymphoma, *Am. J. Med.*, 58, 300, 1975.
81. Gajl-Peczalska, K. J., Chartrand, S. L., and Bloomfield, C. D., Abnormal immunoregulation in patients with non-Hodgkin's malignant lymphomas. I. Increased helper function of peripheral T lymphocytes, *Clin. Immunol. Immunopathol.*, 23, 366, 1982.
82. Alexanian, R., Monoclonal gammopathy in lymphoma, *Arch. Intern. Med.*, 135, 62, 1974.
83. Leonard, R. C. F., MacLennan, I. C. M., Smart, Y., Vanhegan, R. I., and Cuzick, J., Light chain isotype-associated suppression of normal plasma cell numbers in patients with multiple myeloma, *Int. J. Cancer*, 24, 385, 1979.
84. Rosset, G., Farquet, J-J., and Gruchaud, A., The serum immunoglobulins in lymphoproliferative malignancies, *Eur. J. Cancer*, 14, 369, 1978.
85. Galton, D. A. G. and MacLennan, I. C. M., Clinical patterns in B lymphoid malignancy, *Clin. Haematol.*, 11, 561, 1982.
86. Amlot, P. L. and Green, L., Serum immunoglobulins G,A,M,D, and E concentrations in lymphomas, *Br. J. Cancer*, 40, 371, 1979.
87. Sbarra, A. J., Shirley, W., Selvarji, R. J., Ouchie, E., and Rosenbaum, E., The role of the phagocyte in host-parasite interactions. I. The phagocytic capabilities of leucocytes from lymphoproliferative disease, *Cancer Res.*, 24, 1958, 1964.

88. Groch, G. S., Oerillis, P. E., and Finch, S. C., Reticuloendothelial phagocytic function in patients with leukaemia, lymphoma and multiple myeloma, *Blood*, 26, 489, 1965.
89. Sokol, R. J., Durrant, T. E., and Hudson, G., Skin window cellularity and macrophage changes in Hodgkin's and non-Hodgkin's lymphomas, *Acta Haematol.*, 64, 209, 1980.
90. Fu, S. M., Winchester, R. J., Feizi, T., Walzer, P. D., and Kunkel, H. G., Idiotypic specificity of surface immunoglobulin and the maturation of leukaemic bone marrow derived lymphocytes, *Proc. Natl. Acad. Sci. U.S.A.*, 71, 4487, 1974.
91. Stevenson, F. K., Hamblin, T. J., Tutt, A. L., and Stevenson, G. T., Idiotypic immunoglobulin production by human neoplastic B lymphocytes: its use in monitoring chemotherapy and immunotherapy, in *B and T Cell Tumors*, U.C.L.A. Symp. Mol. Cell. Biol., Vol. 24, Vitetta, E. S., Ed., Academic Press, New York, 1982, 507.
92. Chiorazzi, N., Fu, S. M., Montazeri, G., Kunkel, H. G., Rai, K., and Gee, T., T cell helper defect in patients with chronic lymphocytic leukaemia, *J. Immunol.*, 122, 1087, 1979.
93. Dhaliwal, H. S., Ling, N. R., Bishop, S., and Chapel. H., Expression of immunoglobulin G on blood lymphocytes in chronic lymphocytic leukaemia, *Clin. Exp. Immunol.*, 31, 226, 1978.
94. Burns, G. F., Cawley, J. C., Worman, C. P., Karpas, A., Barker, C. R., Coldstone, A. H., and Hayhoe, F. G. J., Multiple heavy chain isotypes on the surface of the cells of hairy-cell leukaemia, *Blood*, 52, 1132, 1978.
95. Dameshek, W., Chronic lymphocytic leukaemia — an accumulative disease of immunoglobically incompetent lymphocytes, *Blood*, 29, 566, 1967.
96. Robert, K.-H., Induction of monoclonal antibody synthesis in malignant human B cells by polyclonal B cell activators, *Immunol. Rev.*, 48, 123, 1979.
97. Catovsky, D., Lauria, F., Matutes, E., Foa, R., Mantovani, V., Tura, S., and Galton, D. A. G., Increase in T gamma lymphocytes in B cell chronic lymphocytic leukaemia. II. Correlation with clinical stage and findings in B prolymphocytic leukaemia, *Br. J. Haematol.*, 47, 539, 1981.
98. Maino, V. C., Kurnick, J. T., Kubo, T., and Grey, M., Mitogen activation of human chronic lymphatic leukaemia cells, *J. Immunol.*, 118, 742, 1977.
99. Cone, L. and Uhr, J. W., Immunological deficiency disorders associated with chronic lymphocytic leukaemia and multiple myeloma, *J. Clin. Invest.*, 43, 2241, 1964.
100. Block, J. B., Haynes, H. A., Thompson, W. L., and Neiman, P. E., Delayed hypersensitivity in chronic lymphocytic leukaemia, *J. Natl. Cancer Inst.*, 42, 973, 1969.
101. Wybran, J., Chantler, S., and Fudenberg, H. H., Isolation of normal T cells in chronic lymphatic leukaemia, *Lancet*, 1, 126, 1973.
102. Foa, R., Catovsky, D., Lauria, F., Zafar, M. N., and Galton, D. A. G., T lymphocytes in B cell chronic lymphocytic leukaemia, *Haematologica*, 66, 105, 1981.
103. Callery, R. T., Strelkauskas, A. J., Yanovich, S., Marks, S., Rosenthal, O., and Schlossman, S. F., Functional abnormalities associated with T-lymphocytes from patients with chronic lymphocytic leukaemia, *Clin. Immunol. Immunopathol.*, 17, 451, 1980.
104. Smith, M. J., Browne, E., and Slungaard, A., The impaired responsiveness of chronic lymphatic leukaemia (CLL) lymphocytes to allogeneic lymphocytes, *Blood*, 41, 505, 1973.
105. Pentycross, C. R., Chronic lymphocytic leukaemia and the mixed lymphocyte reaction, *Lymphology*, 7, 7, 1974.
106. Kasakura, S., MLC stimulatory capacity and production of blastogenic factor in patients with chronic lymphatic leukaemia and Hodgkin's disease, *Blood*, 45, 833, 1975.
107. Wolos, J. A. and Davey, F. R., Depressed stimulation in the MLR by B lymphocytes in chronic lymphocytic leukaemia: failure to demonstrate a suppressor cell, *Clin. Immunol. Immunopathol.*, 14, 77, 1979.
108. Halper, J. R., Fu, S. M., Gottilieb, A. B., Winchester, R. J., and Kunkel, H. G., Poor mixed lymphocyte reaction stimulatory capacity of leukaemic B cells of chronic lymphocytic leukaemia patients despite the presence of Ia antigens, *J. Clin. Invest.*, 64, 1141, 1979.
109. Howell, K. M., Failure of antibody formation in leukaemia, *Arch. Intern. Med.*, 26, 706, 1920.
110. Barr, M. and Fairley, G. H., Circulating antibodies in reticuloses, *Lancet*, 1, 1305, 1961.
111. Heath, R. B., Fairley, G. H., and Malpas, J. S., Production of antibodies against viruses in leukaemia and related diseases, *Br. J. Haematol.*, 10, 365, 1964.
112. Hamblin, T. J., Verrier-Jones, J., and Peacock, D. B., The immune response to 0174 in man. IV. Primary and secondary antibody production in patients with chronic lymphatic leukaemia, *Clin. Exp. Immunol.*, 21, 101, 1975.
113. Jim, R. T. S. and Reinhard, E. H., Agammaglobulinemia and chronic lymphocytic leukaemia, *Ann. Intern. Med.*, 44, 790, 1956.
114. Leoncini, D., Forni, A., Korngold, L., and Miller, D. G., A comparison of paper electrophoretic and immunoelectrophoretic studies of serum proteins of patients with lymphomas and leukaemias, *Oncology*, 22, 81, 1968.

115. Fiddes, P., Penney, R., and Wells, J. Z., Clinical correlations with immunoglobulin levels in chronic lymphatic leukaemia, *Aust. N.Z. J. Med.,* 4, 346, 1972.
116. Foa, R., Catovsky, D., Brozovic, M., Marsh, G., Ooyirilangkumaran, T., Cherchi, M., and Galton, D. A. G., Clinical staging and immunological findings in chronic lymphocytic leukaemia, *Cancer,* 44, 483, 1979.
117. Dhaliwal, H. S., Cell Surface Markers in Chronic Lymphatic Leukaemia, M.D. thesis, 1983.
118. Shaw, R. K., Szwed, C., Boggs, D. R., Fahey, J. L., Frei, E., III, Morrison, E., and Utz, J. P., Infection and immunity in chronic lymphocytic leukaemia, *Arch. Intern. Med.,* 57, 703, 1960.
119. Miller, D. G. and Karnofsky, D. A., Immunologic factors and resistance to infection in chronic lymphatic leukaemia, *Am. J. Med.,* 3, 748, 1961.
120. Hansen, M. M., Chronic lymphocytic leukaemia: clinical studies based on 189 cases followed for a long time, *Scand. J. Haematol.,* 18, 1, 1973.
121. Ben-Bassat, I., Many, A., Modan, M., Peretz, C., and Ramot, B., Serum immunoglobulins in chronic lymphocytic leukaemia, *Am. J. Med. Sci.,* 278, 4, 1979.
122. Jayaswal, U., Roath, S., Hyde, R. S., Chisholm, D. M., and Smith, J. L., Blood lymphocyte surface markers and clinical findings in chronic lymphoproliferative disorders, *Br. J. Haematol.,* 37, 207, 1977.
123. Phillips, E. A., Kempin, S., Passe, S., Mike, V., and Clarkson, B., Prognostic factors in chronic lymphocytic leukaemia and their implications for therapy, *Clin. Haematol.,* 6, 203, 1977.
124. Chandra, R. K., Immunocompetence as a functional index of nutritional status, *Br. Med. Bull.,* 37, 89, 1981.
125. Butler, W. T. and Rossen, R. D., Effects of corticosteroids on immunity in man, *J. Clin. Invest.,* 52, 2629, 1973.
126. Johnstone, A. P., Chronic lymphocytic leukaemia and its relationship to normal B lymphopoiesis, *Immunol. Today,* 3, 343, 1982.
127. Hersey, P., Wotherspoon, J., Reid, G., and Gunz, F. W., Hypogammaglobulinaemia associated with abnormalities of both B and T lymphocytes in patients with chronic lymphatic leukaemia, *Clin. Exp. Immunol.,* 39, 698, 1980.
128. Parrott, D. M., Lymphocyte locomotion. The role of chemokinesis and chemotaxis, *Monogr. Allergy.,* 16, 173, 1980.
129. de Sousa, M., Ecotaxis, ecotaxopathy, and lymphoid malignancy: terms, facts, and predictions, in *The Immunopathology of Lymphoreticular Neoplasms,* Twomey, J. J. and Good, R. A., Eds., Plenum Press, New York, 1978, 325.
130. Broder, S., Humphrey, R., Durm, M., Blackman, M., Meade, B., Goldman, C., Strober, W., and Waldmann, T., Impaired synthesis of polyclonal (non-paraprotein) immunoglobulin by circulating lymphocytes from patients with multiple myeloma: role of suppressor cells, *N. Engl. J. Med.,* 293, 887, 1975.
131. Paglieroni, T. and McKenzie, M. R., Studies on the pathogenesis of an immune defect in multiple myeloma, *J. Clin. Invest.,* 59, 1120, 1977.
132. Paglieroni, T. and MacKenzie, M. R., In vitro cytotoxic response to human myeloma plasma cells by peripheral blood leucocytes from patients with multiple myeloma and benign monoclonal gammopathy, *Blood,* 54, 226, 1979.
133. Paglieroni, T. and McKenzie, M. R., Multiple myeloma: an immunologic profile. III. Cytotoxic and suppressive effects of the EA rosette-forming cell, *J. Immunol.,* 124, 2563, 1980.
134. Osmond, D. G., Fahlman, M. T. E., Fulop, G. M., and Rahal, D. M., Regulation and localisation of lymphocyte production in the bone marrow, in microenvironments, in *Haemopoietic and Lymphoid Differentiation, Ciba Foundation Symp.,* Vol. 84, Pitman, London, 1981, 68.
135. Landreth, K. S., Kincade, P. W., and Lee, G., Relationship between phenotypically and functionally defined precursors of B lymphocytes, *Fed. Proc. Fed. Am. Soc. Exp. Biol.,* 40, 4990, 1981.
136. Benner, R., Hijmans, W., and Haaijman, J. J., The bone marrow: the major source of serum immunoglobulins, but still a neglected site of antibody formation, *Clin. Exp. Immunol.,* 46, 1, 1981.
137. Pereira, R. S. and Platts-Mills, T. A. E., Lymphocyte subsets in hypogammaglobulinaemia, *Clin. Haematol.,* 11, 589, 1982.
138. Sutherland, D. C., Dalton, G., and Wilson, J. D., T-lymphocyte colonies in malignant disease, *Lancet,* 2, 1113, 1976.
139. Nogueira Costa, R., Davis, F., Kusyk, C., Verma, D. S., and Spitzer, G., E-rosette forming cell colonies (ERFC-C) with malignant markers in B cell neoplasms and myeloid leukaemia, *A. A. C. R. Abstr.,* 103, 1982.
140. Layward, L., Levinsky, R. J., and Butler, M., Long-term abnormalities in T and B lymphocyte function in children following treatment for acute lymphoblastic leukaemia, *Br. J. Haematol.,* 49, 251, 1981.

141. Ballester, O. F., Shurafa, M., Toben, H., Kumar, K. S., and Burek, C. L., Impaired antibody responses to a pneumonial polysaccharide vaccine in patients with non-Hodgkin's lymphoma in remission, *J. Clin. Immunol.*, 1, 90, 1981.
142. Jaffe, E. S., Hypothesis: follicular lymphomas — are they benign tumours of the lymphoid system?, in *B and T Cell Tumors, U.C.L.A. Symp. Mol. Cell. Biol.*, Vol. 24, Vitetta, E. S., Ed., Academic Press, New York, 1982, 91.
143. Habeshaw, J. A., Catley, P. F., Stansfeld, A. G., and Brearley, R., Surface phenotyping, histology and the nature of non-Hodgkin's lymphoma in 157 patients, *Br. J. Cancer,* 40, 11, 1979.
144. Faguet, G. B. and Davis, H. C., Survival in Hodgkin's disease: the role of immunocompetence and other major risk factors, *Blood,* 59, 938, 1982.
145. Bjorkholm, M., Wedelin, C., Ogenstad, S., Johansson, B., and Mellstedt, H., Immune status of untreated patients with Hodgkin's disease and prognosis, *Cancer Treat. Rep.,* 66, 701, 1982.
146. Leikin, S., Miller, D., Sather, H., Albo, V., Esber, E., Johnson, A., Rogentine, N., and Hammond, D., Immunologic evaluation in the prognosis of acute lymphoblastic leukaemia. A report from Children's Cancer Study Group, *Blood,* 58, 501, 1981.
147. Lazarus, H. M., Lederman, M., Lubin, A., Herzig, R. H., Schiffman, G., Jones, P., Wine A., and Rodman, H. M., Pneumococcal vaccination: the response of patients with multiple myeloma, *Am. J. Med.,* 69, 419, 1980.
148. Miller, R. A., Maloney, D. G., Warnke, R., and Levy, R., Treatment of a B cell lymphoma with monoclonal anti-idiotype antibody, *N. Engl. J. Med.,* 306, 517, 1982.
149. Nadler, M., Stashenko, P., Hardy, R., Kaplan, W. D., Button, L. N., Kufe, D. W., Antman, K. H., and Schlossman, S. F., Serotherapy of a patient with a monoclonal antibody directed against a human lymphoma-associated antigen, *Cancer Res.,* 40, 3147, 1980.
150. Vitetta, E. S., Krolick, K. A., and Uhr, J. W., Neoplastic B cells as targets for antibody-ricin A chain immunotoxins, *Immunol. Rev.,* 62, 159, 1982.
151. Walker, L., personal communication.

Chapter 5

# CLINICAL UTILITY OF MONOCLONAL ANTIBODIES

John M. Pesando

## TABLE OF CONTENTS

| | | |
|---|---|---|
| I. | Introduction | 108 |
| II. | Production of Polyclonal and Monoclonal Antibodies | 108 |
| III. | Advantages and Disadvantages of Monoclonal Antisera | 110 |
| IV. | Diagnostic Applications of Serologic Reagents | 113 |
| | A. Acute Leukemias | 113 |
| | B. Lymphomas | 114 |
| V. | Etiology of Cancer | 115 |
| | A. Clonal Origin | 115 |
| | B. Tumor-Specific Antigens | 116 |
| VI. | Therapeutic Applications | 117 |
| | A. Serotherapy | 117 |
| | B. Autologous Transplantation | 120 |
| | C. Drug-Antibody Conjugates | 121 |
| VII. | Concluding Remarks | 121 |
| Acknowledgments | | 122 |
| References | | 122 |

## I. INTRODUCTION

Application of the technique of somatic cell hybridization for the production of monoclonal antisera is one of the most active areas of research in medicine. In addition to replacing conventional antisera with relatively pure, inexpensive, and well-characterized reagents, monoclonal antisera have proven to be extremely useful for the previously difficult study of the surfaces of both normal and malignant cells. As a result, a voluminous literature based on the use of monoclonal antisera to phenotype cell types has already emerged. However, despite the power of the technique, the clinical impact of the use of monoclonal antisera for the study and treatment of hematologic diseases remains limited. The purpose of this chapter will be to introduce the reader to the subject of monoclonal antisera and to provide an overview of those applications of this methodology most relevant to the diagnosis and therapy of the lymphomas. The goal of this approach is to facilitate independent evaluation of current and future clinical applications of these reagents. For more comprehensive discussions of these subjects, the reader is referred to specialized reviews.[1-8]

## II. PRODUCTION OF POLYCLONAL AND MONOCLONAL ANTIBODIES

The differences between monoclonal and conventional or polyclonal antisera are best understood by reviewing the process of antibody production at the cellular level. While all antibody-producing or B lymphocytes derive from common precursor cells, each individual B cell develops the capacity to produce a unique antibody through the processes of somatic DNA recombination of the common gene pool and of selective RNA transcription and splicing.[9,10] Each antibody molecule contains a constant region which is shared with other antibody molecules and a unique antigen-binding or variable region. As they develop, B lymphocytes express their unique antibodies on the cell surface. The antigen-binding portions of these different immunoglobulins are capable of specifically binding small molecules or portions of large molecules. That portion of a three-dimensional molecule which is recognized by a specific antibody is called an antigenic determinant or epitope, and a large molecule serving as an antigen may have hundreds or even thousands of epitopes (although the capacity of these different epitopes to elicit an antibody response may vary greatly).[11] When a foreign molecule or antigen binds to the antigen-binding site of the immunoglobulin molecule of a particular B lymphocyte, that cell proliferates and differentiates to produce a clone of immunoglobulin-secreting plasma cells. In addition, some of the initial B lymphocytes remain as effectively nonsecretory, surface immunoglobulin-positive memory cells. Each plasma cell of the clone produces identical immunoglobulin molecules, and each of these antibodies binds specifically to that epitope of the original antigen that triggered the clonal proliferation. Thus, only those B lymphocytes whose surface antibodies are fortuitously capable of binding to the epitopes of a particular antigen to which the animal has been exposed are induced to secrete antibody. The number of antibody-producing cells formed, and hence the number of antibodies produced and the titer of serologic response, is carefully controlled by the immune system of the immunized animal.

When an animal is immunized, it produces a polyclonal or conventional antiserum. In response to the epitopes of the immunizing material, hundreds or even thousands of B lymphocytes are clonally selected to proliferate and differentiate in order to secrete biologically useful amounts of specific antibodies. Each of these B cells makes antibody molecules capable of binding to a single epitope of the immunogen. The serum of the animal thus contains hundreds or thousands of different antibodies, of different avidities and immunoglobulin subtypes. In contrast, a monoclonal antiserum is made up of the immunoglobulin molecules produced by the progeny of the clonal expansion of but a single B cell. As a result, all antibodies produced bind to the same epitope, and all have the same avidity and immunoglobulin subtype. This type of antiserum is not normally produced in nature, and it has only recently become possible to produce it in the laboratory.

The expansion of a single clone of B lymphocytes, and the increased production of the immunoglobulin molecules they make, is achieved through the technique of somatic cell hybridization, as embodied in the hybridoma method for the production of monoclonal antibodies as first described by Köhler and Milstein [12,13] and modified by Kennett.[7,14,15] In this method B lymphocytes from the spleen of an immunized mouse are fused with cells from a mouse plasma cell line in the presence of polyethylene glycol to produce a hybridoma (Sendai virus is also used as a fusing agent but is less popular then polyethylene glycol).[4,12-17] Each hybrid cell is then cultured separately, leading to the generation of a large number of identical cells producing the specific immunoglobulin encoded by an original B lymphocyte of the mouse spleen. Each hybridoma resembles both of its parents. It shares with the parental B cell the capacity to produce immunoglobulin specific for an epitope contained on the material used for immunization. At the same time it shares with its parental myeloma or plasma cell the capacity to proliferate indefinitely in tissue culture and to secrete large amounts of immunoglobulin. The result is an immortal cell line producing large quantities of antibody of predetermined specificity. Since this cell line grows continuously in culture and is tumorigenic in syngeneic mice, it is not governed by normal immune control mechanisms which regulate the total amount of antibody produced.

After the initial cell fusion, normal nonfused B cells from the mouse spleen will fail to replicate in tissue culture and will eventually all die. To prevent overgrowth of cultures by plasma cells from the parent myeloma cell line, myeloma cell lines have been developed which can be selectively killed by certain cytotoxins.[4-18] Specifically, a mutant myeloma cell line has been developed which lacks the enzyme (hypoxanthine-guanine phosphoribosyltransferase) necessary to convert hypoxanthine to DNA precursors using the so-called alternate or salvage pathway. In the presence of aminopterin, which blocks the endogenous synthesis of purines and pyrimidines (the DNA precursors), a cell must use the salvage pathway or die. Normal splenic B cells are capable of using the salvage pathway and of growing in media containing aminopterin (and usually supplemented with hypoxanthine and thymidine), as are the cell hybrids, but cells of the mutant plasma cell line cannot. As a result, the only cells capable of growing in this HAT (hypoxanthine-aminopterin-thymidine) medium will be the cell hybrids or hybridomas.

In a typical cell fusion experiment, it is possible to produce hundreds of hybrid cell lines from a single mouse spleen, and these hybrid cell lines reflect a cross section of the immunologic repertoire of the splenic B lymphocytes of that animal. Many of the B cells, and hence the cell hybrids, will recognize epitopes or binding sites on the material used for immunization, but many will not, presumably because their immune functions pertain to the day-to-day activities of protecting the mouse from its environment or because they as yet serve no specific immune function. Since the cell fusion process is apparently more efficient for cells undergoing clonal expansion[19,20] more hybrids specific for the immunizing material are obtained than would be predicted from studies on the simple hybridization frequency of unfractionated spleen cells. This unexpected finding greatly increases the power of the cell fusion method by reducing the number of hybrids that must be screened in order to find one producing antibody of interest.

Following the cell fusion process, the mixture of normal B lymphocytes, plasma cells, and fused cells is typically aliquoted into a 96-well plate containing the selecting HAT media. After 2 to 3 weeks, cell colonies are seen in many of the wells, and supernatants from these wells can be tested for the production of mouse immunoglobulin specific for the materials used for immunization and of interest to the investigator. Those wells containing clones of interest are expanded and subcloned to ensure that they contain but a single clone of cells.

## III. ADVANTAGES AND DISADVANTAGES OF MONOCLONAL ANTISERA

The advantages of monoclonal antisera over conventional polyclonal antisera are many. The antibodies produced by these permanent hybridoma cell lines constitute a homogeneous population of immunoglobulin molecules that can be well defined chemically. The epitopes and/or antigens which they recognize can also be carefully studied. Virtually unlimited supplies of these high-titered antibodies can be inexpensively produced, making it possible for all investigators to work with standardized reagents. In addition, it is now possible to perform experiments where an excess of antibody over antigen is desired, as in the quantitative and/or serial extraction of molecules from a mixed population.[21,22] In contrast, conventional antisera, particularly those directed to cell surface antigens, are low in titer, often poorly characterized, and of limited availability.

Monoclonal antibodies are ideally suited for the study of new and/or impure antigens. In the past, molecular species have been isolated and studied only after some of their properties, usually functional, were known. Such knowledge not only made the molecules worth investigating but also provided the basis for assays used to monitor their purification. Since each monoclonal antibody recognizes a single epitope and frequently but a single antigen, they can be used to affinity-purify the antigen(s) bearing a particular epitope using the immune precipitation method. A molecule can therefore now be identified and purified without any knowledge of its function, by first preparing a monoclonal antibody specific for it. Use of monoclonal antibodies in this fashion has virtually revolutionized the study of cell surfaces, leading to the identification of a host of new molecules with monoclonal antisera raised to whole and frequently mixed cell populations. The function of at least some of these molecules may be determined following their isolation and chemical characterization.[23-26] In contrast, unless pure material is used for immunization, extensive absorption procedures are required to make a polyclonal antiserum even relatively specific for a given antigen since the immunized animal will produce antibodies to all antigens presented to it (Figure 1).[27-29]

Less obvious are the limitations of monoclonal antibodies. Chief among these is that a monoclonal antibody recognizes an epitope, rather than an antigen. The latter may be composed of hundreds or even thousands of epitopes. When a monoclonal antibody binds to two different samples, it may be recognizing identical antigens (molecules) or merely identical epitopes, since identical epitopes can be shared by unrelated macromolecules (Figure 2). This limitation may be particularly relevant to the study of cell surface proteins, since the majority of these appear to be glycoproteins often having highly antigenic and frequently common antigenic structures.[30,31] Confirmation of identity or near identity of the antigens being detected would have to be determined biochemically, beginning with a molecular weight determination.

In practice, binding of a monoclonal antibody to two different cell populations has usually meant that those cells express identical or closely related antigens. However,

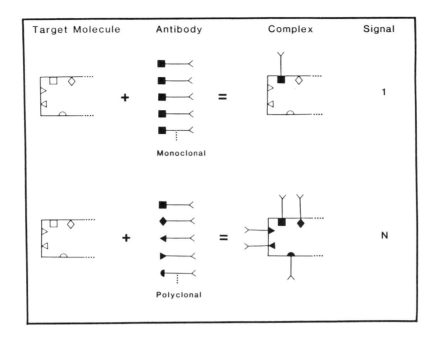

FIGURE 1. Use of monoclonal antibodies to study impure antigens. An animal immunized with a lymphoma cell will make antibodies to many of the epitopes (antigenic determinants) on the multiple antigens to which it has been exposed. The resulting polyclonal antiserum will therefore not be specific for individual surface molecules. The somatic cell hybridization technique for the production of monoclonal antibodies permits the effective purification and clonal expansion of those individual B lymphocytes whose antibodies contribute to the polyclonal antiserum. Since the daughter cells of a single B lymphocyte all make the same antibody, the antiserum so produced is specific for a single epitope (and frequently a single antigen). This figure compares the specificities of monoclonal and polyclonal antisera raised to the same target molecule or cell. While the monoclonal antibody recognizes but a single component, the polyclonal one recognizes many.

there are several reports of a single monoclonal antibody recognizing two distinct antigens. For example, a monoclonal antibody recognizing a fucose-containing carbohydrate structure has been reported to identify antigens having markedly different molecular weights on two neuroblastoma cell lines.[32] In addition, Garson and co-workers[33] have reported that two monoclonal antibodies which identify an antigen on human T cells react exclusively with Purkinje cells in the vertebrate central nervous system. Since the antigen recognized on T cells is on the cell surface, while that recognized in Purkinje cells resides within the cytoplasm, this appears to be another example of unrelated molecules which share a common antigenic determinant. A similar cross reactivity between the Thy-1 antigen and a component of intermediate filaments detected by a monoclonal antibody has been reported by Dulbecco and co-workers.[34] Cross reactivities with unrelated cytoskeletal proteins have been observed with monoclonal antibodies directed to defined epitopes of a synthetic peptide.[35]

A second potential disadvantage of monoclonal antibodies is that all of the antibodies produced by a given hybridoma have the same avidity or binding constant. Depending on the test conditions, low avidity antibodies could present problems. In contrast, a polyclonal antiserum to a particular antigen will be comprised of a mixture of high and low avidity antibodies derived from different cell populations. In addition there have been reports that the ability of some monoclonal antibodies to bind to their spe-

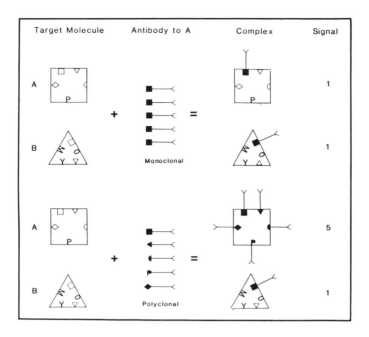

FIGURE 2. Specificity of monoclonal antibodies. A monoclonal antiserum may be less specific than a polyclonal one raised to a pure antigen since individual antibodies recognize antigenic determinants rather than antigens. A large molecule serving as an antigen may have many antigenic determinants or antibody binding sites, some of which may not be unique to that molecule. The exquisite specificity of many polyclonal antisera for molecules is therefore a statistical phenomenon. While few if any antigenic determinants may be specific for a particular molecule, it is improbable that two unrelated molecules (A and B) will share significant numbers of antigenic determinants. With monoclonal antisera, recognition is an all-or-none process. As a result, a monoclonal antiserum might react equally well with two unrelated molecules sharing but a single antigenic determinant. A polyclonal antiserum could reliably discriminate between the two.

cific epitopes may be sensitive to pH and temperature,[36] leading to alterations of their apparent specificity. While some of the antibodies in a polyclonal mixture may be equally affected, there are usually enough unaffected antigen-specific antibodies to mediate effective and specific binding. Similarly, all of the antibody in a monoclonal serum will be of the same immunoglobulin subtype. Thus it may or may not be effective in complement-mediated lysis (IgM antibodies are good for this purpose) or be detectable in assays employing protein A (IgM antibodies as a rule do not bind to protein A). Finally, since all of the components of a monoclonal antiserum have the same specificity, these antisera cannot form extensively cross-linked lattices with target molecules. As a result, monoclonal antibodies fail to form precipitation bands with most antigens in the agar diffusion method of Ouchterlony.

While these limitations of the monoclonal antibody technique require that these tools be used with caution, there is little doubt but that the method has served to revolutionize both the study and methods of immunology. Further, it appears probable that most of the limitations of the monoclonal antibody method with respect to conventional antisera can be overcome by simply pooling a group of well-characterized monoclonal antibodies recognizing different epitopes on the same antigen. This would create a new polyclonal antiserum with defined components available in virtually limitless amounts.

Table 1
POLYCLONAL ANTISERA AS DIAGNOSTIC AIDS

| HTA | Anti-Ia | Anti-CALLA | Diagnosis |
|---|---|---|---|
| + | − | −[a] | T cell ALL |
| − | + | + | Common ALL |
| − | + | − | ANNL[b] or "uncommon" ALL |

[a] Leukemic cells from approximately 10% of patients with what appears to be T cell ALL are HTA$^+$ and CALLA$^+$.
[b] Leukemic cells from approximately 10% of patients with ANNL (for example those with promyelocytic leukemia) are Ia$^-$.

From Pesando, J. M. et al., *Blood*, 54, 1240, 1979. With permission.

## IV. DIAGNOSTIC APPLICATIONS OF SEROLOGIC REAGENTS

### A. Acute Leukemias

Serologic methods are currently widely employed to facilitate the diagnosis of clinically important subtypes of human hemotologic malignancies.[2,27,29,37-53] The utility of this approach was first demonstrated for the acute lymphoblastic leukemias (ALL) when it became apparent that clinical prognosis correlated with the cellular origin of the disease.[54,55] For example, leukemic cells from approximately 20% of patients with ALL share with normal peripheral T lymphocytes the fortuitous ability to clump or rosette sheep red blood cells. These patients are referred to as having T cell ALL and have a much worse prognosis than the rest when treated with conventional therapies for ALL. However, it is possible that cell surface phenotype and circulating leukemic cell count at diagnosis are not independent variables.[56-58]

The polyclonal antisera initially employed as diagnostic aids included those which are operationally specific for T cells (HTA), the Ia-like antigen, and the common ALL antigen (CALLA). Within the hematopoietic series, antisera to human T cells react with all T cells and, to a first approximation, no others. The Ia-like antigen is present on B lymphocytes, most macrophages, early myeloid cells, and on leukemic cells of most patients with non-T cell ALL, but is found only on activated T cells. CALLA is found primarily on leukemic cells of patients with non-T cell ALL and with chronic myelogenous leukemia (CML) in lymphoid blast crisis. The utility of these antisera as diagnostic aids in acute leukemia is shown in Table 1. For example, cells seropositive with HTA but which are Ia$^-$ and CALLA$^-$ characterize patients with T cell ALL. Cells seronegative with HTA but Ia$^+$ and CALLA$^+$ are typical of the majority of patients with non-T cell ALL. Leukemic cells positive only for the Ia-like antigen presently define either acute nonlymphocytic leukemia (ANNL) or an uncommon serologic subtype of ALL. The T cell antisera are used to positively identify T cells, while the Ia antiserum negatively corroborates this assignment, allowing T cell malignancies to be distinguished from all others. Antisera to the common ALL antigen reliably discriminate ALL from ANNL and most cases of non-T cell ALL from T cell ALL. Identification of patients with T cell ALL at the time of diagnosis will permit an organized search for more effective therapies. It has also been suggested that patients with CALLA$^-$HTA$^-$Ia$^+$ ALL (CALLA$^-$ non-T cell ALL) may constitute a clinically important group of individuals having a cure rate better than that of patients with T cell ALL but worse than that of patients with CALLA$^+$ non-T cell ALL.[57,59] However, since this group is negatively defined, there may well exist heterogeneity within it, and further work in this area is needed. In addition, patients with CALLA$^+$Ia$^+$HTA$^-$ lymphoid blast crisis of CML respond better than those of the CALLA$^-$ myeloid variety to vincristine and prednisone, making this a useful clinical distinction. Unfortunately, these responses are short-lived.[60-62]

The advent of monoclonal antibodies having the same specificities as these polyclonal reagents makes possible the use of inexpensive standard reagents to better correlate clinical observations in different treatment centers. Monoclonal antibodies specific for the common ALL (CALLA) and Ia antigens have been described.[63-69] In addition, the development of monoclonal antisera which react preferentially with leukemia cells from some patients with ANLL now makes it possible to effect positive serological identification of many of these individuals.[70-75] However, efforts to produce monoclonal antibodies having the same utility as HTA for the identification of patients with T cell leukemia have only recently been successful.[75a] In retrospect this difficulty is not surprising since immune precipitation experiments, wherein an antibody is used to isolate the antigen(s) which it recognizes, indicate that HTA contains antibodies to several T cell antigens.[76,77] These studies, and subsequent work with monoclonal antibodies specific for various T antigens, indicate that all T cells do not necessarily express the full repertoire of T antigens.[78,79] In short, only a polyclonal antiserum, either made in an animal or prepared by mixing available monoclonal antibodies specific for T antigens, can provide the specificities now encompassed by HTA. However, monoclonal antisera to T cell antigens are now proving to be useful diagnostic reagents.[75a] There is also a preliminary report[80] which suggests that there may exist serologically definable and clinically important subsets of patients with T cell ALL. Specifically, patients with leukemic T cells of the helper phenotype may have a poorer prognosis than those with leukemic T cells of the suppressor phenotype. Confirmation of these tentative findings would indicate an important diagnostic role for at least some monoclonal antibodies specific for T-cell-associated antigens.

Similarly, monoclonal antibodies specific for Ia antigens may also have limited utility as replacements for polyclonal antisera made in the usual fashion. While monoclonal antisera specific for Ia antigens and which react with virtually all Ia positive cells have been prepared by several laboratories, recent work indicates that the Ia antigen is part of a complex molecular system.[22,66-69,81,82] In the mouse, two nonallelic genetic loci coding for Ia molecules have been identified.[83,84] In the guinea pig there are three.[85] Multiple alleles are thought to exist within each of these loci. Multiple nonallelic genes also appear to encode Ia-like complexes in man.[22,66-68,82] This discovery was made in part by extracting from a sample all of the Ia-like complexes recognized by one antibody and then showing that the sample still contained Ia-like complexes recognized by additional Ia-specific monoclonal antibodies.[22] Reciprocal experiments produced identical results. Therefore it cannot be assumed that a monoclonal antibody specific for an Ia antigen will in fact react with all Ia+ cell populations. However, it has recently been proposed that Ia phenotype may be correlated with the duration of disease-free survival,[86] implying that some of the differences detected by monoclonal antisera may prove to be clinically relevant.

B. Lymphomas

The morphologic and clinical diversity of non-Hodgkin's lymphoma, as well as its frequency in the population, has long inspired hope that there might also exist clinically important and serologically definable subsets of this disease. For example, patients having diffuse histiocytic lymphoma of the Rappaport classification are a clinically heterogeneous group.[87-89] Some do very well on conventional therapies for this disease while many do not. Attempts are being made to define histologic and immunologic classification schemes which will be of value in treating such patients.[90-92] For example, if those patients who do well on conventional therapies could be identified at the time of diagnosis, they could be treated as a group. Optimal therapy for patients within that group could be further refined with less risk that a therapeutic innovation which benefits those patients would be less than harmless for unappreciated subgroups within the total population. Similarly, a systematic search for effective therapies could be undertaken for those patients who do not do well on conventional treatments.

Despite a host of reports on the study of lymphomas using serologic reagents,[79,93-103] monoclonal antisera have as yet failed to provide new diagnostic insights. Those studies with monoclonal antibodies reported to date have revealed an enormous and often bewildering array of surface phenotypes for these malignant cells, the significance of which remains to be determined. This failure does not imply either that clinically relevant serologic patient subgroups do not exist or that monoclonal antisera will not be of value in identifying them. Rather, the difficulties encountered to date may simply reflect the capacity of monoclonal antibodies to greatly amplify small and often functionally irrelevant differences between antigens and the cells bearing them. There may simply be much more work to be done. In addition, relative inaccessibility and greater admixture with normal cells make malignant cells in lymphoma more difficult to phenotype than in leukemia.

## V. ETIOLOGY OF CANCER

### A. Clonal Origin

Studies of malignant cells using monoclonal antibodies have already provided elegant confirmation of the clonal origin of human tumors. Most of the initial work in this area was based on studies of X chromosome inactivation mosaicism. Although individual somatic cells of women who carry alleles for two identifiable forms of glucose-6-phosphate dehydrogenase can express either of the two isoenzymes, malignant cells from tumors in such individuals all express the same isoenzyme.[104,105] Mosaicism in the expression of surface immunoglobulin molecules (light chains and variable regions or idiotypes) has been similarly employed.[106-109] With monoclonal antibodies it has become possible to phenotype the surface molecules of a large number of cells using a panel of reagents, thereby providing a serologic fingerprint for different cell types. Using this approach, it has been shown that most tumor cells in patients with hematopoietic malignancies express the same surface markers, although this may not always be the case with nonhematopoietic tumors.

Following the pioneering work in the mouse and then in man using polyclonal reagents,[28,110-112] several laboratories have developed a panel of monoclonal antibodies to surface antigens on human T lymphocytes.[113-126] Some of these antibodies discriminate between functional subsets of T cells. (While most of the epitopes defined by these antibodies are now known not to be cell-lineage-specific[122] according to Pesando,[219] their operational utility has not been diminished.) Tentative proposals for T cell differentiation have been made based on the distribution of these epitopes on thymocytes and peripheral T lymphocytes. For example, Reinherz et al.[127,128] have described three discrete stages of intrathymic differentiation based on the distribution of the epitopes defined by the OKT reagents.

Using monoclonal antibodies to phenotype malignant T lymphocytes, many investigators have reported that these malignancies reflect the clonal expansion of cells at discrete stages of normal T cell differentiation. For example, most malignant cells of patients with acute lymphoblastic leukemia express antigens found on early thymocytes and prothymocytes, but not those found on more mature T cells.[56,122,127,129-131] In contrast, malignant cells of most patients with T cell chronic lymphocytic leukemia (CLL) express surface markers characteristic of mature circulating T lymphocytes of either the helper or suppressor phenotype.[122,132] Several groups have reported that the malignant T cells in Sezary's syndrome have the surface phenotype of mature T cells of only the helper phenotype.[133-135]

Efforts to use monoclonal antisera to explore B lymphocyte heterogeneity and differentiation have met with more limited success. Present models for B lymphocyte differentiation are based on the cellular expression of immunoglobulin chains as determined using polyclonal antisera.[136,137] The earliest detectable B lymphocytes express the μ or heavy chain of IgM in their cytoplasm. These cells subsequently express surface μ chain, surface IgM, surface IgM plus IgD, and surface IgG with or without other classes of immunoglobulin.[138]

Probably the most interesting B cell antigen to be identified by monoclonal antibodies to date is that defined by the B1 antibody.[139,140] This antigen is highly associated with cells of the B cell lineage but is absent on plasma cells as well as on resting and activated T lymphocytes, monocytes, and granulocytes. It appears to define that cell population which can be stimulated to secrete immunoglobulin by pokeweed mitogen. Not only is the B1 antigen expressed on all surface immunoglobulin positive B cells, but its expression on leukemic cells of 30 to 50% of patients having non-T cell ALL suggests that many of these leukemias derive from early B lymphocytes. A similar proposal based on the cytoplasmic expression of the μ chain of IgM had been made earlier.[141] Korsmeyer et al. have recently confirmed the B cell nature of non-T cell ALL by study of immunoglobulin gene rearrangements.[141a] A second B-cell-associated antigen termed B2 has also been described.[142] This second antigen is weakly expressed on circulating B cells but is strongly expressed on B cells of lymphoid organs. However, the proposal that B1 and B2 are B cell differentiation antigens requires careful scrutiny since the models so developed place the cells of Burkitt's lymphoma and B cell CLL in positions at odds with the surface immunoglobulin data. For example, B2 is expressed on cells of CLL but not on those of Burkitt's lymphoma, yet it has been proposed that B2 is lost as B lymphocytes mature. Malignant cells of Burkitt's lymphoma express surface IgM almost exclusively,[143] while those of CLL usually bear both IgM and IgD.[108,144]

### B. Tumor-Specific Antigens

For many years it was the hope and belief of those doing cancer research that malignant cells were characterized by the presence on their surface of unique molecules that somehow mediated their asocial behavior. The discovery of such putative tumor-specific antigens might lead to the development of methods for the selective elimination of tumor cells. Extensive study of the surfaces of malignant cells using serologic methods has cast considerable doubt on the existence of such tumor-specific surface markers. Despite numerous reports of the discovery of tumor-specific antigens over the years,[66,145,146] none of these discoveries has withstood the tests of time and scrutiny.[21,23-25,147-151] Most of the antigens reported have proved to be correlates of cellular differentiation, proliferation, and/or function. Studies of malignant cells with monoclonal antisera by and large support these observations. Not only are tumor-specific antigens proving to be scarce to nonexistent, but it is now becoming apparent that there are relatively few antigens which are even tissue-specific.[122,219] This repeated failure to identify tumor-specific surface antigens is consistent with the proposal that malignancy reflects the abnormal expression of specific normal genes which control cellular growth and differentiation rather than the introduction or creation of new genetic material.[152-157]

The common ALL antigen or CALLA is a case in point. This antigen was initially found on malignant cells from the majority of patients with non-T cell ALL, and from many patients with Burkitt's lymphoma and both nodular and diffuse lymphocytic lymphoma. The antigen was not readily detected on normal cells using extensively absorbed polyclonal antisera, raising the possibility that the antigen might be tumor-specific.[29,146] The first reports[147,148] that CALLA was weakly expressed by some normal cells as revealed by immunofluorescence studies were viewed with some suspicion, since none of the initial absorbed polyclonal antisera were monospecific. In addition, it was not possible to characterize the antigen chemically using an impure antiserum. With the development of monoclonal antibodies specific for epitopes on CALLA, the antigen could finally be isolated by the technique of immune precipitation and characterized.[21,63,158,159] It then became rapidly apparent that the antigen not only was not tumor-specific but that it was also not tissue-specific, being present on normal fibroblasts in tissue culture as well as on a number of nonhematopoietic cell lines.[160] The epitope and probably the antigen defined by one of these anti-CALLA monoclonal antibodies has been reported to be on or in normal renal tubular and glomerular cells, cells of fetal small intestine, and myoepithelial cells of adult breast.[150] There is also a report that it is transiently expressed on PHA-stimulated lymphocytes.[149] All of these data indicate that this tumor-associated antigen is not primarily linked to cell differentiation, as had been proposed.[1]

While the existence of antigens whose expression is specific for a particular type of malignant cell seems increasingly improbable, cell-specific antigens do exist. Every B lymphocyte has a unique idiotype or antigen binding site on the immunoglobulin molecules expressed on its surface. Since malignant tumors are thought to arise from the proliferation of a single clone of cells, then all cells of such a malignant B cell population should share this unique marker. Efforts to exploit these cell-specific antigens for therapeutic purposes have already been reported by Levy and co-workers (vide infra). The major difficulty with this approach is that these antigens are by definition both cell- and patient-specific, so that unique anti-idiotype antibodies would have to be developed for the B cell tumors of each patient.

## VI. THERAPEUTIC APPLICATIONS

### A. Serotherapy

Recently there has been much interest in the use of monoclonal antibodies for serotherapy in patients with malignancies. The specificity, purity, titer, and availability of these antisera suggest that they might prove to be useful as therapeutic agents, despite the fact that similar approaches with conventional or polyclonal antisera have met with limited success.[161-163] However, studies in animals using monoclonal antibodies indicate that such an approach may have therapeutic potential.[164,165] For those antibodies which do not define tumor-specific epitopes, there appears to be a tacit assumption by those working in the field that the elimination of normal cells sharing the tumor-associated epitope would not be injurious to the patient and/or that such cells would be rapidly replaced by the proliferation and differentiation of antigen-negative precursor cells with tolerable clinical side effects. Alternatively, selective toxicity might be achieved by reduced antigen density and/or antigen accessibility to antibody on normal cells relative to leukemic ones.

The results of the first clinical trials involving the use of monoclonal antibodies to treat lymphoid malignancies in man have now been reported. Although only one of the monoclonal antisera employed to date was tumor-specific (the anti-idiotype antibody of Miller et al.),[166] toxicity to normal tissues appears to have been minimal. Toxicity also closely paralleled therapeutic effect: for the most part clinically significant responses were not observed. Nadler et al.[167] treated a patient with diffuse, poorly differentiated lymphoma in leukemic phase with a lytic monoclonal antibody raised to the patient's malignant cells. At the time of serotherapy the patient had a circulating lymphoma cell population of 400,000/mm$^3$. Despite the administration of a total of 2 g of antibody in two courses separated by a 3-week interval, only transient reductions in the number of circulating malignant cells were observed. The presence of large amounts of circulating free antigen which may have neutralized the monoclonal antibody appeared at least to partially explain this phenomenon. Ritz et al.[168] treated four patients with non-T cell ALL in relapse with a lytic monoclonal antibody specific for the common ALL antigen (CALLA). Transient but marked decreases in the number of circulating leukemic cells were observed in all three patients in whom this parameter could be monitored. In addition, reversible antibody-induced loss of the expression of the epitope detected by the antibody was observed (antigenic modulation or more correctly epitope modulation) in all four patients. This process rendered the cells effectively antigen-negative and perforce resistant to the cytotoxic effects of CALLA-specific antibody. Subsequent in vitro studies revealed that the process is rapid, specific, and reversible and that it is dependent on both temperature and antibody concentration.[173] Dillman et al.[169] treated two patients with B cell CLL with a lytic monoclonal antibody that reacted with normal T lymphocytes. In both patients there was a rapid but transient drop in the number of circulating CLL cells. Both patients became systemically ill during treatment but subsequently recovered. The cause of their difficulties was never clear. Miller et al.[170] treated a patient with T cell leukemia with a monoclonal antibody to an antigen present on normal T cells. Again there was a dramatic but brief drop in the number of circulating leukemic cells, after which antibody-induced partial modulation of the target epitope was noted. Although circulating free antigen was not detectable prior to therapy, it was observed following the first dose of antibody. Later host antibodies to mouse antibody were detected. The patient tolerated therapy well. A second patient having T cell cutaneous lymphoma received 17 treatments over 10 weeks without evidence of toxicity.[171] While antigenic modulation was again observed, each treatment resulted in a reduction in the number of circulating leukemic cells as well as regression in the size of lymph nodes and cutaneous lesions. Complete clinical remission was not achieved.

The most exciting serotherapy trial reported to date has been that of Miller et al.[166] in which they treated a patient with a B cell lymphoma with a monoclonal antibody specific for the variable region of the surface immunoglobulin expressed by these cells. The resulting antibody was therefore not only tumor-specific but specific for that patient's clone of malignant cells. Following eight doses of antibody over 4 weeks, an objective clinical remission was induced with disappearance of all detectable tumor cells and of fevers and night sweats. Treatment was well tolerated, and the remission lasted for more than 27 months without further therapy. The precise fate of the patient's tumor cells remains a mystery. These cells may have been killed via destructive immune mechanisms. Alternatively, the anti-idiotype antibody employed for therapy may have induced these tumor cells to undergo terminal differentiation to a nonproliferative state, thereby mimicking the capacity of specific antigens to initiate a comparable physiologic response in normal B lymphocytes. Unfortunately, the necessity of tailoring monoclonal antibodies of this type to each patient precluded both rapid confirmation of the efficacy of this approach and early insight into the cell biology underlying this remission. Recent experience using this method has been less promising.[166a]

While these studies demonstrate that monoclonal antibodies can be used for passive serotherapy with relative safety, antibody-mediated killing of tumor cells in vivo has not been demonstrated. Reports of transient reductions in the number of circulating malignant cells may reflect nothing more than sequestration of antibody-coated cells. Failure to demonstrate unequivocal killing of tumor cells no doubt reflects the fact that human complement is minimally effective in mediating cell lysis. In addition, the efficacy of cell-mediated clearance of antibody-coated malignant cells in this setting remains to be shown.[172]

Problems previously reported in the animal literature were also encountered in the course of these trials. The presence of circulating antigen in one patient served to neutralize large amounts of antibody.[167] Whether the antigen was being secreted by viable cells or reflected endogenous turnover of malignant cells remains to be determined. For those patients in whom this problem is encountered, it may prove necessary to remove circulating antigens before initiating serotherapy. For example, the patient's blood might be passed through a matrix containing bound antibody. Alternatively, it may be necessary to treat these patients with conventional therapies in order to reduce the tumor cell burden before initiating serotherapy.

The problem of antibody-induced loss of antibody binding sites (antigenic modulation) also proved troublesome. While once thought to be a rare phenomenon, antigenic modulation by specific antibody occurs to some extent for many human cell surface antigens, with the notable exception of HLA-A, B, C, and D molecules.[21,173] As a result of modulation, target cells become effectively antigen-negative and resistant to killing mediated by specific antibody. Antigenic modulation can result in shedding, internalization, or simple blocking of the antigen,[174-181] depending on the system being examined. Both surface immunoglobulin and CALLA are internalized during modulation, as are their respective antibodies.[21,160,176,177,182] Since monoclonal antibodies recognize only a portion of a surface antigen, supporting biochemical data are needed to determine the fate of the antigen bearing the epitope being monitored. Efforts are currently under way to circumvent or exploit the process of antibody-mediated antigenic modulation to achieve selective destruction of target cells.[183] For example, potent cytotoxins might be coupled to an antibody to deliver selectively these poisons to the intracellular compartment during the internalization of antibody.

Additional problems will doubtless be encountered in the course of efforts to treat human hematologic malignancies using monoclonal antibodies.[182] For example, it has long been assumed that all malignant cells of a tumor in a patient have the same surface phenotype, yet there is evidence in the animal literature that this is not the case. For example, in the murine Lewis lung tumor system, Olsson et al.[184] have shown that cells from a metastatic focus express an antigen not found on the primary tumor. Antigenic heterogeneity of tumors has also been shown in methylcholanthrene-induced mouse sarcomas[185] and in AKR mouse thymic lymphomas.[186] Karyotypic heterogeneity in metastatic lesions arising from implanted murine melanomas has also been reported.[187] In man, variation in the expression of a surface antigenic determinant in cells derived from a melanoma has been observed.[188] The implications of these observations for the use of monoclonal antibodies in the treatment of human tumors are readily apparent, although it is possible that this problem might be overcome to some extent by using a pool of monoclonal antibodies specific for different tumor-associated antigens.[188]

A related problem is that the clonigenic or replicating cell which maintains a cancer may not be the phenotypically predominant cell in a tumor. The progeny of the true malignant cell may be capable of at least limited differentiation in vivo, resulting in the observed accumulation of abnormal cells.[1] The phenotype and drug sensitivity of the clonigenic cell rather than those of its more numerous progeny ultimately determines the clinical efficacy of any therapeutic approach. Perhaps the best illustration of this process is found in chronic myelogenous leukemia. While the predominant cell types in this disease are granulocytes and their immediate precursors, the Philadelphia chromosome abnormality characteristic of this disease has also been found in precursors of erythrocytes, platelets, and monocytes.[104,105] Recently it has also been found in apparent precursors of the lymphoid lineage.[189-191]

On a more positive note, the production of antibodies to mouse immunoglobulin was not a major problem in these trials, although anti-mouse antibodies were detected in one asymptomatic patient. This potential problem was avoided in part by the tendency of investigators to restrict antibody therapy to short intensive courses. In addition to their capacity to induce systemic anaphylactoid reactions, such anti-mouse antibodies could effectively neutralize monoclonal antibodies used for therapy. This observation may force a reassessment of the potential clinical superiority of human vs. murine monoclonal antibodies for serotherapy, particularly when development of the former is still in its early stages. While patients can be immunized to foreign immunoglobulins, they can also be expected to mount an immune response to at least the idiotypic portions of human monoclonal antibodies administered in a similar fashion.

## B. Autologous Transplantation

To circumvent some of the problems encountered in these serotherapy trials, efforts are being made to develop additional strategies for the use of monoclonal antibodies. One such approach is to attempt to use these reagents to rid bone marrow of malignant cells in vitro prior to autologous bone marrow transplantation. The efficacy of syngeneic and allogeneic bone marrow transplantation for the treatment of patients with hematologic malignancies has been clearly established.[192-196] In this procedure the patient receives massive doses of chemotherapy and radiation to eradicate his malignant cells. Since this treatment is lethal both to malignant and normal hematopoietic cells, patients are given tumor-free bone marrow from an HLA-matched normal donor. Bone marrow transplantation therefore provides a means of intensifying cancer therapy without concern for dose-limiting toxicity to normal marrow elements. Unfortunately, most patients do not have suitable donors. For those who do, the often serious complication of graft-vs.-host disease is frequently a problem. Only those patients fortunate enough to have an HLA-identical twin are spared. With autologous marrow transplantation, each patient receives his or her own marrow. Every patient therefore has a perfectly matched donor.[197] In addition, the potential problem of graft-vs.-host disease would be eliminated. Autologous marrow can be treated to remove malignant cells. By using antibodies to treat bone marrow in the controlled environment of the laboratory, the number of tissues exposed to the potentially toxic effects of antibody is reduced, diminishing though not necessarily eliminating the need for tissue- if not tumor-specific antibodies. Similarly, antigenic modulation can be effectively eliminated by lowering the temperature, and blocking factors can be removed by washing the sample. Lytic animal complement can be repeatedly employed in lieu of human complement to rid marrow of malignant cells. By washing the sample before infusion, the likelihood of inducing allergic reactions to foreign proteins should be reduced. The potential of this approach has already been demonstrated in an animal model using a polyclonal antiserum.[198]

While the preliminary results of a report by Ritz et al.[199] on the use of a monoclonal antibody to CALLA to rid remission marrow samples of leukemic cells prior to autologous transplantation are somewhat encouraging, there exist many potential problems with this approach. Chief among these is the approximately 50% relapse rate now seen in ALL patients who are recipients of allogeneic bone marrow transplants. This figure indicates failure of the ablative procedure to rid the patient of his own leukemic cells, since the bone marrow cells of the donor are normal. Since recipients of autologous marrow transplants would not benefit from the reported anti-leukemic effect of graft-vs.-host disease,[200] the relapse rate in these patients may be still higher. Therefore, regardless of the efficacy of the in vitro serologic treatment of autologous marrow, no more than 50% of patients could benefit from this procedure. In addition, it is highly unlikely that present in vitro techniques for antibody-mediated cell depletion can completely rid the marrow sample of all malignant cells. Even if this treatment is 99.99% effective, it is not known whether the patient can control and eliminate his reduced tumor burden when it is given back to him. (Moreover the long-term survival of several patients with non-Hodgkin's lymphoma treated by use of intensive chemotherapy and/or irradiation followed by autologous transplantation with untreated remission bone marrow supports the idea that such marrow can be used with curative intent, it also seriously questions the need for specific in vitro marrow treatment in this setting.[197,201] Stewart et al. have recently reported that 3 of 13 (23%) patients with ANLL in first remission transplanted with autologous untreated remission bone marrow remain disease-free greater than 600 days post-transplant, further emphasizing the need for appropriate controls to evaluate the efficacy of autologous transplant regimens involving manipulation of donor marrow.[201a] Heterogeneity of antigen expression by individual tumor cells would mean that some cells would not be eliminated even with multiple treatments of a single antibody. If the numerically and phenotypically predominant cell is not the clonigenic one, then eradication of antigen-positive cells by these methods would not cure the disease. Finally, toxicity to normal cells remains a potential risk even when bone marrow is treated with antibodies in vitro to eliminate malignant cells. While in vitro assays for certain progenitor cell types exist (myeloid, erythroid) and can be employed to suggest that these cells are not epitope- or antigen-positive (the two being operationally identical in this context),[202,203] useful assays for other progenitor cell types (lymphoid) are not yet available. It is therefore not possible to know whether or not these cells are antigen-negative. Should important antigen-positive normal cells exist in bone marrow, it remains possible that they might express sufficiently less antigen than malignant cells such that they would be relatively unaffected by antibody-mediated lytic processes. However, as the latter are made more efficient, toxicity to normal cells may well be seen.

## C. Drug-Antibody Conjugates

To make monoclonal antibodies more effective therapeutic agents, many laboratories are now coupling them to potent cytotoxins.[204-208] Such drug-antibody conjugates should, in theory, selectively deliver lethal doses of drug to antigen-positive cells while sparing antigen-negative ones. Use of these conjugates might not only supplant possibly ineffective host immune mechanisms but also exploit the internalization of antibody that occurs during modulation of some antigens. Use of extremely potent toxins such as ricin and diphtheria toxin appears to be required to ensure the selective delivery of lethal doses of drug despite the presence of relatively small numbers of specific antibody binding sites on target cells. Since ricin and related protein toxins are both bifunctional and bimolecular, being composed of both toxic and cell-binding subunits, the cell-binding subunit of the toxin can be replaced by an antibody molecule linked via a disulfide bond. While such toxin-antibody conjugates have proven capable of selectively killing target cell populations in vitro,[183,209-215] they have produced disappointing results in vivo.[213-215] Several explanations of these in vivo results are possible. For example, following therapy a few surviving tumor cells could eventually kill the animal, while such cells might go virtually unnoticed in vitro. Alternatively, access of conjugates to tumor cells may be impaired. In addition, drug-antibody conjugates may be more rapidly inactivated in vivo than in vitro. While these and related technical problems will no doubt be mastered in time, ultimate success in these endeavors may lead to unexpected clinical toxicities. The successful in vivo elimination of tumor cells by such drug-antibody hybrids may well be accompanied by the wholesale elimination of those normal cells bearing similar epitopes or antigens, cells which were previously spared and possibly even undetected because of the very impotence of earlier approaches. However, drug-antibody conjugates might ultimately prove useful for the in-vitro elimination of antigen positive tumor cells.

## VII. CONCLUDING REMARKS

The use of monoclonal antibodies for the study, diagnosis, and treatment of lymphomas is only beginning. Ultimately, application of this technology may have a profound impact on how we perceive and treat these diseases. Systematic application of the somatic cell fusion technique to produce hybridomas secreting monoclonal antisera is already providing the cell biologist with unparalleled tools with which to dissect and study the myriad components of the cell membrane. This increased understanding of the biology of cell membranes in general, and of the structure and function of the surface components of lymphoma cells in particular, will constitute the ultimate payoff of this technique. It is not unrealistic to expect that this knowledge will ultimately improve our ability to identify clinically important subtypes of this disease and thereby select and devise optimum treatment programs. At the same time, certain antibodies may themselves serve as therapeutic tools, not necessarily for the destruction of malignant cells, but, based on an increased understanding of cell and membrane biology, to regulate the abnormalities of proliferation and differentiation that are the hallmarks of malignant disease.

## ACKNOWLEDGMENTS

This work was supported by PHS grant number CA15704, CA30924, and CA34206, DHHS, and by a grant from the Cancer Research Institute, New York, New York.

## REFERENCES

1. Greaves, M. and Janossy, G., Patterns of gene expression and the cellular origins of human leukemias, *Biochim. Biophys. Acta,* 516, 193, 1978.
2. Brouet, J. C. and Seligmann, M., The immunologic classification of acute lymphoblastic leukemias, *Cancer,* 42, 817, 1978.
3. Ritz, J. and Schlossman, S. F., Utilization of monoclonal antibodies in the treatment of leukemia and lymphoma, *Blood,* 59, 1, 1982.
4. Goding, J., Antibody production by hybridomas, *J. Immunol. Methods,* 39, 285, 1980.
5. Nadler, L. M., Ritz, J., Griffin, J. D., Todd, R. F., Reinherz, E. L., and Schlossman, S. F., Diagnosis and treatment of human leukemias and lymphomas utilizing monoclonal antibodies, in *Progress in Hematology,* Vol. 12, Brown, E. B., Ed., Grune & Stratton, New York, 1981, 187.
6. Diamond, B. A., Yelton, D. E., and Scharff, M. D., Monoclonal antibodies: a new technology for producing serologic reagents, *N. Engl. J. Med.,* 304, 1344, 1981.
7. Kennett, R. H., McKearn, T. J., and Bechtol, K. B., Eds., *Monoclonal Antibodies,* Plenum Press, New York, 1980.
8. Greaves, M. F., Clinical applications of cell surface markers, *Progr. Hematol.,* 9, 255, 1975.
9. Leder, P., Max, E. E., and Seidman, J. G., The organization of immunoglobulin genes and the origin of their diversity, in *Immunology 80,* Fougereau, M. and Dausset, J., Eds., Academic Press, New York, 1980.
10. Hozumi, N. and Tonegawa, S., Evidence for somatic rearrangement of immunoglobulin genes coding for variable and constant regions, *Proc. Natl. Acad. Sci. U.S.A.,* 73, 3628, 1976.
11. Lerner, R. A., Tapping the immunological repertoire to produce antibodies of predetermined specificity, *Nature (London),* 299, 592, 1982.
12. Köhler, G. and Milstein, C., Continuous cultures of fused cells secreting antibody of pre-defined specificity, *Nature (London),* 256, 495, 1975.
13. Köhler, G. and Milstein, C., Derivation of specific antibody-producing tissue culture and tumor lines by cell fusion, *Eur. J. Immunol.,* 6, 511, 1976.
14. Kennett, R. H., Denis, K. A., Tung, A. S., and Klinman, N. R., Hybrid plasmacytoma production: fusions with adult spleen cells, monoclonal spleen fragments, neonatal spleen cells and human spleen cells, *Curr. Top. Microbiol. Immunol.,* 81, 77, 1978.
15. Kennett, R. H., Cell fusion, in *Methods in Enzymology,* Vol. 58, Jakoby, W. B. and Pastan, I. M., Eds., Academic Press, New York, 1979, 345.
16. Gefter, M. L., Margulies, D. H., and Scharff, M. D., A simple method for polyethylene glycol-promoted hybridization of mouse myeloma cells, *Somatic Cell Genet.,* 3, 231, 1977.
17. Margulies, D. H., Kuehl, W. M., and Scharff, M. D., Somatic cell hybridization of mouse myeloma cells, *Cell,* 8, 405, 1976.
18. Littlefield, J. W., Selection of hybrids from matings of fibroblasts in vitro and their presumed recombinants, *Science,* 145, 709, 1964.

19. Hansen, D. and Stadtler, J., Increased polyethylene glycol-mediated fusion competence in mitotic cells of a mouse lymphoid cell line, *Somatic Cell Genet.*, 3, 471, 1977.
20. Galfre, G., Howe, S. C., Milstein, C., Butcher, G. W., and Howard, J. C., Antibodies to major histocompatibility antigens produced by hybrid cell lines, *Nature (London)*, 266, 550, 1977.
21. Pesando, J. M., Ritz, J., Lazarus, H., Tomaselli, K. J., and Schlossman, S. F., Fate of a common acute lymphoblastic leukemia antigen during modulation by specific antibody, *J. Immunol.*, 126, 540, 1981.
22. Pesando, J. M., Nadler, L. M., Lazarus, H., Tomaselli, K. J., Stashenko, P., Ritz, J., Levine, H., Yunis, E. J., and Schlossman, S. F., Human cell lines express multiple populations of Ia-like molecules, *Hum. Immunol.*, 3, 67, 1981.
23. Sutherland, R., Delia, D., Schneider, C., Newman, R., Kemshead, J., and Greaves, M., Ubiquitous cell-surface glycoprotein on tumor cells is proliferation-associated receptor for transferrin, *Proc. Natl. Acad. Sci. U.S.A.*, 78, 4515, 1981.
24. Trowbridge, I. S. and Omary, M. B., Human cell surface glycoprotein related to cell proliferation is the receptor for transferrin, *Proc. Natl. Acad. Sci. U.S.A.*, 78, 3039, 1981.
25. Trowbridge, I. S. and Lopez, F., Monoclonal antibody to transferrin receptor blocks transferrin binding and inhibits human tumor cell growth in vitro, *Proc. Natl. Acad. Sci. U.S.A.*, 79, 1175, 1982.
26. Goding, J. W. and Burns, G. F., Monoclonal antibody OKT-9 recognizes the receptor for transferrin on human acute lymphocytic leukemia cells, *J. Immunol.*, 127, 1256, 1981.
27. Greaves, M. F., Brown, G., Rapson, M. J., and Lister, T. A., Antisera to acute lymphoblastic leukemia cells, *Clin. Immunol. Immunopathol.*, 4, 67, 1975.
28. Evans, R. L., Breard, J. M., Lazarus, H., Schlossman, S. F., and Chess, L., Detection, isolation and functional characterization of two human T cell subclasses bearing unique differentiation antigens, *J. Exp. Med.*, 145, 221, 1977.
29. Pesando, J. M., Ritz, J., Lazarus, H., Baseman-Costello, S., Sallan, S. E., and Schlossman, S. F., Leukemia associated antigens in ALL, *Blood*, 54, 1240, 1979.
30. Gahmberg, C. G., Cell-surface proteins: changes during cell growth and malignant transformation, in *Dynamic Aspects of Cell Surface Organization*, Vol. 3, Poste, G. and Nicholson, G. L., Eds., Elsevier, Amsterdam, 1977, 371.
31. Fukuda, M. N., Fukuda, M., and Hakomori, S. I., Cell surface modification by Endo-β-galactosidase: change of blood group activities and release of oligosaccharides from glycoproteins and glycosphingolipids of human erythrocytes, *J. Biol. Chem.*, 254, 5458, 1979.
32. Jonak, Z., Smith, A., Glick, M. C., Feder, M., and Kennett, R. H., Wandering around the cell surface: monoclonal antibody against human neuroblastoma and leukemia cell surface antigens, in *Hybridomas and Cellular Immortality*, Allison, J. P. and Tom, C. H., Eds., Plenum Press, New York, in press.
33. Garson, J. A., Beverley, P. C. L., Coakham, H. B., and Harper, E. I., Monoclonal antibodies against human T lymphocytes label Purkinje neurones of many species, *Nature (London)*, 298, 375, 1982.
34. Dulbecco, R., Unger, M., Bologna, M., Battifora, H., Syka, P., and Okada, S., Cross-reactivity between Thy-1 and a component of intermediate filaments demonstrated using a monoclonal antibody, *Nature (London)*, 292, 772, 1981.
35. Nigg, E. A., Walter, G., and Singer, S. J., On the nature of crossreactions observed with antibodies directed to defined epitopes, *Proc. Natl. Acad. Sci. U.S.A.*, 79, 5939, 1982.
36. Mosmann, T. R., Gallatin, M., and Longenecker, B. M., Alteration of apparent specificity of monoclonal (hybridoma) antibodies recognizing polymorphic histocompatibility and blood group determinants, *J. Immunol.*, 125, 1152, 1980.
37. Brown, G., Greaves, M. F., Lister, T. A., Rapson, N., and Papamichael, M., Expression of human T and B lymphocyte cell surface markers on leukemic cells, *Lancet*, 2, 753, 1974.
38. Schlossman, S. F., Chess, L., Humphreys, R. E., and Strominger, J. L., Distribution of Ia-like molecules on the surface of normal and leukemic human cells, *Proc. Natl. Acad. Sci. U.S.A.*, 73, 1288, 1975.
39. Humphrey, G. B. and Lankford, J., Acute leukemia: the use of surface markers in classification, *Semin. Oncol.*, 3, 243, 1976.
40. Kaplan, J., Ravindranath, Y., and Peterson, W. D., T and B lymphocyte antigen-positive null cell leukemias, *Blood*, 49, 371, 1977.
41. Borella, L., Sen, L., and Casper, J. T., Acute lymphoblastic leukemia (ALL) antigens detected with antisera to E rosette-forming and non-E rosette-forming ALL blasts, *J. Immunol.*, 118, 309, 1977.
42. Metzgar, R. S. and Mohanakumar, T., Tumor-associated antigens of human leukemia cells, *Semin. Hematol.*, 15, 139, 1978.

43. Smyth, J. F., Poplack, D. G., Holiman, B. J., Leventhal, B. G., and Yarbo, G., Correlation of adenosine deaminase activity with cell surface markers in acute lymphoblastic leukemia, *J. Clin. Invest.*, 62, 710, 1978.
44. Koshiba, H., Minowada, J., and Pressman, D., Rabbit antiserum against a non-T, non-B leukemia cell line that carries the Ph' chromosome (NALM-1): antibody specific to a non-T, non-B acute lymphoblastic leukemia antigen, *J. Natl. Cancer Inst.*, 61, 987, 1978.
45. Billing, R., Minowada, J., Cline, M., Clark, B., and Lee, K., Acute lymphocytic leukemia associated cell membrane antigen, *J. Natl. Cancer Inst.*, 61, 423, 1978.
46. LeBien, T. W., Hurwitz, R. L., and Kersey, J. H., Characterization of a xenoantiserum produced against three molar KCl-solubilized antigens obtained from a non-T, non-B (pre-B) acute lymphoblastic leukemia cell line, *J. Immunol.*, 122, 82, 1979.
47. Anderson, J. K., Moore, J. O., Faldetta, J. M., Terry, W. F., and Metzgar, R. S., Acute lymphoblastic leukemia: classification and characterization with antisera to human T-cell and Ia antigens, *J. Natl. Cancer Inst.*, 62, 294, 1979.
48. Koziner, B., Kempin, S., Passe, S., Gee, T., Good, R. A., and Clarkson, B. D., Characterization of B-cell leukemias: immunomorphological scheme, *Blood*, 56, 815, 1980.
49. Thiel, E., Rodt, H., Huhn, D., Netzel, B., Grosse-Wilde, H., Ganeshaguru, K., and Thierfelder, S., Multimarker classification of acute lymphoblastic leukemia: evidence for further T subgroups and evaluation of their clinical significance, *Blood*, 56, 759, 1980.
50. Greaves, M. F., Verbi, W., Kemshead, J., and Kennett, R., A monoclonal antibody identifying a cell surface antigen shared by common acute lymphoblastic leukemia and B lineage cells, *Blood*, 56, 1141, 1980.
51. Abramson, C., Kersey, J., and LeBien, T., A monoclonal antibody (BA-1) reactive with cells of human B lymphocyte lineage, *J. Immunol.*, 126, 83, 1981.
52. Kersey, J. H., LeBien, T. W., Abramson, C. S., Newman, R., Sutherland, D. R., and Greaves, M., p24: a human leukemia-associated and lymphohemopoietic progenitor cell surface structure identified with monoclonal antibody, *J. Exp. Med.*, 153, 726, 1981.
53. Schroff, R. W., Foon, K. A., Billing, R. J., and Fahey, J. L., Immunologic classification of lymphocytic leukemias based on monoclonal antibody-defined cell surface antigens, *Blood*, 59, 207, 1982.
54. Tsukimoto, I., Wong, K. Y., and Lampkin, B. C., Surface markers and prognostic factors in acute lymphoblastic leukemia, *N. Engl. J. Med.*, 294, 245, 1976.
55. Sen, L. and Borella, L., Clinical importance of lymphoblasts with T markers in childhood acute leukemia, *N. Engl. J. Med.*, 292, 828, 1975.
56. Greaves, M. F., Analysis of the clinical and biological significance of lymphoid phenotypes in acute leukemia, *Cancer Res.*, 41, 4752, 1981.
57. Sallan, S. E., Ritz, J., Pesando, J. M., Gelber, R., O'Brien, C., Hitchcock, S., Coral, F. S., and Schlossman, S. F., Cell surface antigens: prognostic implications in childhood acute lymphoblastic leukemia, *Blood*, 55, 395, 1980.
58. Bloomfield, C. D., and Gajl-Peczalska, K. J., The clinical relevance of lymphocyte surface markers in leukemia and lymphoma, in *Current Topics in Hematology*, Vol. 3, Piomelli, S. and Yachnin, S., Eds., Alan R. Liss, New York, 1980, 175.
59. Chessels, J. M., Hardisty, J. M., Rapson, N. T., and Greaves, M. F., Acute lymphoblastic leukaemia in children: classification and prognosis, *Lancet*, 2, 1307, 1977.
60. Rosenthal, S., Canellos, G. P., Whang-Peng, J., and Gralnick, H. R., Blast crisis of chronic granulocytic leukemia: morphologic variants and therapeutic implications, *Am. J. Med.*, 63, 542, 1977.
61. Marks, S. M., Baltimore, D., and McCaffrey, R., Terminal transferase as a predictor of initial responsiveness to vincristine and prednisone in blastic chronic myelogenous leukemia, *N. Engl. J. Med.*, 298, 812, 1978.
62. Janossy, G., Woodruff, R. K., Pippard, M. J., Prentice, G., Hoffbrand, A. V., Paxton, A., Bunch, C., and Greaves, M. F., Relation of "lymphoid" phenotype and response to chemotherapy incorporating vincristine-prednisone in the acute phase of Ph' positive leukemia, *Cancer*, 43, 426, 1979.
63. Ritz, J., Pesando, J. M., Notis-McConarty, J., Lazarus, H., and Schlossman, S. F., A monoclonal antibody to human acute lymphoblastic leukemia antigen, *Nature (London)*, 382, 583, 1980.
64. Knapp, W., Majdic, O., Bettelheim, P., and Liska, K., V1L-A1, a monoclonal antibody reactive with common acute leukemia cells, *Leukemia Res.*, 6, 137, 1982.
65. Reinherz, E. L., Kung, P. C., Pesando, J. M., Ritz, J., Goldstein, G., and Schlossman, S. F., Ia determinants on human T cell subsets defined by monoclonal antibody: activation stimuli required for expression, *J. Exp. Med.*, 150, 1472, 1979.
66. Charron, D. J. and McDevitt, H. O., Analysis of HLA-D region associated molecules with monoclonal antibody, *Proc. Natl. Acad. Sci. U.S.A.*, 76, 6567, 1979.
67. Shackelford, D. A. and Strominger, J. L., Demonstration of structural polymorphism among HLA-DR light chains by two-dimensional gel electrophoresis, *J. Exp. Med.*, 151, 144, 1980.

68. Lampson, L. A. and Levy, R., Two populations of Ia-like molecules on a human B cell line, *J. Immunol.*, 125, 293, 1980.
69. Nadler, L. M., Stashenko, P., Hardy, R., Pesando, J. M., Yunis, C. J., and Schlossman, S. F., Monoclonal antibodies defining serologically distinct HLA-D/DR related Ia-like antigens in man, *Hum. Immunol.*, 2, 77, 1981.
70. Griffin, J. D., Ritz, J., Nadler, L. M., and Schlossman, S. F., Expression of myeloid differentiation antigens on normal and malignant myeloid cells, *J. Clin. Invest.*, 68, 932, 1981.
71. Todd, R. F., Nadler, L. M., and Schlossman, S. F., Antigens on human monocytes identified by monoclonal antibodies, *J. Immunol.*, 126, 1435, 1981.
72. Linker-Israeli, M., Billing, R. J., Foon, K. A., Fitchen, J. M., and Terasaki, P. I., Monoclonal antibodies reactive with acute myelogenous leukemia (AML) cells, *Fed. Proc. Fed. Am. Soc. Exp. Biol.*, 40, 1118, 1981.
73. Perussia, B., Lebman, D., Lange, B., Faust, J., Trinchieri, G., and Rovera, G., Expression of lineage-specific surface antigens in human non-lymphocytic leukemia, in *Differentiation of Neoplastic Cells*, Revoltelle, R. and Pontieri, R., Eds., Raven Press, New York, 1981.
74. Bernstein, I. D., Andrews, R. G., Cohen, S. F., and McMaster, B. E., Normal and malignant human myelocytic and monocytic cells identified by monoclonal antibodies, *J. Immunol.*, 128, 876, 1982.
75. Civin, C. I., Mirro, J., and Banquerigo, M. L., MY1, a new myeloid specific antigen identified by a mouse monoclonal antibody, *Blood*, 57, 842, 1981.
75a. Link, M., Warnke, R., Finlay, J., Amylon, M., Miller, R., Dilley, J., and Levy, R., A single monoclonal antibody identifies T-cell lineage of childhood lymphoid malignancies, *Blood*, 62, 722, 1983.
76. Pratt, D. M., Schlossman, S. F., and Strominger, J. L., Human T lymphocyte surface antigens: partial purification and characterization utilizing a high-titer heteroantiserum, *J. Immunol.*, 124: 1449, 1980.
77. Niaudet, P. and Greaves, M., Diversity of cell surface polypeptides that are recognized by heteroantisera to human T cells, *J. Immunol.*, 124, 1203, 1980.
78. Martin, P. J., Giblett, E. R., and Hansen, J. A., Phenotyping human leukemic T-cell lines: enzyme markers, surface antigens, and cytogenetics, *Immunogenetics*, 15, 385, 1982.
79. Minowada, J., Sagawa, K., Trowbridge, I. S., Kung, P. C., and Goldstein, G., Marker profiles of 55 human leukemia-lymphoma cell lines, in *Malignant Lymphomas: Etiology, Immunology, Pathology, Treatment*, Rosenberg, S. A. and Kaplan, H. S., Eds., Academic Press, New York, 1982, 53.
80. Nadler, L. M., Reinherz, E. L., Weinstein, H. J., D'Orsi, C. J., and Schlossman, S. F., Heterogeneity of T lymphoblastic malignancies, *Blood*, 55, 806, 1980.
81. Tosi, R., Tanigaki, N., Center, D., Ferrara, G. B., and Pressman, D., Immunologic dissection of human Ia molecules, *J. Exp. Med.*, 148, 1592, 1978.
82. Markert, M. L. and Cresswell, P., Polymorphism of human B cell alloantigens: evidence for three loci within the HLA system, *Proc. Natl. Acad. Sci. U.S.A.*, 77, 6101, 1980.
83. Uhr, J. W., Capra, J. D., Vitteta, E. S., and Cook, P. G., Organization of the immune response genes, *Science*, 206, 292, 1979.
84. Klein, J., The major histocompatibility complex of the mouse, *Science*, 203, 516, 1979.
85. Schwartz, B. D., Kask, A. M., Paul, W. E., Gerzy, A. F., and Shevach, E. M., The guinea pig I region. I. A structural and genetic analysis, *J. Exp. Med.*, 146, 547, 1977.
86. Casper, J. T., Marrari, M., Piaskowski, V., Lauer, S. J., and Duquesnoy, R. J., Association between HLA-D region antigens and disease-free survival in childhood non-T, non-B acute lymphocytic leukemia, *Blood*, 60, 698, 1982.
87. Schein, P. S., DeVita, V. T., Jr., Hubbard, S., Chabner, B. A., Canellos, G. P., Berard, C., and Young, R. C., Bleomycin, adriamycin, cyclophosphamide, vincristine and prednisone (BACOP) combination chemotherapy in the treatment of advanced diffuse histiocytic lymphoma, *Ann. Int. Med.*, 85, 417, 1976.
88. Armitage, J. O., Dick, F. R., Corder, M. P., Garneau, S. C., Platz, C. E., and Slymen, D. J., Predicting therapeutic outcome in patients with diffuse histiocytic lymphoma treated with cyclophosphamide, adriamycin, vincristine and prednisone (CHOP), *Cancer*, 50, 1695, 1982.
89. Rosenberg, S. A., Current concepts in cancer: non-Hodgkin's lymphoma — selection of treatment on the basis of histologic type, *N. Engl. J. Med.*, 301, 924, 1979.
90. Strauchen, J. A., Young, R. C., DeVita, V. T., Anderson, T., Fatone, J. C., and Berard, C. W., Clinical relevance of the histopathological subclassification of diffuse ''histiocytic'' lymphoma, *N. Engl. J. Med.*, 299, 1382, 1978.
91. Mann, R. B., Jaffe, E. S., and Berard, C. W., Malignant lymphomas — a conceptual understanding of morphologic diversity, *Rev. Am. J. Pathol.*, 94, 104, 1979.
92. Lukes, R. J. and Collins, R. D., Immunologic characterization of human malignant lymphomas, *Cancer*, 34, 1488, 1974.

93. Aisenberg, A. C. and Long, J. C., Lymphocyte surface characteristics in malignant lymphoma, *Am. J. Med.*, 58, 300, 1975.
94. Gajl-Peczalalska, K. J., Bloomfield, C. D., Coccia, P. F., Sosin, H., Brunning, R. D., and Kersey, H. J., B and T cell lymphomas: analysis of blood and lymph nodes in 87 patients, *Am. J. Med.*, 59, 674, 1975.
95. Brouet, J. C., Preud'homme, J. L., Flandrin, G., Cheloul, N., and Seligmann, M., Membrane markers in "histiocytic" lymphomas (reticulum cell sarcoma), *J. Natl. Cancer Inst.*, 56, 631, 1976.
96. Minowada, J., Janossy, G., Greaves, M. F., Tsubota, T., Srivastava, B. I. S., Morikawa, S., and Tatsumi, E., Expression of an antigen associated with acute lymphoblastic leukemia in human leukemia-lymphoma cell lines, *J. Natl. Cancer Inst.*, 60, 1269, 1978.
97. Bloomfield, C. D., Gajl-Peczalska, K. J., Frizzera, G., Kersey, J. H., and Goldman, A., Clinical utility of lymphocyte surface markers combined with the Lukes-Collins histologic classification in adult lymphoma, *N. Engl. J. Med.*, 301, 512, 1979.
98. Habeshaw, J. A., Catley, P. F., Stansfeld, A. G., and Brearley, R. L., Surface phenotyping, histology and the nature of non-Hodgkin's lymphoma in 157 patients, *Br. J. Cancer*, 40, 11, 1979.
99. Murphy, S. B., Melvin, S. L., and Mauer, A. M., Correlation of tumor cell kinetic studies with surface marker results in childhood non-Hodgkin's lymphoma, *Cancer Res.*, 39, 1534, 1979.
100. Warnke, R., Miller, R., Grogan, T., Pederson, M., Dilley, J., and Levy, R., Immunologic phenotype in 30 patients with diffuse large-cell lymphoma, *N. Engl. J. Med.*, 303, 293, 1980.
101. Ritz, J., Nadler, L. M., Bhan, A. K., Notis-McConarty, J., Pesando, J. M., and Schlossman, S. F., Expression of common acute lymphoblastic leukemia antigen (CALLA) by lymphomas of B cell and T cell lineage, *Blood*, 58, 648, 1981.
102. Aisenberg, A. C. and Wilkes, B. M., Lymph node T cells in Hodgkin's disease: analysis of suspensions with monoclonal antibody and rosetting techniques, *Blood*, 59, 522, 1982.
103. Bernard, A., Murphy, S. B., Melvin, S., Bowman, P., Cailland, J., Lemerle, J., and Boumsell, L., Non-T, non-B lymphomas are rare in childhood and associated with cutaneous tumor, *Blood*, 59, 549, 1982.
104. Fialkow, P. J., Clonal origin of human tumors, *Biochim. Biophys. Acta*, 458, 283, 1976.
105. Fialkow, P. J., Jacobson, R. J., and Papayannopoulou, T., Chronic myelocytic leukemia: a clonal origin in a stem cell common to the granulocyte, erythrocyte, platelet and monocyte/macrophage, *Am. J. Med.*, 63, 125, 1977.
106. Salsano, F., Froland, S. S., Natvig, J. B., and Michaelson, T. E., Same idiotype of B-lymphocyte membrane IgD and IgM. Formal evidence for monoclonality of chronic lymphocyte leukemia cells, *Scand. J. Immunol.*, 3, 841, 1974.
107. Schroer, K. R., Briles, D. E., van Boxel, J. A., and Davie, J. M., Idiotypic uniformity of cell surface immunoglobulin in chronic lymphocytic leukemia: evidence for monoclonal proliferation, *J. Exp. Med.*, 140, 1416, 1974.
108. Fu, S. M., Winchester, R. J., Feizi, T., Walzer, P. D., and Kunkel, H. G., Idiotypic specificity of surface immunoglobulin and the maturation of leukemic bone-marrow-derived lymphocytes, *Proc. Natl. Acad. Sci. U.S.A.*, 71, 4487, 1974.
109. Aisenberg, A. C. and Bloch, K. J., Immunoglobulins on the surface of neoplastic lymphocytes, *N. Engl. J. Med.*, 287, 272, 1972.
110. Bach, M.-A., and Bach, J.-F., The use of monoclonal anti-T cell antibodies to study T cell imbalances in human diseases, *Clin. Exp. Immunol.*, 45, 449, 1981.
111. Strelkauskas, A. J., Schauf, V., Wilson, B. S., Chess, L., and Schlossman, S. F., Isolation and characterization of naturally occurring subclasses of human peripheral blood T cells with regulatory functions, *J. Immunol.*, 120, 1278, 1978.
112. Cantor, H. and Boyse, E. A., Functional subclasses of T lymphocytes bearing different Ly antigens. I. The generation of functionally distinct T cell subclasses is a differentiative process independent of antigen, *J. Exp. Med.*, 141, 1376, 1975.
113. Reinherz, E. L., Nadler, L. M., Sallan, S. E., and Schlossman, S. F., Subset derivation of T cell acute lymphoblastic leukemia in man, *J. Clin. Invest.*, 64, 392, 1979.
114. Kung, P. C., Goldstein, G., Reinherz, E. L., and Schlossman, S. F., Monoclonal antibodies defining distinctive human T cell surface antigens, *Science*, 206, 347, 1979.
115. Levy, R., Dilley, J., Fox, R. I., and Wernke, R., A human thymus-leukemia antigen defined by hybridoma monoclonal antibodies, *Proc. Natl. Acad. Sci. U.S.A.*, 76, 6552, 1979.
116. Royston, I., Majda, J. A., Baird, S. M., Meserve, B. L., and Griffiths, J. C., Human T cell antigens defined by monoclonal antibodies: the 65,000 dalton antigen on T cells (T65) is also found on chronic lymphocytic leukemia cells bearing surface immunoglobulin, *J. Immunol.*, 125, 725, 1980.
117. McMichael, A. J., Pilch, J. R., Galfre, G., Mason, D. Y., Fabre, J. W., and Milstein, C., A human thymocyte antigen defined by a hybrid myeloma monoclonal antibody, *Eur. J. Immunol.*, 9, 205, 1979.

118. Hansen, J. A., Martin, P. J., and Nowinski, R. C., Monoclonal antibodies identifying a novel T-cell antigen and Ia antigens of human lymphocytes, *Immunogenetics*, 10, 247, 1980.
119. Reinherz, E. L., Kung, P. C., Goldstein, G., and Schlossman, S. F., A monoclonal antibody reactive with the human cytotoxic/suppressor T cell subset previously defined by a heteroantiserum termed TH2, *J. Immunol.*, 124, 1301, 1980.
120. Kamoun, M., Martin, P. J., Hansen, J. A., Brown, M. A., Siadak, A. W., and Nowinski, R. C., Identification of a human T lymphocyte surface protein associated with the E-rosette receptor, *J. Exp. Med.*, 153, 207, 1981.
121. Ledbetter, J. A., Evans, R. L., Lipinski, M., Cunningham-Rundles, C., Good, R. A., and Herzenberg, L. A., Evolutionary conservation of surface molecules that distinguish T lymphocyte helper/inducer and cytotoxic/suppressor subpopulations in mouse and man, *J. Exp. Med.*, 153, 310, 1981.
122. Greaves, M., Delia, D., Sutherland, R., Rao, J., Verbi, W., Kemshead, J., Hariri, G., Goldstein, G., and Kung, P., Expression of the OKT monoclonal antibody defined antigenic determinants in malignancy, *Int. J. Immunopharmacol.*, 3, 283, 1981.
123. Evans, R. L., Wall, D. W., Platsoucas, C. D., Siegal, F. P., Fikrig, S. M., Testa, C. M., and Good, R. A., Thymus-dependent membrane antigens in man: inhibition of cell-mediated lympholysis by monoclonal antibodies to the $TH_2$ antigen, *Proc. Natl. Acad. Sci. U.S.A.*, 78, 544, 1981.
124. Fox, R., Baird, S., Kung, P., Levy, R., and Royston, I., Lymphoid cell surface antigens on human cells, in *Differentiation Antigens of Lymphocytes*, Warner, N., Ed., Academic Press, New York, in press.
125. Engleman, E. G., Warnke, R., Fox, R. I., and Levy, R., Studies on a human T lymphocyte antigen recognized by a monoclonal antibody, *Proc. Natl. Acad. Sci. U.S.A.*, 78, 1791, 1981.
126. Fox, R. I., Harlow, D., Royston, I., and Elder, J., Structural characterization of the human T cell surface antigen (p67) isolated from normal and neoplastic lymphocytes, *J. Immunol.*, 129, 401, 1982.
127. Reinherz, E. L., Kung, P. C., Goldstein, G., Levy, R. H., and Schlossman, S. F., Discrete stages of human intrathymic differentiation: analysis of normal thymocytes and leukemic lymphoblasts of T lineage, *Proc. Natl. Acad. Sci. U.S.A.*, 77, 1588, 1980.
128. Reinherz, E. L. and Schlossman, S. F., The differentiation and function of human T lymphocytes: a review, *Cell*, 19, 821, 1980.
129. Foon, K. A., Billing, R. J., Terasaki, P. I., and Cline, M. J., Immunologic classification of acute lymphoblastic leukemia: implications for normal lymphoid differentiation, *Blood*, 56, 1120, 1980.
130. Koziner, B., Gebhard, D., Denny, T., McKenzie, S., Clarkson, B. D., Miller, D. A., and Evans, R. L., Analysis of T-cell differentiation antigens in acute lymphocytic leukemia using monoclonal antibodies, *Blood*, 60, 752, 1982.
131. Bernard, A., Boumsell, L., Reinherz, E. L., Nadler, L. M., Ritz, J., Coppin, H., Richard, Y., Valensi, F. M., Dausset, J., Flandrin, G., Lemerle, J., and Schlossman, S. F., Cell surface characterization of malignant T cells from lymphoblastic lymphoma using monoclonal antibodies, *Blood*, 57, 1105, 1981.
132. Boumsell, L., Bernard, A., Reinherz, E. L., Nadler, L. M., Ritz, J., Coppin, H., Richard, Y., Dubertret, L., Degos, L., Lemerle, J., Flandrin, G., Dausset, J., and Schlossman, S. F., Surface antigens on malignant Sezary and T cell CLL cells correspond to those of mature T cells, *Blood*, 57, 526, 1981.
133. Haynes, B. F., Metzgar, R. S., Minna, J. D., and Bunn, P. A., Phenotypic characterization of cutaneous T-cell lymphoma, *N. Engl. J. Med.*, 304, 1319, 1981.
134. Kung, P. C., Berger, C. L., Goldstein, G., LoGerfo, P., and Edelson, R. L., Cutaneous T cell lymphoma: characterization by monoclonal antibodies, *Blood*, 57, 261, 1981.
135. Wood, G. S., Deneau, D. G., Miller, R. A., Levy, R., Hoppe, R. T., and Wernke, R. A., Subtypes of cutaneous T-cell lymphoma defined by expression of Leu-1 and Ia, *Blood*, 59, 876, 1982.
136. Gathings, W. E., Lawton, A. R., and Cooper, M. D., Immunofluorescent studies of the development of pre-B cells, B lymphocytes and immunoglobulin isotype diversity in humans, *Eur. J. Immunol.*, 7, 804, 1977.
137. Nilsson, K. and Ponten, J., Classification and biological nature of established human hematopoietic cell lines, *Int. J. Cancer*, 15, 321, 1975.
138. Vitetta, E. S., Melcher, U., McWilliams, M., Lamm, M. E., Phillips-Quagliata, J. M., and Uhr, J. W., Cell surface immunoglobulin. XI. The appearance of an IgD-like molecule on murine lymphoid cells during ontogeny, *J. Exp. Med.*, 141, 206, 1975.
139. Stashenko, P., Nadler, L. M., Hardy, R., and Schlossman, S. F., Characterization of a human B lymphocyte specific antigen, *J. Immunol.*, 125, 1678, 1980.
140. Nadler, L. M., Stashenko, P., Ritz, J., Hardy, R., Pesando, J. M., and Schlossman, S. F., A unique cell surface antigen identifying lymphoid malignancies of B cell origin, *J. Clin. Invest.*, 67, 134, 1981.

141. Vogler, L. B., Crist, W. M., Bockman, D. E., Pearl, E. R., Lawton, A. R., and Cooper, M. D., Pre-B-cell leukemia: a new phenotype of childhood lymphoblastic leukemia, *N. Engl. J. Med.*, 298, 872, 1978.
141a. Korsmeyer, S. J., Arnold, A., Bakhshi, A., Ravetch, J. V., Siebenlist, U., Hieter, P. A., Sharrow, S. O. LeBien, T., Kersey, J. H., Poplack, D. G., Leder, P., and Waldmann, T. A., Immunoglobulin gene rearrangement and cell surface antigen expression in acute lymphocytic leukemias of T cell and B cell precursor origins, *J. Clin. Invest.*, 71, 301, 1983.
142. Nadler, L. M., Stashenko, P., Hardy, R., van Angthoven, A., Terhorst, C., and Schlossman, S. F., Characterization of a human B cell specific antigen (B2) distinct from B1, *J. Immunol.*, 126, 1941, 1981.
143. Klein, G., The role of Epstein-Barr virus in the etiology of Burkitt's lymphoma and nasopharyngeal carcinoma, in *Malignant Lymphomas: Etiology, Immunology, Pathology, Treatment*, Rosenberg, S. A. and Kaplan, H. S., Eds., Academic Press, New York, 1982, 155.
144. Fu, S. M., Winchester, R. J., and Kunkel, H. G., Occurrence of surface IgM, IgD, and free light chains on human lymphocytes, *J. Exp. Med.*, 139, 451, 1974.
145. Bramwell, M. E. and Harris, H., An abnormal membrane glycoprotein associated with malignancy, *Proc. R. Soc. London B*, 201, 87, 1978.
146. Brown, G., Hogg, N., and Greaves, M. F., Candidate leukemia-specific antigen in man, *Nature (London)*, 258, 454, 1975.
147. Greaves, M., Delia, D., Janossy, G., Rapson, N., Chessells, J., Woods, M., and Prentice, G., Acute lymphoblastic leukemia associated antigen. IV. Expression on non-leukemic 'lymphoid' cells, *Leukemia Res.*, 4, 15, 1980.
148. Janossy, G., Bollum, F. J., Bradstock, K. F., McMichael, A., Rapson, N., and Greaves, M. F., Terminal transferase-positive human bone marrow cells exhibit the antigenic phenotype of common acute lymphoblastic leukemia, *J. Immunol.*, 123, 1525, 1979.
149. Jager, G., Lau, B., and Dormer, P., Induction to cALL antigen and terminal deoxynucleotidyl transferase in normal peripheral lymphocytes during PHA stimulation, *Leukemia Res.*, 6, 421, 1982.
150. Metzgar, R. S., Borowitz, M. J., Jones, N. H., and Dowell, B. L., Distribution of a common acute lymphoblastic leukemia antigen in nonhematopoietic tissues, *J. Exp. Med.*, 154, 1249, 1981.
151. Reisfeld, R. A., Monoclonal antibodies to human malignant melanoma, *Nature (London)*, 298, 325, 1982.
152. Pierce, G. B. and Johnson, L. D., Differentiation and cancer, *In Vitro*, 7, 140, 1971.
153. Stehelin, D., Varmus, H. E., Bishop, J. M., and Vogt, P. K., DNA related to the transforming gene(s) of avian sarcoma viruses is present in normal avian DNA, *Nature (London)*, 260, 170, 1976.
154. Spector, D. H., Varmus, H. E., and Bishop, J. M., Nucleotide sequences related to the transforming gene of avian sarcoma virus are present in DNA of uninfected vertebrates, *Proc. Natl. Acad. Sci. U.S.A.*, 75, 4102, 1978.
155. Hayward, W. S., Neel, B. G., and Astrin, S. M., Activation of a cellular oncogene by promoter insertion in ALV-induced lymphoid leukosis, *Nature (London)*, 290, 475, 1981.
156. Klein, G., The role of gene dosage and genetic transpositions in carcinogenesis, *Nature (London)*, 294, 313, 1981.
157. Rowley, J. D., Identification of the constant chromosome regions involved in human hematologic malignant disease, *Science*, 216, 749, 1982.
158. Pesando, J. M., Ritz, J., Levine, H., Terhorst, C., Lazarus, H., and Schlossman, S. F., Human leukemia-associated antigen: relation to a family of surface glycoproteins, *J. Immunol.*, 124, 2794, 1980.
159. Newman, R. A., Sutherland, R., and Greaves, M. F., The biochemical characterization of a cell surface antigen associated with acute lymphoblastic leukemia and lymphocyte precursors, *J. Immunol.*, 126, 2024, 1981.
160. Pesando, J. M., Tomaselli, K. J., Lazarus, H., and Schlossman, S. F., Distribution and modulation of a human leukemia-associated antigen (CALLA), *J. Immunol.*, 131, 2038, 1983.
161. Fisher, R. I., Kubota, T. T., Mandell, G. L., Broder, S., and Young, R. C., Regression of a T cell lymphoma after administration of anti-thymocyte globulin, *Ann. Int. Med.*, 88, 799, 1978.
162. Currie, G. A., Eighty years of immunotherapy: a review of immunobiological methods used for the treatment of human cancer, *Br. J. Cancer*, 26, 141, 1972.
163. Rosenberg, S. A. and Terry, W. D., Passive immunotherapy of cancer in animals and man, *Adv. Cancer Res.*, 25, 323, 1977.
164. Young, W. W. and Hakomori, S. I., Therapy of mouse lymphoma with monoclonal antibodies to glycolipid: selection of low antigenic variants in vivo, *Science*, 211, 487, 1981.
165. Bernstein, I. D., Tam, M. R., and Nowinski, R. C., Mouse leukemia: therapy with monoclonal antibodies against a thymus differentiation antigen, *Science*, 207, 68, 1980.
166. Miller, R. A., Maloney, D. G., Warnke, R., and Levy, R., Treatment of B-cell lymphoma with monoclonal anti-idiotype antibody, *N. Engl. J. Med.*, 306, 517, 1982.

166a. Meeker, T. C., Maloney, D. G., Theilemans, K., Miller, R. A., Lowder, J., and Levy, R., Anti-idiotype monoclonal antibody therapy of human B lymphocyte malignancy, *Blood*, 62, 214a, 1983 (abstr.).
167. Nadler, L. M., Stashenko, P., Hardy, R., Kaplan, W. D., Button, L. N., Kufe, D. W., Antman, K. H., and Schlossman, S. F., Serotherapy of a patient with a monoclonal antibody directed against a human lymphoma-associated antigen, *Cancer Res.*, 40, 3147, 1980.
168. Ritz, J., Pesando, J. M., Sallan, S. E., Clavell, L. A., Notis-McConarty, J., Rosenthal, P., and Schlossman, S. F., Serotherapy of acute lymphoblastic leukemia with monoclonal antibody, *Blood*, 58, 141, 1981.
169. Dillman, R. O., Shawler, D. L., Sobol, R. E., Collins, H. A., Beauregard, J. C., Wormsley, S. B., and Royston, I., Murine monoclonal antibody therapy in two patients with chronic lymphocytic leukemia, *Blood*, 59, 1036, 1982.
170. Miller, R. A., Maloney, D. G., McKillop, J., and Levy, R., In vivo effects of murine hybridoma monoclonal antibody in a patient with T-cell leukemia, *Blood*, 58, 78, 1981.
171. Miller, R. A. and Levy, R., Response of cutaneous T cell lymphoma to therapy with hybridoma monoclonal antibody, *Lancet*, 2, 226, 1981.
172. Lanier, L. L., Babcock, G. F., Raybourne, R. B., Arnold, L. W., Warner, N. L., and Haughton, G., Mechanism of B cell lymphoma immunotherapy with passive xenogeneic anti-idiotype serum, *J. Immunol.*, 125, 1730, 1980.
173. Ritz, J., Pesando, J. M., Notis-McConarty, J., and Schlossman, S. F., Modulation of human acute lymphoblastic leukemia antigen induced by monoclonal antibody in vitro, *J. Immunol.*, 125, 1506, 1980.
174. Boyse, E. A., Stockert, E., and Old, L. J., Modification of the antigenic structure of the cell membrane by thymus-leukemia (TL) antibody, *Proc. Natl. Acad. Sci. U.S.A.*, 58, 954, 1967.
175. Old, L. J., Stockert, E., Boyse, E. A., and Kim, J. H., Antigenic modulation: loss of TL antigens from cells exposed to TL antibody. Study of the phenomenon in vitro, *J. Exp. Med.*, 127, 523, 1968.
176. Taylor, R. B., Duffus, W. P. H., Raff, M. C., and dePetris, S., Redistribution and pinocytosis of lymphocyte surface immunoglobulin molecules induced by anti-immunoglobulin antibody, *Nature (London) New Biol.*, 233, 225, 1971.
177. Unanue, E. R., Perkins, W. D., and Karnovsky, M. J., Endocytosis by lymphocytes of complexes of anti-Ig with membrane-bound Ig, *J. Immunol.*, 108, 569, 1972.
178. Stackpole, C. W., Jacobsen, J. B., and Landis, M. P., Antigenic modulation in vitro. I. Fate of thymus-leukemia (TL) antigen-antibody complexes following modulation of TL antigenicity from the surfaces of mouse leukemia cells and thymocytes, *J. Exp. Med.*, 140, 939, 1974.
179. Joseph, B. S. and Oldstone, M. B. A., Immunologic injury in measles virus infection. II. Suppression of immune injury through antigenic modulation, *J. Exp. Med.*, 142, 864, 1975.
180. Calafat, J., Hilgers, J., van Blitterswijk, W. J., Verbeet, M., and Hageman, P. C., Antibody-induced modulation and shedding of mammary tumor virus antigens on the surfaces of GR ascites leukemia cells as compared with normal antigens, *J. Natl. Cancer Inst.*, 56, 1019, 1976.
181. van Blitterswijk, W. J., Hilgers, J., Feltkemp, C. A., and Emmelot, P., Mammary tumor virus expression and dynamics in the cell surface, in *Mammary Tumors in the Mouse*, Hilgers, J. and Sluyser, T., Eds., Biomedical Press, New York, 1981, 574.
182. Pesando, J. M. and Conrad, T. A., Nonhuman primates express human leukemia-associated antigens, *Blood*, in press.
183. Raso, V., Ritz, J., Basala, M., and Schlossman, S. F., Monoclonal antibody-ricin A chain conjugate selectively cytotoxic for cells bearing the common acute lymphoblastic leukemia antigen, *Cancer Res.*, 42, 457, 1982.
184. Olsson, L., Kiger, N., and Kronstom, H., Sensitivity of cloned high-metastatic and low-metastatic murine Lewis lung-tumor cells to lysis by cytotoxic autoreactive cells, *Cancer Res.*, 41, 4706, 1981.
185. Prehn, R. T., Analysis of antigenic heterogeneity within individual 3-methylcholanthrene-induced mouse sarcomas, *J. Natl. Cancer Inst.*, 45, 1039, 1970.
186. Olsson, L. and Ebbesen, P., Natural polyclonality of spontaneous AKR leukemia and its consequences for so-called specific immunotherapy, *J. Natl. Cancer Inst.*, 62, 623, 1979.
187. Talmadge, J. E., Wolman, S. R., and Fidler, I. J., Evidence for the clonal origin of spontaneous metastases, *Science*, 217, 361, 1982.
188. Yeh, M. Y., Hellström, I., and Hellström, K. E., Clonal variation in expression of a human melanoma antigen defined by a monoclonal antibody, *J. Immunol.*, 126, 1312, 1981.
189. Janossy, G., Roberts, M., and Greaves, M. F., Target cell in chronic myeloid leukemia and its relationship to acute lymphoid leukemia, *Lancet*, 2, 1058, 1976.
190. Prchal, J. T., Throckmorton, D. W., Carroll, A. J., Fuson, E. W., Gams, R. A., and Prchal, J. F., A common progenitor for human myeloid and lymphoid cells, *Nature (London)*, 274, 590, 1978.
191. Martin, P. J., Najfeld, V., Hansen, J. A., Penfold, G. K., Jacobson, R. J., and Fialkow, P. J., Involvement of the B lymphoid system in chronic myelogenous leukemia, *Nature (London)*, 287, 49, 1980.

192. Thomas, E. D. and Storb, R., Technique for human marrow grafting, *Blood,* 36, 507, 1970.
193. Fefer, A., Cheever, M. A., Thomas, E. D., Appelbaum, F. R., Buckner, C. D., Clift, R. A., Glucksberg, H., Greenberg, P. D., Johnson, F. L., Kaplan, H. G., Sanders, J. E., Storb, R., and Weiden, P. L., Bone marrow transplantation for refractory acute leukemia in 34 patients with identical twins, *Blood,* 57, 421, 1981.
194. Johnson, F. L., Thomas, E. D., Clark, B. S., Chard, R. L., Hartman, J. R., and Storb, R., A comparison of marrow transplantation with chemotherapy for children with acute lymphoblastic leukemia in second or subsequent remission, *N. Engl. J. Med.,* 305, 846, 1981.
195. Thomas, E. D., Sanders, J. E., Fluornoy, N., Johnson, F. L., Buckner, C. D., Clift, R. A., Fefer, A., Goodell, B. W., Storb, R., and Weiden, P. L., Marrow transplantation for patients with acute lymphoblastic leukemia in remission, *Blood,* 54, 468, 1979.
196. Thomas, E. D., The role of marrow transplantation in the eradication of malignant disease, *Cancer,* 49, 1963, 1982.
197. Herzig, G. P., Autologous marrow transplantation in cancer therapy, in *Progress in Hematology,* Vol. 12, Brown, E. B., Ed., Grune & Stratton, New York, 1981, 1.
198. Feeney, M., Knapp, R. C., Greenberger, J. S., and Bast, R. C., Elimination of leukemic cells from rat bone marrow using antibody and complement, *Cancer Res.,* 41, 3331, 1981.
199. Ritz, J., Sallan, S. E., Bast, R. C., Lipton, J. M., Clavell, L. A., Feeney, M., Hercend, T., Nathan, D. G., and Schlossman, S. F., Autologous bone marrow transplantation in CALLA-positive acute lymphoblastic leukemia after in vitro treatment with J5 monoclonal antibody and complement, *Lancet,* 2, 60, 1982.
200. Weiden, P. L., Fluornoy, N., Thomas, E. D., Prentice, R., Fefer, A., Buckner, C. D., and Storb, R., Antileukemic effect of graft-versus-host disease in human recipients of allogeneic-marrow grafts, *N. Engl. J. Med.,* 300, 1068, 1979.
201. Appelbaum, F. R., Herzig, G., Graw, R. G., and Ziegler, J., Accelerated hemopoietic recovery following the infusion of cryopreserved autologous bone marrow in humans, *Exp. Hematol.,* 7, (Suppl. 5), 297, 1979.
201a. Stewart, P., Buckner, D., Bensinger, B. W., Appelbaum, F., Fefer, A., Clift, R. A., Storb, R., Sanders, J., Meyers, J., Hill, R., and Thomas, E. D., Autologous marrow transplant in patients with acute nonlymphocyte leukemia in firt remission, *Exp. Hematol.,* in press.
202. Janossy, G., Francis, G., Capellaro, D., Goldstone, A. H., and Greaves, M. F., Cell sorter analysis of leukemia-associated antigens on human myeloid precursors, *Nature (London),* 276, 176, 1978.
203. Clavell, L. A., Lipton, J. M., Bast, R. C., Kudisch, M., Pesando, J. M., Schlossman, S. F., and Ritz, J., Absence of common ALL antigen on normal bipotent myeloid, erythroid and granulocyte progenitors, *Blood,* 58, 333, 1981.
204. Olsnes, S. and Pihl, A., Chimaeric toxins, in *Pharmacology of Bacterial Toxins,* Drews, J. and Dorner, F., Eds., Pergamon Press, New York, in press.
205. Olsnes, S. and Pihl, A., Chimeric toxins, *Pharmacol. Ther.,* 15, 355, 1981.
206. Olsnes, S. and Pihl, A., Toxic lectins and related proteins, in *The Molecular Actions of Toxins and Viruses,* Cohen, P. L. and van Heyningen, S., Eds., Elsevier, Amsterdam, in press.
207. Ghose, T., Antibody-linked cytotoxic agents in the treatment of cancer: current status and future prospects, *J. Natl. Cancer Inst.,* 61, 657, 1978.
208. Gregoriadis, G., Targeting of drugs, *Nature (London),* 265, 407, 1977.
209. Masuho, Y., Hara, T., and Noguchi, T., Preparation of a hybrid of fragment Fab' of antibody and fragment A of diphtheria toxin and its cytotoxicity, *Biochem. Biophys. Res. Commun.,* 90, 320, 1979.
210. Raso, V. and Griffin, T., Specific cytotoxicity of a human immunoglobulin-directed FAB'-ricin A chain conjugate, *J. Immunol.,* 125, 2610, 1980.
211. Gilliland, D. G., Steplewski, Z., Collier, R. J., Mitchell, K. F., Chang, T. H., and Koprowski, H., Antibody-directed cytotoxic agents: use of monoclonal antibody to direct the action of toxin A chains to colorectal carcinoma cells, *Proc. Natl. Acad. Sci. U.S.A.,* 77, 4539, 1980.
212. Krolick, K. A., Villemez, C., Isakson, P., Uhr, J. W., and Vitetta, E. S., Selective killing of normal or neoplastic B cells by antibodies coupled to the A chain of ricin, *Proc. Natl. Acad. Sci., U.S.A.,* 77, 5419, 1980.
213. Blythman, H. E., Casellas, P., Gros, O., Gros, P., Jansen, F. K., Paolucci, F., Pau, B., and Vidal, H., Immunotoxins: hybrid molecules of monoclonal antibodies and a toxin subunit specifically kill tumor cells, *Nature (London),* 290, 145, 1981.
214. Olsnes, S., Directing toxins to cancer cells, *Nature (London)*, 290, 84, 1981.
215. Trowbridge, I. S. and Domingo, D. L., Anti-transferrin receptor monoclonal antibody and toxin-antibody conjugates affect growth of human tumour cells, *Nature (London),* 294, 171, 1981.
216. Coffino, P., Baumal, R., Laskov, R., and Scharff, M. D., Cloning of mouse myeloma cells and detection of rare variants, *J. Cell. Physiol.,* 79, 429, 1972.
217. Kearney, J. F., Radbruch, A., Liesegang, B., and Rajewsky, K., A new mouse myeloma line which has lost immunoglobulin expression but permits the construction of antibody secreting hybrid cell lines, *J. Immunol.,* 123, 1548, 1979.

218. Shulman, M., Wilde, C. D., and Kohler, G., A better cell line for making hybridomas secreting specific antibodies, *Nature (London)*, 276, 269, 1978.
219. Pesando, J. M., unpublished observations.

Chapter 6

# THE SPECTRUM OF T CELL NEOPLASMS

David T. Rowlands, Jr. and Peter C. Nowell

## TABLE OF CONTENTS

| | | |
|---|---|---|
| I. | Introduction | 134 |
| II. | Identification, Enumeration, and Functional Markers of T Cells | 134 |
| III. | Development of T Cells | 136 |
| IV. | Functions of T Cell Antigens | 137 |
| V. | Monoclonal Antibodies in Human Disorders | 138 |
| VI. | Phenotyping Lymphomas and Leukemias | 138 |
| VII. | Classification of T Cell Neoplasms | 139 |
| | A. Cutaneous T Cell Lymphomas (Skin-Related Neoplasms) | 140 |
| |     1. Mycosis Fungoides | 140 |
| |     2. Sézary's Syndrome | 141 |
| |     3. Other | 142 |
| |     4. Natural History of CLCL | 143 |
| | B. Acute Lymphoblastic Leukemia | 144 |
| | C. Adult T Cell Leukemia (Japanese Experience) | 144 |
| | D. Chronic Lymphocytic Leukemia | 145 |
| | E. Chronic Lymphocytic Leukemia of T Cell Origin | 146 |
| | F. Immunoblastic Lymphadenopathy | 146 |
| | G. Lymphomas | 147 |
| VIII. | Discussion and Conclusions | 147 |
| References | | 148 |

## I. INTRODUCTION

The panoply of T cell leukemias and lymphomas is only now being recognized. Our state of knowledge is still sufficiently primitive that a classification acceptable to morphologists, biologists, and therapists is not at hand. In searching for a useful understanding of these tumors it will be necessary to consider the development and interrelationships of T cells with other mononuclear cells as well as identifying the methods currently used for identification and enumeration of lymphocyte populations.

The modern concept that lymphoid tissues are heterogeneous is barely two decades old; having its origins in the reports of Good[1] and Miller.[2] They, working independently, showed that removal of the thymus from very young mice resulted in defective development of lymphoid tissues in other organs with failure of these animals to display cellular immunity. The studies were initially interpreted as showing equally deficient humoral immunity but later research initiated by Glick[3] demonstrated control of humoral immunity by other parts of what has come to be known as central lymphoid tissues.

An improved understanding of the relationship of T cells to humoral immunity was established by Claman and associates.[4] Both thymic and bone marrow cells were found necessary to reconstitute the immune system of sublethally irradiated mice. Bone marrow cells were responsible for synthesis of immunoglobulins and T cells were necessary for expression of the humoral immune response to most antigens. It has since been recognized that monocytes are required for the full functioning of T cells. Other investigators amplified the concept of cellular cooperation by showing that T cells have multiple functions in the humoral immune response. Some subpopulations of T cells aid the humoral immune response while other subpopulations of T cells suppress it. Adding support to the interpretation of the experimental results in mice, was recognition that deficiencies of immunity in humans could be associated with specific defects in development of their lymphoid tissues. The earliest of these descriptions was that of Bruton's agammaglobulinemia relating to B cells.[5] Subsequently, the work of DiGeorge showed that defects in thymic development (T cells) could be observed in humans.[6]

Following these observations a great deal of effort has gone into the study of those mechanisms by which T cells act either in cellular immunity or as modulators in humoral immunity. A growing number of lymphokines have been described which help to account for the attraction of lymphoid cells and macrophages to sites of inflammation, their maintenance and activation in these sites, and have direct effects on the vasculature.[7] More significant from our point of view, was the discovery that various of the lymphocyte subpopulations had cell surface markers permitting their enumeration. Several such groups of cells correspond to T cells having discrete functions (e.g., helper and suppressor/cytotoxic).

## II. IDENTIFICATION, ENUMERATION, AND FUNCTIONAL MARKERS OF T CELLS

Proper interpretation of data relevant to lymphocyte subpopulations depends on an appreciation of the technical limitations of available methods for isolating and characterizing subpopulations of lymphocytes. A two-step process is generally required. The first, separation, depends on the size or density of the cell or on cell surface properties determining binding of cells to foreign materials such as glass, plastic, or lectins. The second process relies on cell surface characteristics which are distinctive for the cell population under study. Often a substance (e.g., sheep red blood cells, specific antibodies) can be used having the capacity to bind with a subset of lymphocytes.

Isolation of lymphocytes is now most often done by density gradient centrifugation using the Ficoll® -Hypaque technique.[8,9] Blood collected in heparin free of preservatives is diluted 1:3 with a balanced salt solution and the cells are placed in a Ficoll® - Hypaque gradient. After centrifugation lymphoid cells are harvested from the interface of the gradient and then washed in calcium-free saline.

It should be anticipated that 90% of the cells applied to gradients will be recovered. Either faulty technique in recovery of cells at the gradient interface or improper washing accounts for lesser recoveries. This and other separation techniques have been developed using peripheral blood obtained from normal subjects. The techniques are generally applicable to separation of leukemic cells and cells from single-cell suspensions of solid lymphoid tissues or tumors.

Monocytes may make up as much as 40% of the mononuclear cells recovered from the gradients when peripheral blood is the starting material. Because there are C3 and Fc receptors on monocytes, these cells may be expected to cause difficulty in estimating B cells among the lymphocytes, but monocytes are less likely to cause significant errors in estimates of T cells. Should there be concern about monocytes one may choose to attempt their removal or to correct for their presence.

Enumeration of T cells may be done by formation of rosettes with sheep erythrocytes (Srbc). These rosettes, designated as E rosettes, provide a good, inexpensive measure of total T cells. Washed mononuclear cells are mixed with a 1% suspension of Srbc with best results being when the ratio of Srbc to lymphocytes is 50: to 100:1. The tube is then placed at 4° C for 16 or more hr. Cells resuspended from the pellet which forms are pipetted into a hemocytometer and the ratio of rosetting cells to total mononuclear cells is calculated. Normal values of E rosetting cells in the peripheral blood varies from 60 to 80% of mononuclear cells depending on the laboratory.

The availability of an array of anti-T cell sera has begun to revolutionize laboratory methodology permitting more precise identification of an increasing number of T cell subsets as well as the total T cell population. Development of cellular hybridization (hybridomas) and consequent generation of monoclonal antibodies has been especially helpful in the study of T cells. The reagents must be carefully titered prior to use, with optimal activity being most often obtained at a dilution of 1:50. An equal volume of antiserum is incubated with 50 $\mu\ell$ of lymphocytes at a concentration of cells of 5 × $10^6/m\ell$ for 30 min at 4° C after which the cells are washed two times in PBS. Appropriately fluoresceinated antibodies specific for mouse immunoglobulins are then added in a volume of 100 $\mu\ell$ at a dilution of 1:20. The stained cells are washed again after incubation at 4° C for 30 min.

These cells may be analyzed using a fluorescence microscope. The intensity of staining is often relatively low so that more accurate and rapidly available results can be expected using a commercially available apparatus for flowcytometry.[10] Several are sufficiently sophisticated to permit sorting of labeled cells.

The repertoire of antisera is increasing rapidly. Those specific for various stages of maturation will be described in a later section, but two deserve specific comment at this time. The T11 antiserum (Ortho®) reacts with all T cells and values obtained with this reagent compare favorably with results using the E-rosetting technique. The T11 antiserum seems to recognize the srbc receptor. The second antiserum deserving comment is that against Ia antigens. Although these antigens are most obvious on B cells, monocytes, and endothelial cells, they can be found on certain "activated" T cells.

It has been clearly recognized that Fc receptors appear characteristically on B cells and monocytes. It was observed that such receptors may also appear on activated T cells and that the receptors for particular Fc components of immunoglobulins correlate, to some degree, with helper and suppressor T cell activities. More recently T cells with Ig receptors have been largely discarded for such identification. This in large part reflects the transient and hence unreliable nature of such receptors as well as the obvious fact that monoclonal antibodies may well detect more meaningful antigens for the specific identification of functional T cell subsets.

When dealing with tumor masses of T cells whether in skin, lymph nodes, thymus, or spleen, other techniques are required. In some instances, the masses can be minced and single-cell preparations be made. Enumeration of subpopulations of lymphocytes can then be carried out exactly as outlined above. In other cases identification of subsets of lymphocytes within intact lymphoid tissues is desired. Adaptations of rosetting techniques on frozen sections may be useful in some cases.[11] However, more sophisticated technology using immunoperoxidase or biotin-avidin complexes[12] may better serve the investigator. This is especially true in cutaneous T cell lymphomas (CTCL) and in lymphomas made up of heterogeneous cell populations.

## III. DEVELOPMENT OF T CELLS

As has been mentioned and will become increasingly evident in this discussion, a satisfactory classification of T cell tumors is not at hand. However, those studies which are available suggest that ultimately a classification will evolve based on the stages of normal differentiation of the lymphoid system. It is, therefore, pertinent to consider differentiation of T cells in some detail.

Although appearing first as an epithelial organ, the thymus is soon the seat of proliferation of abundant cells recognized readily as lymphocytes. These lymphocytes are presumed to originate as "prothymocytes" in the bone marrow, but processing in the thymus is required to permit full expression of their functional capacities. Peripheralization of lymphocytes into other centers (e.g., lymph nodes) and formation of clearly defined thymic cortex and medulla are relatively late embryologic developments. The relationship between parturition and development of the thymus as well as the peripheral distribution of lymphocytes is inconstant, varying significantly from species to species. In some (e.g., certain strains of mice), the process is late, becoming evident only after birth but in others (e.g., guinea pigs) peripheral migration of lymphocytes precedes parturition. The situation in man is like the latter case, with lymph nodes being evident at the time of birth. The relationship between epithelial elements of the thymus and its lymphocytes is not fully clarified. That epithelial cells are required for maturation of lymphocytes in the thymus seems evident from morphologic studies and experimental analyses. However, whether such a relationship depends entirely on humoral factors or requires cellular contact has not been determined unambiguously.

Extensive work in mice has shown clearly that thymic and peripheral blood T cells are heterogeneous in form and function. It has been demonstrated that there are sequential changes of antigens on cell surfaces during normal development of lymphocytes.[13] The antisera recognizing such differentiation antigens were largely prepared by immunization of carefully selected congenic strains of mice. It was also demonstrated that certain populations of lymphocytes identified in this way have unique functions. In mice, initial differentiation from stem cell to thymocytes was characterized by acquisition of TL, Thy1, and Ly 1, 2, 3 antigens on cell surfaces. Further differentiation saw a loss of TL and a reduction of Thy 1 antigens. The Ly antigens were characteristic of peripheral T cells which could be further divided as helper and suppressor cells. The former were characterized by Ly 1 and the latter by Ly 2, 3 surface markers.

Similar efforts to define differentiation antigens of humans have been in progress. Heteroantisera were first applied to this problem[14,15] with it soon being recognized that an antigen (HTL) was lost as thymocytes emerged into the peripheral circulation. Subsequently, an ever-expanding array of monoclonal antibodies has permitted definition of several steps in intrathymic and extrathymic maturation of T lymphocyte subpopulations of human cells with helper and suppressor functions.[16]

Thus far the antigen T10 has been recognized on the most primitive thymic lymphocytes.[16,17] This antigen persists throughout intrathymic maturation, being lost only after T cells enter the peripheral circulation. A second antigen, T9, appears on primitive T cells transiently.[16,17] Cells in what is regarded as the middle or second stage of maturation may be characterized as having a more elaborate cell surface phenotype with T10, T6, T4, T5, and T8 antigens. Further modification of cell surface antigens is observed in the final phase of intrathymic maturation of cell surface antigens, with helper and suppressor T cells being found. Intrathymic helper cells have the phenotype T10, T1, T3, T4[18] and intrathymic suppressor cells display T10, T1, T3, T5/T8 surface antigens.[19] Emergence of these cells from the thymus into the peripheral circulation is accompanied by loss of the T10 antigen but the other markers are retained. At first glance it would seem that the entire complement of surface antigens has been changed from the most primitive, prothymocyte stage, to T cells appearing in the peripheral blood. That such is not the case is now clear with the development of the T11 antiserum *(vide supra)* which seems to react with all thymocytes regardless of their differentiation. As mentioned earlier, this antiserum (T11) seems to react with the E receptor.

Maturation of T cells in mice is characterized by reduction in the concentration of certain antigens prior to their loss. It is not now clear whether or not similar phenomena are to be observed in human thymocytes during their maturation.

Antigenic markers for helper and suppressor cell subpopulations have been established, but their true relationship to these functions in man is not understood. The nature of the biophysical relationships between cell surface markers and processes operative in cell functions remains to be determined and should be a fertile area for investigation.

## IV. FUNCTIONS OF T CELL ANTIGENS

The structure and functions of T cell antigens detected by monoclonal antibodies are currently subject to extensive and detailed analyses. Substantial work has been done on antigens detected with T3, T4, T5, T9, T10, T11, and Ia antisera.

The T3 antiserum recognizes an antigen which appears to have profound functional importance in lymphocyte biology. Binding of T3 antiserum is a strong mitogenic stimulus and this antigen is to be found on nearly all peripheral T cells.[20]

Antigens recognizing T4 and T5/T8 antigens are of special interest since they are found together on lymphocytes in relatively early stages of T cell differentiation only to appear separately on populations of lymphocytes having discrete helper and suppressor functions.[17] The antigens detected by these antisera are distinct. As analyzed on SDS polyacrylamide gels, the T4 antigen is a glycoprotein with a molecular weight of 62,000. Antigens of the T5 type are composed of 30,000 and 32,000 mol wt glycoproteins.[21] The glycoproteins obtained with antisera to T4 and T5 antigens correspond in size with those isolated as Lyt 1 and Lyt 2,3 antigens, for murine T cells having functions like those of human T cells. T8 antigens are probably like T5 antigens and currently can be regarded as synonymous with each other for purposes of subpopulation recognition.

The T9 antigen was originally believed confined to T cells in early stages of development. However, its specificity for T cells now appears less certain, with binding to B cells having been demonstrated.[22] More recently antisera to this antigen have been found to react with a large molecular weight (200,000) compound having two subunits of equal size. Based on considerations of size, peptide mapping, and reactivity with transferrin, this protein is believed to be a transferrin receptor.[23]

Studies using antiserum to T11 have shown the corresponding antigen to be present in small amounts on T cells. When this antiserum was added to lymphocytes within 2 hr of stimulation, it completely inhibited antigen-induced cellular proliferation but was only partially effective in limiting polyclonal responses to agents such as Con A and PHA. T11 antiserum was also shown to inhibit stimulation with T3 antiserum. Quantitative considerations led to the conclusion that T11 antiserum, T3 antiserum, and Srbc receptors are each present in relatively small numbers on T cells.[24]

The Ia antiserum is notable for its normal reactivity with B cells, monocytes, and endothelial cells. It also reacts with cell surfaces of activated T cells. Because the reactivity is with T cells from many individuals, it is reasonable to suppose that this antiserum recognizes a framework receptor for antigens.[25]

## V. MONOCLONAL ANTIBODIES IN HUMAN DISORDERS

The growing array of monoclonal antibodies can detect and enumerate discrete populations of lymphocytes. They are especially effective in identifying stages of maturation and cells with discrete functional capacities (e.g., helper and suppressor cells).

Alterations in T cell number, functional class, and the presence of autoantibodies to T cells have been recognized in many human disorders.[17] Such studies have proven useful in explaining several cases of acquired agammaglobulinemia,[26] and excesses of suppressor cells or deficiencies of helper cells have been found in autoimmune disorders.[17] In systemic lupus erythematosus[27] and multiple sclerosis,[28] the extent of deficits of suppressor cells has been correlated with activity of these diseases.

Autoantibodies to lymphocytes in these and other disorders of immunity have been of interest. Antibodies to T cells found in patients with sarcoidosis may contain the naturally occurring counterpart of the T11 antisera since antibodies in sarcoidosis were demonstrated to inhibit Srbc rosettes.[29] The role(s) of such autoantibodies in sarcoidosis and other disease is not at all clear. It is tempting to speculate that these autoantibodies are involved directly in suppression of cellular imunity in sarcoidosis and in the pathogenesis of autoimmune disorders. However, it can by no means be discounted that autoantibodies to T cells may simply be byproducts of extensive injury to lymphocytes from other causes. This viewpoint is supported by the ubiquitous appearance of similar antibodies in a host of disorders affecting lymphocytes.

T cell subsets are altered in transplantation.[30] Increases in numbers of helper cells are important markers of renal graft rejection. Similarly, a relative excess of helper cells has been identified in acute graft vs. host disease.[31] In fact, suppressor cells, as identified by heteroantisera, were virtually undetectable in these patients. The mechanisms operative in such drastic changes are poorly understood. It may well be that agents such as cytoxan, used to ensure suitable immunosuppression, acted on short-lived suppressor cells to cause the observed changes, or these changes may represent a more integral part of the disease itself.

## VI. PHENOTYPING LYMPHOMAS AND LEUKEMIAS

A primary purpose of this discussion is to emphasize the extent to which neoplasms of T cell origin can be defined with the tools currently at hand. Extension of this process should improve our understanding of such neoplasms and provide prognostic and therapeutic aid to the physician.

Phenotypic characterization of lymphomas and leukemias is done using E-rosetting,[32] enzyme histochemistry,[11] cell surface immunoglobulins,[33] Fc receptors,[34] and complement receptors.[35] Fc and complement receptors as well as surface immunoglobulins have been used to enumerate B cells and monocytes. E-rosetting, enzyme histochemistry, and monoclonal antibodies to cell surface antigens have found special use in defining T cell malignancies.

T cells may be separated from other lymphocytes by various techniques — most commonly filtration through nylon wool[11] and E-rosetting with sedimentation centrifugation.[11] Although not extensively reported as yet, it seems likely that cell sorting using fluorescent activated instrumentation will become important in this regard in the near future.[10] These techniques are only useful in dealing with cells in the peripheral blood or with cell suspensions from solid tumors.

Many of the neoplastic lymphocytes to be discussed in this paper have a predilection for concentrating in tissues such as lymph nodes and skin. At present they can only be adequately evaluated in most laboratories by preparing cellular suspensions and applying the techniques described above. However, a growing number of methods are becoming available to study these cells in tissues.[36] These methods, as mentioned previously, include fluorescence and enzymatic staining, often with techniques such as the biotin-avidin complex which permits increased ease in visualizing the cell surface reaction. Such techniques are especially promising for demonstrating structural relationships between neoplastic lymphocytes and other tissue elements. In a similar way, E-rosetting can be employed.[11] As yet, none of the measures with intact tissues is quantitative.

Measurements of functional characteristics of neoplastic lymphoid cells have been used relatively infrequently. Stimulation of lymphocytes in vitro with lectins such as phytohemagglutinin (PHA) have been most extensively applied. In the case of PHA, T cells are usually stimulated selectively.[37] Their proliferation and maturation can be estimated by light microscopic identification of blast cells, and by incorporation of radioactive thymidine evaluated by radioautography. As will be emphasized later, care must be taken in evaluating these studies since dilutional effects can cause an inaccurate interpretation of proliferation studies. Quantitation of T cells can be had by introducing colchicine into the cultures to block mitoses and permit enumeration of responding cells at various times after stimulation.[38]

Function can be measured more directly. For example, helper cells added to appropriately stimulated B cells increase their antibody production as measured by plaque assays.[39] Similarly, cytotoxicity of lymphocytes can be used to identify the helper cells. In this case, release of radioactivity from damaged target cells serves as a quantitative measure of function.

## VII. CLASSIFICATION OF T CELL NEOPLASMS

Morphologic classification of lymphoid neoplasms is needed because it offers the clinician a modicum of guidance as to therapy and prognosis. However, the subjectivity of morphologic diagnosis is demonstrated by the not-infrequent differences of opinion among panels of pathologists regarding the proper placement of a given case. Hence, a more objective means of classification is badly needed.

Phenotyping of lymphoid malignancies using cell surface markers is the current best hope for obtaining such objectivity. Early efforts suggest that such phenotyping will permit provision of a meaningful prognosis and selection of appropriate therapy. However, such efforts have not reached the point where one can feel secure in using this as the sole indicator of the nature of the neoplasm.

In the present paper it is intended to use the principal morphologic classes of lymphoid tumors as the basis for discussion, to emphasize those varieties in which T cell neoplasms are more than a rarity, and to emphasize the differences in natural history of the T cell forms. Table 1 lists the neoplasms to be discussed.

T cell neoplasms are not uniform in their morphology. One large group, cutaneous T cell lymphomas (CTCL) stands out as the archetype of malignant T cell disease. T cell neoplasms have been identified as subsets of nearly all morphologic types of

Table 1
T CELL NEOPLASMS
DISCUSSED

Cutaneous T cell lymphomas
   Mycosis fungoides
   Sézary's syndrome
   Other
Acute lymphoblastic leukemia
Adult T cell leukemia
Chronic lymphocytic leukemia — T cell variant
Immunoblastic lymphadenopathy
Lymphomas — non-Hodgkin's

lymphoid leukemias and non-Hodgkin's lymphomas, but in few of these is the T cell form dominant. Those neoplasms which have more than a rare occurrence of T cell forms include ALL, CLL, and diffuse non-Hodgkins lymphomas. Even in these cases, fewer than 20% of patients have disease represented by T cell variants of the tumor in question.

## A. Cutaneous T Cell Lymphomas (Skin-Related Neoplasms)

There is a current trend to regard T cell tumors of the skin as a single constellation, "cutaneous T cell lymphomas" (CTCL), with each of the syndromes being part of a continuum. Those who accept this concept consider mycosis fungoides and Sezary's syndrome as a single entity with different phenotypic expressions. A unitary view of cutaneous lymphomas may be appropriate, but since current prognostic implications and therapeutic decisions rest on classifications, it seems appropriate first to delineate the component entities of CTCL, and only then argue their biologic continuity.

### 1. Mycosis Fungoides

Mycosis fungoides derives its name from the gross appearance of skin neoplasms first recognized over a century ago.[40] That these lesions followed more benign-appearing, often undiagnosable, skin lesions was not appreciated until the end of the last century.[41] Finally, dermatopathologists grew accustomed to recognizing premycotic lesions progressing to plaque lesions before giving rise to the full-blown tumors of mycosis fungoides. Thus, mycosis fungoides was thought of as a continuum having three distinctive phases: nonspecific dermatitis (erythematous), plaques, and full-blown tumors. A further variant, "d'emblée", was recognized as a cutaneous lymphoma which appeared suddenly without premonitory lesions.[42] Progression from one stage to another of mycosis fungoides requires years and proceeds in an irregular temporal pattern with clinical and morphologic evidence of each of the components of the disease often being evident simultaneously in the same patient.

For the sake of completeness, it is appropriate to discuss the characteristics of skin lesions representing each of the major clinical entities. The erythematous stage is often not recognized clinically as part of mycosis fungoides. The scaling, erythematous patches are readily confused with eczema, psoriasis, and other common skin lesions. Most often microscopic examination is equally nondiagnostic. With inflammatory cellular exudates being localized in the dermis, including the papillae, a clue to the correct diagnosis is provided by "mycosis cells" lying within the cellular exudate or as separate aggregates. The nuclei of these mononuclear cells are hyperchromatic and have irregular shapes.[43,44]

The plaque stage is more readily identified as part of mycosis fungoides. The plaques are sharply demarcated, indurated lesions with centrally cleared areas. Microscopically the cellular infiltrate, although heavily populated with mycosis cells, is polymorphous and includes eosinophils and plasma cells. Although neoplastic cells may be recognized throughout the dermis, their band-like localization in the upper dermis is readily apparent. Pautrier's abscesses are virtually pathognomonic, appearing in more than 50% of plaques. These abscesses are microscopic intraepidermal accumulations of mycosis cells and neutrophils. They are also seen in histiocytic lymphomas in which the neoplastic cells are actually most likely lymphocytes.

Of special interest is that the plaques are spontaneously reversible in a small number of patients. Such self-healing tendencies are not now predictable in an individual patient. It may be that the lesions which are apparently self-healing plaques really represent lymphomatoid papulosis or some variant of this essentially benign, protracted but self-healing eruptive dermatosis. The dermal infiltrates of lymphomatoid papulosis are T cells which are often enlarged and bizarre.[45] The skin eruptions, seen at any age, ordinarily persist for weeks or years. Lymphomatoid papulosis is considered with CTCL because of: (1) its similarity to self healing plaques of mycosis fungoides, (2) its T cell composition, and (3) the observation that it can proceed to a disseminated lymphoma on rare occasions.

The ultimate tumor stage of mycosis fungoides is readily recognized as irregularly shaped, raised, brown to red lesions on the skin. The overlying epidermis is often interrupted by ulceration. The tumors are made up largely of mycosis cells which often have a more anaplastic appearance than was the case in earlier stages of mycosis fungoides. The cells may also be multinucleated so as to resemble Reed-Sternberg cells of Hodgkin's disease. As one might imagine, the polymorphous character of the infiltrate of earlier lesions is often lost with a more homogeneous cellular infiltrate being evident.

Involvement of visceral organs is characteristic of mycosis fungoides.[46] Since mycosis fungoides is most often clearly diagnosed only in the tumor stage, it has been assumed that multisystem involvement is a late event. However, it has been suggested that some therapeutic failures in what appear to be earlier phases of the disease can be accounted for by involvement of other systems earlier than expected.[46] In contrast, the fact that widespread clinical disease is not universal has become evident from autopsies done on patients late in their disease who die from other than neoplastic-related causes. The fact that 1/3 of these patients have no detectable visceral lesions suggests that mycosis fungoides is a heterogeneous disorder at least in terms of its clinical course.

Extracutaneous neoplastic involvement is heavily concentrated in lymph nodes but has been found in virtually all organ systems. Although not often recognized during life, pulmonary involvement, like that of non-Hodgkin's lymphomas, is frequent at autopsy (50%). Tumor in bone marrow is nearly as common as in the lungs and is often associated with pathologic fractures of the bone. A lower but appreciable incidence of oral, gastrointestinal, optic, and central nervous system involvement by neoplastic cells has been described.[46]

*2. Sézary's Syndrome*

Sézary's syndrome,[47] recognized more recently than mycosis fungoides, is characterized by generalized erythema, associated lymphadenopathy, and relative sparing of the bone marrow.[45,48,49] Morphologically, abundant dermal cellular infiltrates composed of lymphoid cells associated with eosinophils, neutrophils, and plasma cells are to be found. Pautrier's abscesses are common, and even from the earliest descriptions, "conversion" to mycosis fungoides was a recognized event in some patients with Sézary's syndrome.

*Establishing the relationships between mycosis fungoides, Sézary's syndrome, and other skin tumors* has been a focus of interest for several groups of investigators.[50,51]

As can be gathered from our earlier discussion, it had long been recognized that there is a group of neoplasms of the skin having in common a possibly unique neoplastic mononuclear cell. Some authors believed that mycosis fungoides simply represented a clinical syndrome with clearly recognizable stages of progression while others used the term to include all lymphomas seeming to originate in the skin. It was also generally accepted that the nonmononuclear elements making up the pleomorphic cellular infiltrate represented inflammatory reactions to the tumor cells.[52] Early lesions then represented a small neoplastic infiltrate with an exuberant inflammatory response with neoplastic cells becoming increasingly dominant with progression of the tumor.

The more recent identification of the neoplastic cells as T lymphocytes has been useful in relating the various cutaneous lymphomas to each other.[12,53] The conclusion that these neoplastic cells are T cells rests on studies of cells isolated from typical lesions with cell surface markers being used to establish their T cell origins[53] and on analyses of biopsies of skin lesions with frozen sections using monoclonal antibodies. One study using the latter method showed that the tumor cells in all 25 patients had the phenotype of helper T cells[13] A small number of suppressor cells (<10% of lymphocytes) were present in each biopsy and were interpreted as reactive to the tumor. About one-third of cells in the infiltrates were Ia$^+$ macrophages and dendritic cells.

A minority view still holds that mycosis fungoides is more likely to be an exuberant inflammatory response since the mycosis cells are not dissimilar to inflammatory cells found in other skin lesions. The increased evidence that the cells in mycosis fungoides represent a single subpopulation of T cells and the clonal proliferation of these cells in response to mitogens tends to speak against the view of this as an inflammatory disorder.

The cells identified in Sézary's syndrome are morphologically indistinguishable from mycosis cells and now, with studies of cell surface markers, they too have been classified as T cells.[54,55] The most likely relationship between Sézary's syndrome and mycosis fungoides is that the former is an erythrodermatous form of the latter. Sézary's syndrome is also marked by a relative wealth of neoplastic cells in the peripheral blood in comparison to what may appear in the bone marrow. Some investigators are of the opinion that the neoplastic cells in Sézary's syndrome arise in lymph nodes where, to be sure, neoplastic cells are very common. Others believe that such cells are formed in the skin itself. There is little hard evidence to permit a choice between these possibilities at present. It should be emphasized that Sézary's syndrome has the feature of masses of circulating neoplastic cells setting it apart from other cutaneous T cell lymphomas. Having reached the conclusion that mycosis fungoides and Sézary's syndrome are most appropriately considered as part of the same complex it remains to be shown why some patients display a leukemic pattern with relatively little visceral involvement, while in other patients visceral involvement predominates. This problem is, of course, not unique to CTCL, being common in lymphomas-leukemias generally.

In summary, support for lumping mycosis fungoides and Sézary's syndrome under the general designation of CTCL include: (1) morphologically identical skin lesions, (2) identity of the neoplastic cells at the ultrastructural level, and (3) characterization of the neoplastic cells as helper T cells in both cases. The relationships between these T cell neoplasms and those to be discussed later are unclear except that they have their origins in the same cell populations but not necessarily at the same site in the body.

*3. Other*

As was mentioned earlier, a minority opinion would suggest that these lesions are inflammatory rather than neoplastic. However, cytogenetic studies are far more supportive of CTCL being a neoplasm. When tumor cells isolated from several different tissues (blood, nodes, skin) of the same patient were evaluated, each showed identical abnormal karyotypes suggesting that CTCL represents a monoclonal growth of T cells with systemic dissemination. A single caveat is necessary to interpret these data; namely, since the chromosome analyses were from patients with advanced lesions, a polyclonal origin with overgrowth by one of several clones of cells cannot be excluded. It should also be emphasized that, as with most other neoplasms, appreciable karyotypic variation between patients was observed.

The relationship between lymphomatoid papulosis and CTCL has already been alluded to in an earlier portion of this discussion. It is most appropriate to consider lymphomatoid papulosis as a benign proliferative lesion of T lymphocytes. The fact that regression of this lesion is usual places it in an inflammatory category. However, the apparent occasional conversion of lymphomatoid papulosis to a lymphoma coupled with descriptions of occasional self-healing of mycosis fungoides may be taken to mean that these lesions can be confused morphologically. Whether this is the case or whether the conversions described indeed reflect progression from inflammatory to malignant lesions will only be defined clearly when cytogenetic studies are applied to lymphomatoid papulosis to establish its monoclonal or polyclonal nature. Unfortunately, preliminary data (unpublished) indicate that both lymphomatoid papulosis and early CTCL typically have normal chromosome patterns.

### 4. Natural History of CTCL

Clinical progression of CTCL from nondiagnostic involvement of the skin to widely disseminated systemic disease has been outlined earlier. The skin lesions are usually first seen in patients 40 to 60 years of age. The rate of progression is variable but most patients have a relatively prolonged course so that it is usual for skin lesions to be present 4 to 10 years before a definitive diagnosis of CTCL can be made. The possibility that progression accelerates during the disease process is suggested by the observation that the mean duration of disease is less after histologic diagnosis than was the length of time between appearance of the first recognizable skin lesions and histologic diagnosis.[56] More recently, studies of series of patients have indicated more prolonged survival after biopsy-proven diagnosis.[57,58] It is uncertain whether this reflects a higher index of suspicion with earlier biopsy or is a consequence of improved therapy.

Prognostic factors in CTCL include age at onset, lymphocyte count, symptomatology, and extent of disease.[59] Among these, extent of disease appears to be the most reliable prognostic indicator.[46] Comparisons of series with regard to extent of disease has been difficult, since until recently there has been striking variability in the methods of presenting these data. It is hoped that the staging program proposed recently by the National Workshop on CTCL will improve this situation.[51]

The most critical point in judging extent of disease may be appraisal of lymphadenopathy, and the number of involved nodes may prove to be significant. Therapeutic responses to topical chemotherapy or electron-beam radiotherapy are lessened in patients with lymphadenopathy.[57,58] For the most part such enlarged nodes are not diagnostic of lymphoma by ordinary light microscopy. The combined use of cytogenetics, electronmicroscopy, and cell surface markers, however, permit diagnosis of malignancy (T cell) in such enlarged nodes.[60-62]

The relationship between lymphocytes and epidermal cells in CTCL is obvious from morphologic studies. It may be significant that normal early differentiation of lymphocytes within the thymus is dependent on a population of epithelioid cells. Similar relationships between B cells and epithelioid cells have been well described in the Bursa of Fabricius and in the mammalian gastrointestinal tract and tonsils. Whether the epithelium of the skin has some special nutritive or other supporting role for neoplastic T cells has not been established. However, the dominant view now is that neoplastic T cells remain localized to the epidermis in the earliest phases of CTCL. It is thought that loss of this epidermotropism is required for dissemination of the cells to other tissues.[63] The mechanisms for this change remain obscure. Reversal of this course, namely, early dissemination of neoplastic cells with later establishment of epidermotropism has been described less often.[63] It has been suggested that such a sequence of events is most apt to be related to therapy.

### B. Acute Lymphoblastic Leukemia

The acute leukemias have been a special target of cell surface marker studies since the recognition that various of these patients respond exceedingly well to therapy.[64,65] Until the development of such tools, there was little to permit identification of subsets of patients who might benefit especially well from therapy. An exception was recognition that childhood ALL associated with high white blood cell counts and a mediastinal mass boded a poor prognosis.

Classification into null cell (75% of cases), T cell (20% of cases), and B cell (5% of cases) on the basis of E- and EAC-rosetting, surface immunoglobulins, and Fc receptors permitted identification of patients who might be especially apt to respond to therapy.[65,66] Only the B cell group (Burkitt's cell leukemia) could be identified by cytology alone.[65] The peripheral blood count is typically low in these patients and few of the circulating cells can be classified as blast cells. Tumor masses are often found in the abdomen and in the central nervous system. Although therapy usually causes disappearance of such B cell tumors, the overall response of the patient is likely to be poor with nearly all patients succumbing to their disease within 6 months of diagnosis.[65] T cell ALL cells are typically positive for acid phosphatase, alpha naphthyl esterase, beta glucuronidase, periodic acid-Schiff, and terminal deoxynucleotydyl transferase (Tdt). Their blood cell counts usually exceed $100,000/mm^3$ and mediastinal masses are especially likely to be present.[65] The patients are usually male and they tend to be in their late 'teens and early twenties. There is no clearly recognized difference between these T cell ALL cases and those of younger children.

The availability of reagents recognizing T cell subsets has made further study of these patients rewarding. The significance of such analyses has already become apparent with T cell leukemias arising from helper cells having been shown to have prognoses different from those of suppressor cell origin.[66] Helper T cell leukemias are usually found in children and are more frequently seen in females. White blood cell counts in these patients are relatively high and the patients are unlikely to have mediastinal masses. Suppressor T cells leukemias make up only 25% of the T cell ALL childhood leukemias but are the rule in patients over 21 years of age. The patients are usually male and mediastinal masses are not common. Overall, patients with helper T cell leukemias are likely to live longer than are those with suppressor T cell tumors.

What has been called childhood lymphocytic lymphoma should be mentioned at this point because of its frequent conversion to ALL.[52,67] Such conversion may be more marked in those patients with associated mediastinal masses (>50%). Lukes and colleagues[68] have described distinctive cytologic details using the term convoluted lymphocytic lymphoma to define this tumor. T cell surface markers have been demonstrated in these cases.

### C. Adult T Cell Leukemia (Japanese Experience)

A T cell lymphoma/leukemia has been well described among the Japanese and deserves special comment because of its inordinately high incidence among patients from Kyushu.[69,70] Genetic factors have been suspected in this adult T cell leukemia (ATL) because of its geographic concentration, family clusters, and the increased incidence of other neoplasms among these patients.

Characteristically, lymph nodes, liver, spleen, skin, and peripheral blood are involved. Thymic or other mediastinal masses are not common. The skin lesions are of particular interest since they may be indistinguishable from those of CTCL. Most often the skin tumors are heavily concentrated in the subepidermal zone of the skin but Pautrier's abscesses are not infrequently seen.

Although the neoplastic cells are characteristically T cells as identified by E-rosetting techniques, there is less satisfactory data as to the subsets involved. Since these neoplastic cells are typically Tdt-negative, they most likely represent peripheral blood T cells. What data are available suggest that these neoplastic cells have suppressor activity.[71]

Patients with this neoplasm are likely to have a poorer prognosis than is true of patients with CTCL or T cell CLL.

Recent attention has been centered on a human type-C T cell lymphoma-leukemia virus (HTLV).[72] This has proven to be especially prevalent among the Japanese patients just described.[73] A T cell disorder similar to ATL, and associated with HTLV, appears also to be endemic in the West Indies and to occur sporadically elsewhere in the world.[74]

### D. Chronic Lymphocytic Leukemia

In most cases of chronic lymphocytic leukemia, the neoplastic cells have the cell surface characteristics now recognized as those of B lymphocytes.[38,75] Cell surface immunoglobulins are present in small amounts, so that they are often difficult to detect. However, when appropriate studies are done, these cells can be shown to be restricted in their surface immunoglobulins with IgM (often associated with IgD) presenting on most of these neoplastic B cells.[76] Because of this and the identification of restricted idiotypic determinants on neoplastic B cells,[77] these neoplasms may be appropriately considered as monoclonal.

Although it is generally agreed that the T cells in B cell CLL are not part of the neoplasm, their role, if any, in the disease is not clear. Early studies suggested that T cells in the usual B CLL patient were functionally abnormal.[78,79] This conclusion was based largely on what seemed to be a proliferative response to PHA which was delayed as compared to the proliferative response in normal subjects. However, when colchicine was added to lectin-stimulated cultures it was demonstrated that peak responses of T cells in B cell CLL coincided with those seen in cells from normal subjects.[38] It, therefore, is likely that earlier studies of the proliferative response of T cells can be best interpreted as a dilutional effect of the neoplastic B cells.

The more recent availability of reagents to T cell subsets has permitted a more detailed analysis of the circulating T cells in B cell CLL.[80] In some studies, suppressor T cells isolated from patients with B cell CLL were superior to normal T suppressor cells in decreasing DNA synthesis by B cells.[39] Similarly, T helper cells from some patients with B cell CLL were not as effective as their normal counterparts in modulating normal B cells.[81] The significance and consistency of these observations is not clearly established. Before concluding that such changes in helper and suppressor T cells are significant in the disease process, it will be necessary to examine the functions of similar cells harvested from other patients with chronic diseases and especially patients with long-term neoplasms. Of equal importance will be evaluation of alterations of helper and suppressor T cells in patients with B cell CLL over the course of their illness. If changes in helper and suppressor cells correlate with changes in clinical course, they may well be considered as influencing the disease process. It is likely that these abnormalities reflect the altered immune responses characteristic of patients with CLL rather than reflecting a change related more directly to the neoplasm. In any case, altered helper and suppressor functions seem certain to be significant for the patients' well being and their status may suggest modification of the patients' therapeutic programs.

### E. Chronic Lymphocytic Leukemia of T Cell Origin

Chronic lymphocytic leukemia of T cell origin is now a clearly defined entity. As seen in Western countries, it is uncommon, making up only a percentage of cases of chronic lymphocytic leukemia. T cell chronic lymphocytic leukemia in the U.S. appears to have a variable presentation. The blood and bone marrow are only modestly involved while the spleen may be greatly enlarged and skin lesions are often extensive. This disease may be related to Sézary's syndrome and other parts of CTCL but, in contrast to these, the lymph nodes seem to be relatively spared. Analyses of T cell subsets in T cell CLL are as yet limited. Those patients who have been studied fail to display evidence of the disease preferentially involving one of the T cell subsets more than the other. Because of the relatively small number of patients whose cells have been analyzed thus far, further studies will be required before reaching any definitive conclusion with regard to the role(s) of T cell subsets in T cell CLL.

The natural history of T cell CLL has still to be understood. Since T cells proliferate in response to mitogens, it has been possible to follow the courses of a small number of these patients with chromosome markers. There are no characteristically altered chromosomes which permit ready identification of T cell CLL as a disease, but most cases of T cell CLL have shown cytogenetically altered clones. Two cases were of particular interest in that 14q$^+$ alterations were seen.[82] Similar alterations have also been found in B cell neoplasms, and involve the chromosomal site of the immunoglobulin heavy chain gene. One surprising observation among the T cell CLL patients studied was that the clones of chromosomally abnormal cells gave variable responses to different mitogens. Two of seven patients showed a superior response to a calcium ionophore A23187 as compared to PHA, and the cells of one patient responded only to PHA. One patient followed for several years displayed progressive expansion of the neoplastic clone so that the cytogenetically altered clone nearly replaced the diploid T cell population over a 2½-year period. This same patient developed new chromosomal changes suggesting that there was clonal evolution with progression of the patient's disease to Richter's syndrome.

A possibly related condition termed "chronic T cell lymphocytosis with neutropenia" deserves comment at this time. A small number of such patients have been reported to-date.[83] They characteristically present with recurrent infections. The circulating T cells are notable for having cytotoxic/suppressor surface phenotypic markers and most of these T cells have Fc receptors. The clonal nature of these lymphocytes has not been demonstrated. Because of this and the prolonged course of the disease, the disorder has been interpreted as inflammatory rather than neoplastic. It is unclear as to what the relationship is between lymphocytosis and neutropenia in these patients.

### F. Immunoblastic Lymphadenopathy

This entity, also called angioimmunoblastic lymphadenopathy, represents a proliferative lesion which may terminate as a malignancy.[84] Most often the proliferating cells are of B cell origin but T cell forms have also been identified and in both cases a morphologic distinction from frank malignancy may be difficult to define. The extensive proliferation has been suggested as representing an elaborate and excessive response to antigenic stimulations.[84,85]

Lennert's lymphoma, a possibly related entity, may prove to be especially valuable in eventually unraveling the intricate relationship of neoplastic cells in lymphomas.[86] Epithelioid cells with some of the characteristics of Reed-Sternberg cells are the key elements in this tumor. The normal nodal architecture is largely replaced, and interspersed between these cells are abundant lymphocytes. Eosinophils and plasma cells are apt to be found in approximately 50% of these patients along with polyclonal hypergammaglobulinemia. It has been suggested that at least some cases of Lennert's lymphoma represent a clonal T cell response to a B cell neoplasm,[87] but objective proof of such a pathogenesis is not available. Evaluations of lymphocyte subpopulations in Lennert's lymphoma are limited, but at least one group has suggested that suppressor/cytotoxic cells may be the tumor cells.[87]

### G. Lymphomas

Solid tissue proliferative lesions have already been referred to on several occasions both in connection with CTCL and chronic lymphocytic lymphomas of childhood. Both cell suspension and frozen section histochemistry can be applied to the study of lymphomas, with the latter method offering considerable advantage in analyses of those tumors made up of heterogeneous cell populations.

Nearly all non-Hodgkin's lymphomas have been found to have T cell variants. For the most part, histologic separations of T and B cell lymphomas are not possible on cytologic grounds but requires cell surface marker analyses. However, in general, the T cell tumors are almost exclusively diffuse rather than nodular.[88] There are relatively few studies of T cell subpopulations in lymphomas but those which have been reported suggest that a large proportion are helper cells.[89]

## VIII. DISCUSSION AND CONCLUSIONS

Technical advances have permitted increasingly sophisticated evaluation of lymphoproliferative disorders. It seems clear now that T cell neoplasms involving the skin reflect a generalized process and should be included in the category of cutaneous T cell lymphomas (CTCL). The reasons for their predilection for growth in the skin are far from clear. It is tempting to speculate that interactions between T cells and epithelial cells are required for growth and proliferation of such neoplasms. In this connection it may be important to recall that normal development of thymic T cells depends on epithelioid cells. In the latter case hormonal factors and possibly cell-cell interactions seem to be important. It has yet to be shown that epithelial cells of the skin have properties which are similar to those of the thymus. It may be important, in this regard, to point out that the neoplastic cells of Pautrier's abscesses lie within epithelial layers of the skin.

There is still much to be done in studying the natural history of CTCL. Chromosomal markers and methods for accurately identifying T cell subsets in tissues should prove to be especially useful in this regard. The fact that certain variants of CTCL appear to be dominated by lymph node as opposed to bone marrow involvement, needs a more staisfactory explanation than is currently available. The same may be said for components of CTCL in which a leukemic phase is often to be found.

The relationship between CTCL as recognized classically and the T cell lymphoma/leukemias described by the Japanese (ATL) has yet to be worked out. Fully 50% of these patients have skin (typically subepidermal) infiltrations of neoplastic cells. A portion of these patients have demonstrable Pautrier's abscesses. It is not clear from available descriptions whether the cutaneous involvement is an early or late event. A major difference between conventional CTCL and ATL is that the former are mostly of helper cell origin while the latter are suppressor cells. The strong relationship between ATL and human T cell leukemia virus may be especially important in this regard.

It seems clear that the minority opinion that CTCL is inflammatory, rather than neoplastic, is incorrect as evidenced by cytogenetic studies as well as by proliferation of a single T cell subset. The suggestion that CTCL may be similar to Hodgkin's disease in having a major component of host inflammatory cells, perhaps reactive to the neoplasm, deserves more attention. The cellular exudate of eosinophils and plasma cells which accompanies proliferation of the neoplastic cells is in some respects like that of Hodgkin's disease and it has been observed that Reed-Sternberg-like cells (the neoplastic component?) are to be found in some neoplastic growths of CTCL. In addition, Rowlands[90] has come across a case in which long-standing CTCL appeared to precede the development of Hodgkin's disease.

At present ALL is best regarded as a heterogeneous disorder. Null cells are usually the dominant elements in these patients and B cell variants are rare. The uncommon T cell ALLs are also heterogeneous. Considered as a whole, patients with helper T cell neoplasms have a better prognosis and are younger than are those with suppressor cell neoplasms. That there is a significant difference in pathogenesis of helper and suppressor cell tumors is suggested by the more frequent occurrence of a mediastinal mass in patients with suppressor cell neoplasms.

Chronic lymphocytic leukemia should also be regarded as several different disorders. The usual B cell CLL is clearly established as a monoclonal proliferation of malignant B cells. The role of the non-neoplastic T cells in B cell CLL remains to be clarified. T cell CLL is an uncommon form of CLL. Cyogenetic studies have been done in relatively few cases of T cell CLL. Emphasis on this phase of research should help to define the clonal characteristics of malignant T cells. Involvement of chromosome 14 in several of these patients is of particular interest since the rearrangement probably includes the gene for immunoglobulin heavy chains.

With the exception of CTCL there has been little systematic study of T cell lymphomas with regard to the relationship between natural history and T cell subsets. With continued development of immunohistochemical technology and monoclonal antibodies, rapid advances in this area may be expected.

## REFERENCES

1. Good, R. A., Dalmasso, A. P., Martinez, C., Archer, O. K., Pierce, J. C., and Papermaster, B. W., The role of the thymus in development of immunologic capacity in rabbits and mice, *J. Exp. Med.,* 116, 773, 1962.
2. Miller, J. F. A. P. and Osoba, D., Current concepts of the immunological function of the thymus, *Physiol. Rev.,* 47, 437, 1967.
3. Glick, B., Chang, T. S., and Jaap, R. G., The bursa of fabricius and antibody production, *Poult. Sci.,* 35, 224, 1956.
4. Clayman, H. N., Chaperon, E. A., and Triplett, R. F., Thymus-marrow cell combinations. Synergism in antibody production, *Proc. Soc. Exp. Biol. Med.,* 122, 1167, 1966.
5. Bruton, O. C., Agammaglobulinemia, *Pediatrics,* 9, 722, 1952.
6. DiGeorge, A., Congenital absence of the thymus and its immunological consequences: concurrence with congenital hypoparathyroidism in immunologic deficiency diseases in man, Bergsma, D. and Good, R. A., Eds., Natl. Found.: *Birth Defects Orig. Art. Ser.,* Vol. 4, No. 1, Williams & Wilkins, Baltimore, 1968.
7. Ruscetti, F. W. and Gallo, R. C., Human T lymphocyte growth factor: regulation of growth and function of T lymphocytes, *Blood,* 57, 379, 1981.
8. Boyum, A., Separation of blood leucocytes from blood and bone marrow: introduction, *Scand. J. Clin. Lab. Invest.,* 21 (Suppl. 97), 77, 1968.
9. Boyum, A., Separation of blood leucocytes, granulocytes, and lymphocytes, *Tissue Antigens,* 4, 269, 1974.
10. Herzenberg, L. A., Sweet, R. G., and Herzenberg, L. A., Fluorescence-activated cell sorting. A new tool for isolating functional cell types, *Sci. Am.,* March, 108, 1976.
11. Rowlands, D. T., Jr., Whiteside, T. L., and Daniele, R. P., *Lymphocytes in Clinical Diagnosis and Management by Laboratory Methods,* Henry, J. B., Ed., W. B. Saunders, Philadelphia, 1983.
12. Wood, G. S., Deneau, D. G., Miller, R. A., Levy, R., Hoppe, R. T., and Warnke, R. A., Subtypes of cutaneous T-cell lymphoma defined by expression of Leu-1 and Ia blood, 59, 876, 1982.

13. Cantor, H. and Weissman, I., Development and function of subpopulation of thymocytes and T lymphocytes, *Progr. Allerg.*, 20, 1, 1976.
14. Smith, R. W., Terry, W. D., Buell, D. N., et al., An antigenic marker for human thymic lymphocytes, *J. Immunol.*, 110, 884, 1973.
15. Aisenberg, A. S., Bloch, K. J., Long, J. C., et al., Reaction of normal human lymphocytes and chronic lymphocytic leukemia cells with an antithymocytes antiserum, *Blood*, 41, 417, 1973.
16. Reinherz, E. L., Kung, P. C., Goldstein, G., Levy, R. H., Schlossman, S. F., Discrete stages of human intrathymic differentation: analysis of normal thymocytes and leukemic lymphoblasts of T-cell lineage, *Proc. Natl. Acad. Sci. U.S.A.*, 77, 1588, 1980.
17. Reinherz, E. L. and Schlossman, S. F., Regulation of the immune response inducer and suppressor T-lymphocyte subsets in human beings, *N. Engl. J. Med.*, 303, 370, 1980.
18. Reinherz, E. L., Kung, P. C., Goldstein, G., and Schlossman, S. F., Further characterization of the human inducer T cell subset defined by a monoclonal antibody, *J. Immunol.*, 123, 2894, 1979.
19. Reinherz, E. L., Kung, P. C., Goldstein, G., Schlossman, S. F., A monoclonal antibody reactive with human cytotoxic/suppressor T cell subset previously defined by a heteroantiserum $TH_2$, *J. Immunol.*, 124, 1301, 1980.
20. Van Wauwe, J. P., De May, J. R., and Goossens, J. G., OKT3: a monoclonal anti-human T lymphocyte antibody with potent mitogenic properties, *J. Immunol.*, 124, 2708, 1980.
21. Terhorst, C., van Agthoven, A., Reinherz, E., Schlossman, S., Biochemical analysis of human T lymphocyte differentiation antigens T4 and T5, *Science*, 209, 520, 1980.
22. Aisenberg, A. C. and Wilkes, B. M., Unusual human lymphoma phenotype defined by monoclonal antibody, *J. Exp. Med.*, 152, 1126, 1980.
23. Goding, J. W. and Burns, G. F., Monoclonal antibody OKT-9 recognizes the receptor for transferrin on human acute lymphocytic leukemia cells, *J. Immunol.*, 127, 1256, 1981.
24. Van Wauwe, J., Goossens, J., Decock, W., Kung, P., and Goldstein, G., Suppression of human T-cell mitogenesis and E-rosette formation by the monoclonal antibody OKT11A, *Immunology*, 44, 865, 1981.
25. Hansen, J. A., Martin, P. J., and Nowinski, R. C., Monoclonal antibodies identifying a novel T-cell antigen and Ia antigens of human lymphocytes, *Immunogenetics*, 10, 247, 1980.
26. Reinherz, E. L., Rubinstein, A., Geha, R. S., Strelkauskas, A. J., Rosen, F. S., and Schlossman, S. F., Abnormalities of immunoregulatory T cells in disorders of immune function, *N. Engl. J. Med.*, 301, 1018, 1979.
27. Morimoto, C., Reinherz, E. L., Schlossman, S. F., Schure, P. H., Mills, J. A., and Steinberg, A. D., Alterations in immunoregulatory T cell subsets in active systemic lupus erythematosis, *J. Clin. Invest.*, 66, 1171, 1980.
28. Reinherz, E. L., Weiner, H. L., Hauser, S. L., Cohen, J. A., Distaso, J. A., and Schlossman, S. F., Loss of suppressor T cells in active multiple sclerosis, *N. Engl. J. Med.*, 303, 125, 1980.
29. Daniele, R. P. and Rowlands, D. T., Jr., Antibodies to T cells in sarcoidosis *Ann. N.Y. Acad. Sci.*, 276, 88, 1976.
30. Cosimi, A. B., Colvin, R. B., Burton, R. C., Rubin, R. H., Goldstein, G., Kung, P. C., Hansen, W. P., Delmonico, F. L., and Russell, P. S., Use of monoclonal antibodies to T-cell subsets for immunologic monitoring and treatment in recipients of renal allografts, *N. Engl. J. Med.*, 305, 308, 1981.
31. Reinherz, E. L., Parkman, R., Rappaport, J., Rosen, F. S., and Schlossman, S. F., Aberrations of suppressor T cells in human graft-versus-host disease, *N. Engl. J. Med.*, 300, 1061, 1979.
32. Gaji-Peczalska, K. J., Bloomfield, C. D., Coccia, P. F., Sosin, H., Brunning, R. D., and Kersey, J. H., B and T cell lymphomas. Analysis of blood and lymph nodes in 87 patients, *Am. J. Med.*, 59, 674, 1975.
33. Gray, H. M., Rabellino, E., and Pirofsky, B., Immunoglobulins on the surface of lymphocytes. IV. Distribution in hypogammaglobulinemia, cellular immune deficiency and chronic lymphotic leukemia, *J. Clin. Invest.*, 50, 2368, 1971.
34. Dickler, H. B. and Kunkel, H. G., Interaction of aggregated γ-globulins with B lymphocytes, *J. Exp. Med.*, 136, 191, 1972.
35. Bianco, C., Patrick, R., and Nussenzweig, V., A population of lymphocytes bearing a membrane receptor for antigen-antibody-complement complexes. I. Separation and characterization, *J. Exp. Med.*, 132, 702, 1970.
36. Edelson, R. L., Smith, R. W., Frank, M. M., et al., Identification of subpopulations of mononuclear cells in cutaneous infiltrates. I. Differentiation between B cells, T cells, and histiocytes, *J. Invest. Dermatol.*, 61, 82, 1973.
37. Greaves, M. and Janossy, G., Elicitation of selective T and B lymphocyte responses by cell surface binding ligands, *Trans. Rev.*, 11, 87, 1972.
38. Rowlands, D. T., Jr., Daniele, R. P., Nowell, P. C., and Wurzel, H. A., Characterization of lymphocyte subpopulations in chronic lymphocytic leukemia, *Cancer*, 34, 1962, 1974.

39. Chiorazzi, N., Fu, S. M., Montazeri, G., Kunkel, H. G., Rai, K., and Gee, T., T cell helper defect in patients with chronic lymphocytic leukemia, *J. Immunol.*, 122, 1087, 1979.
40. Alibert, J. L., Description des maladies de la peau; Observées à l'hôpital St. Louis et exposition des meilleures méthodes suivies pour leur traitement, Barrois L'ainé et Fils, Paris, 1806, 157.
41. Bazin, E., Lecons sur le traitement des maladies chroniques en général affections de la peau en particulier par l'emploi comparé des eaux minérales de l'hydrothérapie et des moyens pharmaceutiques, Adrien Delahaye, Paris, 1870, 425.
42. Vidal, E. and Brocq, L., Etude sur le mycosis fungoide, *La France Médical*, 2, 946, 1885.
43. Lutzner, M. A. and Jordan, H. W., Ultrastructure of an abnormal cell in Sézary's syndrome, *Blood*, 31, 719, 1968.
44. Lutzner, M. A., Hobbs, J. W., and Horvath, P., Ultrastructure of abnormal cells in Sézary syndrome, mycosis fungoides, and parapsoriasis en plaque, *Arch. Dermatol.*, 103, 375, 1971.
45. Lutzner, M., Edelson, R., Schein, P., Green, I., Kirkpatrick, C., and Ahmed, A., Cutaneous T-cell lymphomas: the Sézary syndrome, mycosis fungoides, and related disorders, *Ann. Int. Med.*, 83, 534, 1975.
46. Carney, D. N. and Bunn, P. A., Jr., Manifestations of cutaneous T-cell lymphoma, *J. Dermotol. Surg. Oncol.*, 6, 369, 1980.
47. Sézary, A. and Bourain, Y., Erythrodermie avec presence de cellules monstreuses dans le derme et dans le sang circulant, *Bull. Soc. Fr. Dermatol. Syphiligr.*, 45, 254, 1938.
48. Alderson, W. E., Barrow, G. L., and Turner, R. L., Sézary's syndrome, *Br. Med. J.*, 1, 256, 1955.
49. Edelson, R. L., Kirkpatrick, C. H., Skevach, E. M., et al., Preferential cutaneous infiltration by neoplastic thymus-derived lymphocytes. Morphologic and functional studies, *Am. Int. Med.*, 80, 685, 1974.
50. Edelson, R. L., Cutaneous T cell lymphomas—perspective, *Ann. Int. Med.*, 83, 548, 1975.
51. Lamberg, S. I. and Bunn, P. A., Proceedings of the workshop on cutaneous T cell lymphomas (mycosis fungoides and Sézary syndrome), *Cancer Treat. Rep.*, 63, 561, 1979.
52. Safai, B. and Good, R. A., Lymphoproliferative disorders of the T-cell series, *Medicine*, 59, 335, 1980.
53. Kung, P. C., Berger, C. L., Goldstein, G., Lo Gerfo, P., and Edelson, R. L., Cutaneous T cell lymphoma: characterization by monoclonal antibodies, *Blood*, 57, 261, 1981.
54. Brouet, J. C., Flandrin, G., Seligmann, M., Indication as the thymus-derived nature of the proliferating cells in six patients with Sézary's syndrome, *N. Engl. J. Med.*, 289, 314, 1973.
55. Lutzner, M. A., Edelson, R. L., Smith, R. W., et al., Two varieties of Sézary syndrome, both bearing T-cell markers, *Lancet*, 2, 207, 1973.
56. Epstein, E. H., Jr., Levin, D. L., Croft, J. D., Jr., and Lutzner, M. A., Mycosis fungoides survival, prognostic features, response to therapy, and autopsy findings, *Medicine*, 51, 61, 1972.
57. Vonderheid, E. C., Van Scott, E. J., Wallner, P. E., and Johnson, W. C., A 10-year experience with topical mechlorethamine for mycosis fungoides: comparison with patient treated by total-skin electron-beam radiation therapy, *Cancer Treat. Rep.*, 63, 681, 1979.
58. Hoppe, R. T., Cox, R. S., Fuks, Z., Price, N. M., Bagshaw, M. A., and Farber, E. M., Electron-beam therapy for mycosis fungoides: the Stanford University experience, *Cancer Treat. Rep.*, 63, 691, 1979.
59. Lamborg, S. I., Green, S. B., Byer, D. P., et al., Status report of 376 mycosis fungoides patients at 4 years: mycosis fungoides cooperative group, *Cancer Treat. Rep.*, 63, 701, 1979.
60. Rosas-Uribe, A., Variakojiis, D., Molnar, Z., and Rappaport, H., Mycosis fungoides: an ultrastructural study, *Cancer*, 34, 634, 1974.
61. Erkman-Balis, B. and Rappaport, H., Cytogenetic studies in mycosis fungoides, *Cancer*, 34, 626, 1974.
62. Whang-Peng, J., Bann, P., Knutzen, T., et al., Cytogenetic abnormalities in patients with cutaneous T-cell lymphomas, *Cancer Treat. Rep.*, 63, 575, 1979.
63. Edelson, R. L., Cutaneous T-cell lymphoma, *J. Dermatol. Surg. Oncol.*, 6, 358, 1980.
64. McKenna, R. W., Byrnes, R. K., Nesbit, M. E., Bloomfield, C. D., Kersey, J. H., Spanjers, E., and Brunning, R. D., Cytochemical profiles in acute lymphoblastic leukemia, *Am. J. Pediatr. Hematol./Oncol.*, 1, 263, 1979.
65. Bloomfield, C. D., B and T markers in leukemia and lymphoma, *Minn. Med.*, 499, 1979.
66. Reinherz, E. L., Nadler, L. M., Sallan, S. E., and Schlossman, S. F., Subset derivation of T-cell acute lymphoblastic leukemia in man, *J. Clin. Invest.*, 64, 392, 1979.
67. Kaplan, J., Mastrangelo, R., and Peterson, W. D., Jr., Childhood lymphoblastic lymphoma, a cancer of thymus-derived lymphocytes, *Cancer Res.*, 34, 521, 1974.
68. Barcos, M. P. and Lukes, R. S., *Malignant Lymphoma of Convoluted Lymphocytes: A New Entity of Possible T-Cell Type in Conflicts in Childhood Cancer*, Alan R. Liss, New York, 1975, 147.
69. Uciyama, T., Yodoi, J., Sagawa, K., Takatsuki, K., and Uchino, H., Adult T-cell leukemia: clinical and hematological features of 16 cases, *Blood*, 50, 481, 1977.

70. Watanabe, S., Shimosato, Y., and Shimoyama, M., Lymphoma and leukemia of T-lymphocytes. II, *Pathol. Annu.*, 16, 155, 1981.
71. Uchiyama, T., Sagawa, K., Takatsuki, K., et al., Effect of adult T-cell leukemia cells on pokeweed mitogen-induced normal B-cell differentiation, *Clin. Immunol. Immunopathol.*, 10, 24, 1978.
72. Poiesz, B. J., Ruscetti, F. W., Gazdar, A. F., Bunn, P. A., Minna, J. D., and Gallo, R. C., Detection and isolation of type-C retrovirus particles from fresh and cultured lymphocytes of a patient with cutaneous T-cell lymphoma, *Proc. Natl. Acad. Sci. U.S.A.*, 77, 7415, 1980.
73. Hinuma, Y., Nagata, K., Hanaoka, M., Nakai, M., Matsumoto, T., Kinoshito, K., Shirakawa, S., and Miyoshi, I., Adult T-cell leukemia: antigen in an ATL cell line and detection of antibodies to the antigen in human sera, *Proc. Natl. Acad. Sci. U.S.A.*, 78, 6476, 1981.
74. Gallo, R. C., Blattner, W. A., Reitz, M. S., and Ito, Y., HTLV: the virus of adult T-cell leukemia in Japan and elsewhere, *Lancet*, 1, 1642, 1982.
75. Gray, A. M., Rabellino, E., Schrek, R., and Williams, R. C., Immunoglobulins on the surface of lymphocytes. IV. Distribution in hypogammaglobulinema, cellular immune deficiency and chronic lymphotic leukemia, *J. Clin. Invest.*, 50, 2368, 1971.
76. Aisenberg, A. C., and Bloch, K. J., Immunoglobulins on the surface of neoplastic lymphocytes, *N. Engl. J. Med.*, 287, 272, 1972.
77. Hurley, J. N., Fu, S. M., Kunkel, H. G., McKenna, G., and Scharff, M. D., Lymphoblastoid cell lines from patients with chronic lymphocytic leukemia: identification of tumor origin by idiotypic analysis, *Proc. Natl. Acad. Sci. U.S.A.*, 75, 5706, 1978.
78. Rubin, A. D., Havemann, K., and Dameshek, W., Studies in chronic lymphocytic leukemia: further studies of the proliferative abnormality of the blood lymphocyte, *Blood*, 33, 313, 1969.
79. Han, T., Studies of correlation of lymphocyte response to phytohemagglutinin with the clinical and immunologic status in chronic lymphocytic leukemia, *Cancer*, 31, 280, 1973.
80. Matutes, E., Wechsler, A., Gomez, R., Cherchi, M., and Catovsky, D., Unusual T-cell phenotype in advanced B-chronic lymphocytic leukemia, *Br. J. Hematol.*, 49, 635, 1981.
81. Kay, N. E., Abnormal T-cell subpopulation function in CLL: excessive suppressor (T$\alpha$) and deficient helper (T$\mu$) activity with respect to B-cell proliferation, *Blood*, 57, 418, 1981.
82. Finan, J., Daniele, R., Rowlands, D., Jr., and Nowell, P., Cytogenetics of chronic T cell leukemia, including two patients with a 14q$^+$ translocation, *Virchows Arch. B. Cell Pathol.*, 29, 121, 1978.
83. Aisenberg, A. C., Wilkes, B. M., Harris, N. L., Ault, K. A., and Carey, R. W., Chronic T-cell lymphocytosis with neutropenia: report of a case studied with monoclonal antibody, *Blood*, 58, 818, 1981.
84. Lukes, R. J. and Tindle, B. H., Angio-immunoblastic (immunoblastic) lymphadenopathy, *N. Engl. J. Med.*, 292, 42, 1975.
85. Kessler, E., Angioimmunoblastic lymphadenopathy, *Cancer*, 38, 1587, 1976.
86. Burke, J. S. and Butler, J. J., Malignant lymphoma with a high content of epithelial histiocytes (Lennert's lymphoma), *Am. J. Clin. Pathol.*, 66, 1, 1976.
87. Han, T., Barcos, M., Yoon, J. M., Rakowski, and Minowada, J., Malignant lymphoma with a high content of epithelial histiocytes: report of a T-cell variant of so-called Lennert lymphoma and review of the literature, *Med. Pediatr. Oncol.*, 8, 227, 1980.
88. Bloomfield, C. D., Kersey, J. H., Brunning, R. D., and Gaji-Peczalska, K. J., Prognostic significance of lymphocytic surface markers and histology in adult non-Hodgkin's lymphoma, *Cancer Treat. Rep.*, 61, 963, 1977.
89. Knowles, D. M., II and Halper, J. P., Human T-cell malignancies. Correlative clinical, histiopathologic, immunologic, and cytochemical analysis of 23 cases, *Am. J. Pathol.*, 106, 187, 1982.
90. Rowlands, D. T., Jr., private observation.

Chapter 7

# BIOCHEMICAL MARKERS IN NEOPLASTIC LYMPHOID CELLS

Richard Bell, Ram Prakash Agarwal, Anne Lillquist, and Ronald McCaffrey

## TABLE OF CONTENTS

| | | |
|---|---|---:|
| I. | Introduction | 154 |
| II. | Ecto-5′Nucleotidase | 154 |
| III. | Adenosine Deaminase | 155 |
| IV. | Purine Nucleoside Phosphorylase | 156 |
| V. | Lactate Dehydrogenase | 157 |
| VI. | Hexosaminidase | 157 |
| VII. | Terminal Deoxynucleotidyl Transferase | 158 |
| VIII. | Summary and Future Directions | 161 |
| | Acknowledgments | 161 |
| | References | 162 |

## I. INTRODUCTION

Over the past decade there has been the development of a variety of new techniques to supplement traditional morphology in the analysis of neoplastic lymphoid cells. These techniques include the identification of normal T and B lymphocyte surface properties on malignant cells[1,2] the demonstration of restricted antigenic properties on neoplastic cells, e.g., cALLa reactivity,[3] the characterization of the in vitro growth characteristics and requirements of the malignant cells,[4] the detailed analysis of malignant cell karyotypes,[5] and the identification of a variety of specific intracytoplasmic and intranuclear components in malignant cells using biochemical, histochemical, and immunologic assay systems.[6] These marker studies have resulted in a significant refinement of our ability to group patients with leukemia and lymphoma into therapeutically meaningful categories. The utility of marker data in predicting disease behavior and outcome in response to defined forms of therapy has been repeatedly documented.[1,7] In some instances the marker data have themselves suggested therapeutic approaches.[8,9] Marker studies have also provided a useful substrate for the generation of working hypotheses on the ontogeny of lymphoid cell differentiation. Although one could argue the biologic validity of some of the extrapolations of neoplastic marker data to ontologic theory, in general such studies have provided a very important conceptual scaffolding from which to explore the origin, level of differentiation, and regulation of lymphoid cell populations.[6,10]

This review will summarize some work by the authors and others on certain intracellular enzyme markers which have turned out to provide important information, of both a theoretical and practical nature, on neoplastic lymphoid diseases. This information, considered in the context of the chapters on surface markers in this monograph, indicates the degree to which the understanding of neoplastic lymphoid biology has advanced in the last decade.

## II. ECTO-5′ NUCLEOTIDASE

Lymphocytic 5′-nucleotidase (5′-NT) is an ectoenzyme (EC 3.1.3.5) which catalyzes dephosphorylation of 5′ nucleotides to produce corresponding nucleosides.[11,12] Intact red blood cells, platelets, and monocytes have no detectable 5′-NT activity, although the latter can acquire the activity during in vitro culture.[13] The enzyme is absent from human polymorphonuclear leukocytes.[14] Because of an incomplete enzyme system for *de novo* purine synthesis,[15] lymphocytes depend on this salvage pathway, and 5′-NT could provide nucleoside metabolites for this pathway.[14] However, the extremely low concentrations of 5′-nucleotides found in plasma do not support this hypothesis and the exact function of this enzyme remains open to speculation. In addition to adenosine deaminase (ADA) and purine nucleoside phosphorylase (PNP)[16,17] this is the third enzyme of the purine salvage pathway that has been implicated in immune deficiency states. All patients with congenital agammaglobulinemia[18,19] and the majority of patients with common variable immunodeficiency[20,21] are deficient in 5′-NT. Interestingly, unlike generalized ADA or PNP deficiency, the 5′-NT deficiency is restricted to lymphocytes.[22] This suggests that a specific isotype may be expressed in lymphoid tissues, or that a subpopulation of lymphoid cells rich in 5′-NT is deficient in these diseases.

Initial biochemical measurement of activity in enriched populations failed to reveal any differences between circulating B and T cells in 5′-NT activity,[22,23] but histochemical methods showed that the activity is predominantly in B cells. These histochemical observations were later confirmed by the finding that B cells from normal subjects had about four times the enzyme activity of T cells. Studies of normal and transformed fibroblasts suggested that decreased 5'-NT activity is related to transformation process.[24] Similarly, that 5'-NT activity may represent a marker of human lymphoid maturation was suggested by the findings that human thymic epithelium-conditioned medium and thymosin, induce a two- to three-fold increase in enzymic activity in thymocytes.[25] There is low activity in cord blood T lymphocytes,[26] in malignant lymphocytes of patients with CLL,[27] in cutaneous T-cell lymphoma,[28] and a transient decrease is found in the lymphocytes of patients in infectious mononucleosis.[23] Enzymic activities comparable to unfractionated peripheral blood lymphocytes are found in PHA-stimulated lymphocytes,[23] in lymphoblasts with B cell markers and some Sezary cells[28] and in acute leukemic lymphoblasts that do not have B cell or T cell markers.[29,30] Increased 5'-NT activity has been observed in leukemia cells of four CML patients with lymphoid blast crisis and one of five with myeloid blast crisis, while there was little or no detectable activity in CML in the chronic phase.[30]

Further evidence that 5'-NT may serve as a biochemical marker comes from the studies of Boss et al.,[31] who found an age-related fall in 5'-NT which they ascribed to changes in T cell subsets. Thompson et al.[32] showed that 5'-NT activity defines two subpopulations of T lymphocytes (5'-NT-positive and -negative). OKT8-enriched cells have threefold higher 5'-NT activity than OKT4-enriched preparations, although both are low in comparison to B lymphocytes. In patients with congenital agammaglobulinemia and common variable immunodeficiency, the low 5'-NT activity may thus be explicable on the basis of a reduced OKT8-positive lymphocyte subset.[32] Further studies are required to evaluate and define the role of this intracellular enzyme as a marker within lymphoid malignancies.

## III. ADENOSINE DEAMINASE

Adenosine deaminase (ADA: adenosine aminohydrolase EC. 3.5.5.4.) is an enzyme of purine salvage metabolism which irreversibly deaminates adenosine, deoxyadenosine, and their analogs and is widely distributed among mammalian tissues.[33-37] Elevated levels of ADA have been reported in infectious mononucleosis,[38] in bronchial carcinoma,[39,40] in bladder carcinoma,[41] in lymphocytes of construction workers with asbestos contact,[42] and acute leukemia.[43] These observations and several other developments in the last 10 years suggest that ADA plays an important role in lymphocyte metabolism and may possibly regulate cell-mediated immunity. These developments were: (1) a genetically determined deficiency of ADA in patients with an autosomal recessive form of severe combined immunodeficiency disease with both T and B cell dysfunction provided an important clue to the pathogenesis of immune dysfunction at the molecular level;[16,44-46] (2) in vitro stimulation with mitogen causes two- to ninefold increase in ADA activity in lymphocytes[47,48] and monocytes;[49] (3) inhibition of ADA by specific inhibitors[50,51] prevents cell transformation, particularly in T cells[47,52] and tumor-directed cell-mediated cytotoxicity.[53]

These observations have raised several questions. Is there any relationship between the ontogeny of lymphocytes and ADA activity which may be utilized for classification when taken together with other lymphocytic markers? Are differences in the enzymic activity among various lymphocytic groups quantitative or qualitative or both? Can the difference in ADA activity be exploited for chemotherapeutic purposes?

Smyth and Harrap[54] measured ADA activity in the blast cells on 36 patients with acute leukemia. High levels of activity were found in ALL, AML, and CML blast crisis. These findings have been confirmed recently in a study of a much larger group.[30,55] In studies of human lymphoid cell lines, within T cells the enzymic activity increases during logarithmic growth, but there is no change in activity during the growth cycle of B cells.[56] B cells and cells of B cell origin including normal lymphocytes transformed by Epstein-Barr virus,[57] multiple myeloma, hairy cell leukemia,[58] B cell ALL, and CLL,[59-63] have low ADA activity. On the other hand, except for two conflicting reports,[64,65] the enzymic activity was significantly higher in CML blast crisis,[54] T cell and T cell ALL[63,66] and non-T, non-B lymphoblasts.[62,66]

Some of the studies described above have also determined TdT activity.[55-57,59] Where both TdT and ADA activities were determined it appeared that T, null, and B cell ALL fell into clearly defined separate biochemical groups. B cell disease was characterized by low TdT-low ADA, T cell by high TdT-high ADA, and null cell by low TdT- intermediate ADA activities.[55] Furthermore, it has been suggested that the wide range of ADA activity in the non-B, non-T ALL may represent heterogeneity of this subgroup.[62] Evidence exists that some non-B, non-T cell ALL cases represent T cell progenitors while others have intracytoplasmic IgM.[67] Therefore, it is possible that these non-B, non-T cells with low ADA are pre-B cells, whereas with high activity are pre-T cells. Additional data are needed to further examine this hypotheses.

ADA from human tissues exhibits heterogeneity in the size of molecular species and electrophoretic mobility.[68] Data on the qualitative differences of ADA in malignant lymphoid cells are extremely limited:[69,70] human leukemic granulocytic ADA has slightly different molecular weight and electrophoretic mobility[69] and T cell ADA seems to be more specific to deoxyadenosine.[70] It will be interesting to evaluate further the question of qualitative differences of ADA.

2'-Deoxycoformycin (DCF) is a potent inhibitor of ADA.[50] The lymphocytotoxicity and lymphopenia produced by DCF in man[71] have prompted clinical trials of DCF as a single agent and in combination with an adenosine analog, arabinosyl adenine, in the treatment of lymphoid neoplasms. These studies have demonstrated the effectiveness of this therapy in T cell ALL and mycosis fungoides.[71-79] There appears to be a correlation between ADA activity and therapeutic effectiveness of DCF. Further studies are underway with this drug. It should have clinical use in T cell lymphomas, including mycosis fungoides and Sézary syndrome. From these limited data on ADA, it appears that ADA assays may be of some use in the classification, prognosis, and treatment of lymphoid malignancies.

## IV. PURINE NUCLEOSIDE PHOSPHORYLASE

Another enzyme of the purine salvage pathway which has recently been associated with lymphocytic function is purine nucleoside phosphorylase (PNP: purine nucleoside: orthophosphate ribosyltransferase, EC 2.4.2.1.). PNP catalyzes the reversible phosphorolytic cleavage of the products of ADA reaction, inosine and deoxyinosine, in addition of guanosine and deoxyganosine.[80] Thus it acts sequentially with ADA. PNP is widely distributed among mammalian tissues and exists in a number of polymorphic forms.[80] A partial[81] and complete[17] genetic deficiency of this enzyme in an immunodeficiency disease with defects in T cell activity focused attention on its role in lymphocyte function and regulation.

Despite a large amount of literature on PNP, the enzymic activity in malignat lymphoid cells has not been extensively studied. Normal or low activity reported in CLL and ALL[43] was confirmed by Dietz and Czebotar.[82] In a survey of ADA and PNP in human T cell, B cell, and null cell lines where ADA was clearly higher in T cells as compared to other cell lines, the trend for PNP activity was opposite. The differences in PNP activity among the cell lines, however, were small and not statistically significant.[56] These findings are consistent with those of others[28,83,84] who found comparable PNP activities in normal B cells, B cell CLL, and other lymphoblastoid cell lines of B cell origin, non-T, non-B lymphoblasts, and peripheral T cells. Lower PNP activities have also been reported in the lymphoblast of T cell ALL and in cutaneous T cell lymphoma.[28] An attempt to find electrophoretic variants of PNP failed to distinguish markedly isozymic patterns in B cell and T cell lines. Most positively charged species were present during the growth cycle of both cell lines while negatively charged components remained constant. However, the negatively charged component was always higher than the positively charged components.[56]

On comparison of the specific acivities of PNP and ADA and their ratios in various human tissues, an inverse relationship was found between the thymus and other tissues. The thymus having highest ADA activity and lowest PNP activity had lowest (0.1) ratio of PNP/ADA, whereas the ratios in spleen, brain, kidney, liver, lung, small intestine, heart, peripheral lymphocytes, and granulocytes were in the range of 2 to 100.[85] A similar comparison has been made in rat lymphoid cell populations (thymus, lymph node, spleen, and bone marrow). The thymocytes had the lowest PNP and high ADA activity, whereas spleen and bone marrow lymphocytes had highest PNP and lowest ADA. This type of relationship was also apparent in cells of T lymphocyte lineage at various stages of differentiation suggesting that specific stages of T cell development may be characterized by the levels of PNP and ADA activities.[86] A comparative study of these enzyme markers and their ratios may be useful in further diagnosis and classification of neoplastic lymphoid cells.

## V. LACTATE DEHYDROGENASE

Lactate dehydrogenase is an enzyme of the glycolytic pathway which catalyzes the conversion of lactate to pyruvate. Nicotinamide adenine dinucleotide is cofactor in this reaction. The enzyme is a tetramer composed of A and B subunits yielding five isoenzymes,[87] and these enzyme species are readily distinguishable because of differing electrophoretic mobility. The relative contribution of each isoenzyme type to total intracellular LDH is characteristic of many normal and malignant tissues.[88,89] Different subsets of lymphoid cells have been shown to have characteristic isoenzyme patterns, and LDH isoenzymes have thus been proposed as markers for lymphoid tissues and cells.[90-92] The relative rates of LDH isoenzyme synthesis vary during the cell cycle.[93] In nonmalignant lymphoid tissues, B cells are characterized by a relatively high percentage of intracellular LDH 3 and 5, while T cells have more LDH 1. Immature T cells (thymocytes) have a preponderance of LDH 3, as do non-T non-B lymphoblasts, fetal and immature tissues.[91,92,94,95] LDH 1 increased in thymocytes with maturation,[96] and probably LDH 4 and 5 increase with B cell differentiation.[92] It is likely that the intracellular LDH isoenzymes in malignant lymphoid populations similarly reflect their T or B origin and level of maturation.[91,92,95] Thus LDH isoenzyme studies are of use in the classification of lymphoid malignancies, in conjunction with other marker and enzyme data. An intracellular marker of this nature is of great potential value where manipulations or therapy may have altered or masked cell surface markers.[90]

Plasma LDH is known to be a useful determinant of disease activity, but to date, serum isozyme levels have not been sufficiently studied to assess their value in the classification and prognosis of malignant lymphoma.

## VI. HEXOSAMINIDASE

Hexosaminidase (N acetyl β-glucosaminidase EC 3.2.1.30) is an acid hydrolase which has three isozymes (A, B, and I) with characteristic relative amounts in lymphoid cells. Isozyme I is greatly elevated in common ALL.[97,98] Cytochemical staining for this enzyme is useful in the classification of CLL with T CLL showing uniform polar positivity with absent staining in B CLL.[99] These cytochemical findings have been con-

Table 1
OCCURRENCE OF TERMINAL TRANSFERASE
IN HEMATOLOGIC MALIGNANCY

| Clinical Diagnosis | No. of cases | No. TdT(+) |
|---|---|---|
| Acute lymphoblastic leukemia | 300 | 290 |
| Acute myeloblastic leukemia | 120 | 10 |
| Acute undifferentiated leukemia | 30 | 16 |
| Blastic chronic myelogenous leukemia | 100 | 38 |
| Postpolycythemia vera leukemia | 15 | 3 |
| Postmyeloid metaplasia leukemia | 16 | 10 |
| Postchemo/radiotherapy leukemia | 9 | 2 |
| Stable phase chronic myelogenous leukemia | 30 | 0 |
| B cell chronic lymphocytic leukemia | 15 | 0 |
| T cell chronic lymphocytic leukemia | 3 | 0 |
| Sézary syndrome | 6 | 0 |
| Hairy cell leukemia | 9 | 0 |
| Multiple myeloma | 7 | 0 |
| Hodgkin's disease | 7 | 0 |
| Lymphoblastic lymphoma | 15 | 15 |
| Nodular Diffuse, poorly differentiated lymphocytic lymphoma | 9 | 0 |
| Diffuse histiocytic lymphoma | 6 | 0 |

firmed by biochemical determinations of enzyme content.[99,100] This and other lysosomal enzymes are of greatest use in the differential diagnosis of acute leukemia.[101]

## VII. TERMINAL DEOXYNUCLEOTIDYL TRANSFERASE

It is now slightly more than a decade since the original report of the presence of the enzyme terminal deoxynucleotidyl transferase (TdT) in the blast cells of a child with acute lymphoblastic leukemia.[102] Over the years since then, survey studies on the expression of TdT in malignant cells from a wide spectrum of hematopoietic neoplastic processes have been reported from several centers.[103,104] A summary of some of our original data is given in Table 1.

This distribution of enzyme-positive and -negative cases within the various diagnostic categories in this series is similar to that which has been reported in surveys performed by other groups. Thus, even acknowledging the minor exceptions of TdT-negative lymphoblastic disease and TdT-positive myeloblastic disease, it is clear that TdT activity reliably distinguished between neoplastic lymphoblastic and myeloblastic cells with about 95% confidence. However, among the less common variants of acute leukemia there is an apparent randomness to blast cell TdT expression. As shown in Table 1, TdT can be present in blast cells from a spectrum of apparently diverse, nonlymphoid neoplastic processes — blastic chronic myelogenous leukemia, undifferentiated acute leukemia, and leukemia following a variety of dyspoietic states. At least two interpretations of this "randomness" are possible. One is to agree that randomness, or chance, accounts for TdT expression in leukemic cells; that TdT expression is haphazard and a reflection of a chaotic metabolic cellular state. A second interpretation is to consider the expression of TdT to be an indication of lymphoid origin of neoplastic cell populations. These authors have favored this second interpretation. Data from a variety of sources have emerged, which increasingly support such an interpretation, as discussed below.

The utility of TdT assays in the formulation of clinical decisions derives from the hypothesis that TdT-positive blast cells are lymphoid in nature, irrespective of their

Table 2
BLASTIC CML STUDY — CHARACTERISTICS OF
RESPONDERS AND NONRESPONDERS TO
VINCRISTINE-PREDNISONE THERAPY

|  | TdT(+) (16 cases) | | TdT(−) (14 cases) | |
|---|---|---|---|---|
|  | Responders (11 cases) | Failures (5 cases) | Responders (1 case) | Failures (13 cases) |
| Morphology | | | | |
| Lymphoblastic | 6 | 2 | 1 | 4 |
| Myeloblastic | 5 | 3 | — | 9 |
| Age (years) | | | | |
| Range | 3—78 | 23—75 | 47 | 5—62 |
| Median | 27 | 51 | 47 | 52 |

morphology. (The use of the term lymphoid in this nonmorphologic manner is obviously confusing. Lymphoid is used in this manner here, not to fracture the English language, but to convey a meaning for which there is no suitable alternative term). This TdT-lymphoblast hypothesis was tested directly in a therapeutic trial using the agents vincristine and prednisone in blastic chronic myelogenous leukemia (CML).[105] This variant of acute leukemia was selected for study because it had been traditionally classified as a variant of acute myeloblastic leukemia. Vincristine and prednisone were selected as therapeutic agents because of the high rate (80%) of responsiveness to these agents in authentic lymphoblastic leukemia and the low rate (15%) in authentic myeloblastic leukemia. It was argued that a high rate of responsiveness to this drug combination among the TdT-positive patients would partially validate the hypothesis that such cases were lymphoblastic in nature. An added impetus to this study was the similarity between the incidence of TdT positivity and the proportion of cases reported by Canellos et al. to be responsive to vincristine and prednisone therapy.[106] This study sought to determine whether TdT-positivity and vincristine-prednisone responsiveness would coincide.

A total of 30 patients with Philadelphia-chromosome-positive blastic CML were studied in a multi-institutional cooperative clinical trial. Blast crisis was defined by the presence of at least 25% blast cells in the bone marrow or peripheral blood. Of the 30 patients, 3 had *de novo* blast crisis; the remaining 27 had a well defined preceding chronic phase, ranging in duration from 8 months to 10 years. Patients' ages ranged from 3 to 78 years; 13 were below the age of 50 years. Therapy was limited to vincristine sulfate, 1.5 mg/m² (with a maximum dose of 2 mg) given intravenously each week, and prednisone, 60 mg/m² given by mouth each day. In all cases, at least 2 doses of vincristine and 14 days of prednisone therapy were administered before a patient was considered to be nonresponsive. The results of the TdT assay were not known to the physicians caring for the patients until the chemotherapy had been completed. Complete response was defined as the total elimination of blast cells from the peripheral blood, return of peripheral blood values to normal, and return of normal marrow cellularity with less than 5% blast cells.

Responsiveness to vincristine-prednisone therapy is summarized in Table 2. Only one of the 14 TdT-negative cases responded, whereas 11 of the 16 TdT-positive cases achieved remission ($p < 0.008$). The association of several patient characteristics with responsiveness was analyzed. TdT positivity alone predicted a 67% response rate (11 of 16 TdT-positive patients responded). Only 1 of 14 (7%) TdT-negative patients responded. Where age and TdT status were considered together, 78% of TdT-positive patients under age 50 years responded, whereas only 11% of TdT-negative patients under age 50 years responded. Thus, age and TdT status considered together were extremely significant. Morphology alone was not significantly predictive for either responsiveness or TdT status, a finding which requires emphasis (Table 2).

The copresence with TdT of independent, lymphoid-related surface markers in cells from blastic CML patients also supports the TdT-lymphoblast hypothesis. This association was first shown in 1973 in a small group of blast crisis patients studied simultaneously in London and Boston for TdT expression and common ALL antigen (cALLa) status.[107] Additional reports[108,109] on larger numbers of patients have substantiated this relationship. A practical consequence of these observations is that TdT status (and/or other lymphoid-related markers) can be used *a priori* to recognize blast crisis patients who are likely to respond to vincristine-prednisone therapy. It is also probable that other forms of TdT-positive disease (Table 1), which are not usually considered to be lymphoblastic in nature, would be similarly vincristine-prednisone responsive. This possibility should be directly tested, particularly in those leukemias which emerge in survivors of treated Hodgkin's disease, and following dyspoietic syndromes.

Among the lymphomas, TdT expression is confined to those with lymphoblastic morphology. (A minor subset — probably 5% — of patients with histiocytic lymphoma also have TdT-positive malignant cells). These data and those of others[110,111] on TdT expression in the lymphomas suggest that the finding of TdT-positive cells in lymphomatous tissue is highly suggestive of lymphoblastic lymphoma. Since the unequivocal establishment of the diagnosis of lymphoblastic lymphoma is not a trivial matter for the pathologist,[110] the use of TdT as a reliable marker in this setting represents an important diagnostic advance. Likewise, the recognition of TdT-positive cells in extramedullary sites has facilitated the recognition of leukemic cells in cerebrospinal fluid and testicular biopsies.[113,114] The immunofluorescent assays for TdT have been particularly useful in this regard.

Several attempts have been made to monitor remission status of TdT-positive lymphoblastic disease with serial marrow TdT assays. Despite the development of elegant methodology, there has been a notable lack of success in adapting the assay to this use.[115,116] Bone marrow from these patients can have two types of TdT-positive cells: residual TdT-positive lymphoblasts and TdT-positive normal marrow cells. The TdT-positive normal marrow cell population can fluctuate dramatically in response to a variety of stimuli, including fever, chemotherapy, and certain viral illnesses. Thus, the relative contribution of either class of TdT-positive cell, normal or malignant, to the activity observed in remission marrow cannot be assessed with current assay systems. Only when marrow is largely replaced by blast cells, or when TdT-positive cells are obtained from peripheral blood can the observed TdT activity be termed disease-associated. Thus, the present inability to distinguish normal marrow cell TdT from TdT which is leukemia cell-associated, prevents the use of TdT assays of bone marrow to monitor remission status in TdT-positive leukemia.

Data from several sources are now consistent with a model which states that TdT-positive cells in normal bone marrow may be initially capable of either B or T cell differentiation.[115] As intramedullary B cell differentiation proceeds, TdT expression is curtailed. Cytoplasmic Ig-positive normal marrow cells are TdT-positive; surface Ig-positive cells are TdT-negative.[116] Further, it was not possible to demonstrate TdT-positive cells in chicken bursa, even within hours of hatching.[115] TdT-positive marrow cells which are not programmed for B cell differentiation migrate to the thymus where they undergo a process which results in their ultimate release from this site as functional T cells. Such migration has been reliably observed during the neonatal period in rats.[114] In mature humans 1 to 4 per 10,000 circulating peripheral blood lymphocytes are TdT-positive.[117] In the thymus, TdT expression is progressively curtailed during differentiation; no cells have been identified exiting from the thymus while still expressing TdT.[115] The occurrence of TdT positivity in rare leukemia cells with myeloid characteristics and in exceptional lymphoma cells with histiocytic features, suggest that TdT may be a property of a primitive founder cell population which can differentiate into multiple defined populations. In these unusual neoplastic cells it may be that the primitive founder cell characteristic of TdT positivity has become asynchronously regulated in relation to morphologic development. The factors regulating TdT expression in either normal or neoplastic cells remain largely unknown.

Although the physiological function of TdT is unknown, its major limitation to cells obviously committed to B and T cell differentiation suggest that it has a role in generating the functional properties of circulating B and T cells. Baltimore[118] suggested that since TdT has the properties of an enzyme which would be obligate in any system involving somatic mutation of DNA, it may have a function in the generation of differentiated, functionally mature lymphoid cells, if such differentiation occurs on the basis of somatic mutation. In extending this model, Alt and Baltimore have recently suggested that the somatic rearrangement of germ line DNA elements required to form complete variable region genes of immunoglobulin light and heavy chains may involve TdT;[119] they have suggested a role for TdT in the generation of the extra nucleotides at D-J joints, which may contain multiple dG residues.

## VIII. SUMMARY AND FUTURE DIRECTIONS

The clinical utility of marker data — be it biochemical, immunological, or cytochemical — in predicting disease behavior and outcome to defined forms of therapy has been repeatedly documented. In some instances the marker data have themselves suggested novel therapeutic approaches. For example, a variety of anti-ALL antisera are being tested as potential clinical cytotoxic agents.[8] The enzyme TdT may prove useful as a target for a new class of agents which are showing potential as cytotoxic agents via TdT inhibition.[9] Inhibition of the enzyme ADA by agents such as deoxycoformycin may prove to be a useful therapeutic strategy.

The recognition that small populations of normal primitive lymphoid cells exhibit an identical composite phenotype to that expressed by neoplastic lymphoid cells has caused a fundamental reevaluation of the popular view that neoplastic cells are per se abnormal. The accumulating marker data appear to indicate that no fundamental phenotypic differences exist between subsets of normal primitive lymphoid cells and the cells which are conventionally recognized as neoplastic lymphoid cells. One would thus define the neoplastic abnormality as quantitative; primitive parental cells existing in an abnormally high proportion, and lacking a maturation response, or perhaps lacking a signal to undergo that maturation. In this analysis, the central abnormality of neoplastic lymphoid cells is in this lack of maturation. Marker techniques now make it feasible to harvest normal primitive lymphoid populations with an equivalent composite neoplastic phenotype. The availability of such populations for studies on differentiation and a maturation should prove useful in dissecting the relevance of studies using a variety of maturation inducers in leukemia cell lines.

## ACKNOWLEDGMENTS

This work was supported by grants CA 18662, A-105877, FR-128, CAL-19514, CA15187, and GM21747 from the U.S. National Institute of Health, and by American Cancer Society grant CH-221. Ronald McCaffrey was the recipient of Research Cancer Development Award CA 00099 from the U.S. National Institute of Health.

## REFERENCES

1. Sen, L. and Borella, L., Clinical importance of lymphoblasts with T markers in childhood acute leukemia, *N. Engl. J. Med.*, 292, 828, 1975.
2. Seligman, M., Brout, J. C., and Preud'Homme, J. L., The immunological diagnosis of human leukemias and lymphomas: an overview, in *Hematology and Blood Transfusion*, Vol. 20, Thierfelder, S., Rodt, H., and Thiel, E., Eds., Springer-Verlag, Berlin, 1977, 1031.
3. Greaves, M. F., Cell surface characteristics of human leukemic cells, *Essays Biochem.*, 15, 78, 1979.
4. Moore, M. A. S., Spitzer, N., Williams, N., et al., Agar culture studies in 127 cases of untreated acute leukemia: the prognostic value of reclassification of leukemia according to *in vitro* growth characteristics, *Blood*, 44, 1, 1974.
5. Golomb, H. M., Diagnostic and prognostic significance of chromosome abnormalities in acute non-lymphocytic leukemia, *Cancer Genet. Cytogenet.*, 1, 249, 1980.
6. Greaves, M. F., Analysis of the clinical and biological significance of lymphoid phenotypes in acute leukemia, *Cancer Res.*, 41, 4752, 1981.
7. Marks, S. M., Baltimore, D., and McCaffrey, R. P., Terminal transferase as a predictor of initial responsiveness to vincristine and prednisone in blastic chronic myelogenous leukemia, *N. Engl. J. Med.*, 298, 812, 1978.
8. Ritz, J., Pesando, J. M., Notis-McConorly, J., et al., Use of monoclonal antibodies as diagnostic and therapeutic reagents in acute lymphoblastic leukemia, *Cancer Res.*, 41, 4771, 1981.
9. McCaffrey, R., Bell, R., Lillquist, A., et al., Selective killing of leukemia cells by inhibition of TdT, *Hematol. Blood Transf.*, 28, 24, 1983.
10. Reinhertz, E. L., Kung, P. C., Goldstein, G., Levy, R. H., and Schlossman, S. F., Discrete stages of human intrathymic differentiation: analysis of normal thymocytes and leukemic lymphoblasts of T-cell lineage, *Proc. Natl. Acad. Sci. U.S.A.*, 77, 1588, 1980.
11. Uusitalo, R. J. and Karnovsky, M. J., 5'-Nucleotidase in different populations of mouse lymphocytes, *J. Histochem. Cytochem.*, 25, 97, 1977.
12. Webster, A. D. B., North, M., Allsop, J., Asherson, G. L., and Watts, R. W. E., Purine metabolism in lymphocytes from patients with primary hypogammaglobulinemia, *Clin. Exp. Immunol.*, 31, 456, 1978.
13. Berman, J. D. and Johnson, W. D., Monocyte functions in human neonates, *Infect. Immunol.*, 19, 898, 1978.
14. DePierre, J. W. and Karnovsky, M. L., Ectoenzymes of the guinea pig polymorphonuclear, leukocytes. II. Properties and suitability as markers for the plasma membrane, *J. Biol. Chem.*, 249, 7121, 1974.
15. Scott, J. L., Human leukocyte metabolism *in vitro*. I. incorporation of adenosine-8-$c^{14}$ and formate-$c^{14}$ into nucleic acids of leukemic leukocytes, *J. Clin. Invest.*, 41, 67, 1962.
16. Giblett, E. R., Anderson, J. E., Cohen, F., Pollara, B., and Meuwissen, H. J., Adenosine deaminase deficiency in two patients with severely impaired cellular immunity, *Lancet*, 2, 1067, 1972.
17. Giblett, E. R., Amman, A. J., Wara, D. W., Sandman, R., and Diamond, L. K., Nucleoside phosphorylase deficiency in a child with severely defective T-cell immunity and normal B-cell immunity, *Lancet*, 1, 1010, 1975.
18. Edwards, N. L., Gelfand, E. W., Bunk, L., Dosch, H. M., and Fox, I. H., Distribution of 5'-nucleotidase in human lymphoid tissues, *Proc. Natl. Acad. Sci. U.S.A.*, 76, 3474, 1979.
19. Thompson, L. F., Boss, G. R., Spiegelberg, H. L., Jansen, I. V., O'Connor, R. B., Waldman, T. A., Hamberger, R. N., and Seegmiller, J. E., Ecto 5'-nucleotidase activity in T and B lymphocytes from normal subjects and patients with X-linked agammaglobulinemia, *J. Immunol.*, 123, 2475, 1979.
20. Johnson, S. M., North, M. E., Asherson, G. L., Allsop, J., Watts, R. W. E., and Webster, A. D. B., Lymphocyte purine 5'-nucleotidase deficiency in primary hypogamma-globulinaemia, *Lancet*, 1, 168, 1977.
21. Rich, K. C., Sampson, H., Edwards, L. N., and Fox, I. H., Familial hypogammaglobulinemia with variable serum immunoglobulins, *Am. J. Dis. Child*, 135, 795, 1981.
22. Edwards, N. L., Cassidy, J. T., and Fox, I. H., Lymphocyte 5'-nucleotidase deficiency in hypogammaglobulinemia: clinical characteristics, *Clin. Immunol. Immunopathol.*, 17, 76, 1980.
23. Quagliata, F., Faig, D., Conklyn, M., and Silber, R., Studies on the lymphocytes 5'-nucleotidase in chronic lymphocytic leukemia, infectious mononucleosis, normal subpopulations and phytohemagglutinin stimulated cells, *Cancer Res.*, 34, 3197, 1974.
24. Raz, A., Collard, J. G., and Inbar, M., Decrease in 5'-nucleotidase activity in malignant transformed and normal stimulated cells, *Cancer Res.*, 38, 1282, 1978.
25. Colen, A., Dosch, H. M., and Gelfand, E., Induction of ecto-5' nucleotidase activity in human thymocytes, *Clin. Immunol. Immunopathol.*, 18, 287, 1981.

26. Webster, A. D. B., Rowe, M., Johnson, S. M., Asherson, G. L., and Harkness, A., Ecto 5'-nucleotidase deficiency in primary hypogammaglobulinemia, in *The enzyme defects and immune dysfunctions, Ciba Found. Symp. Ser. 68, Excerpta Medica, New York, 1979, 135.*
27. Lopez, J., Zucker-franklin, D., and Silber, R., Heterogeneity of 5'-nucleotidase activity in lymphocytes in chronic lymphocytic leukemia, *J. Clin. Invest.*, 52, 1297, 1973.
28. Blatt, J., Reaman, G., and Poplack, D. G., Biochemical markers in lymphoid malignancy, *N. Engl. J. Med.*, 303, 918, 1980.
29. Reaman, G. H., Levin, N., Munchmore, A., Holiman, B. J., and Poplack, D. G., Diminished lymphoblast 5'-nucleotidase activity in acute lymphoblastic leukemia with T-cell characteristics, *N. Engl. J. Med.*, 300, 1374, 1979.
30. Koya, M., Kanoh, T., Sawada, H., Uchino, H., and Ueda, K., Adenosine deaminase and ecto 5'-nucleotidase activities in various leukemias with special reference to blast crisis: significance of ecto-5'-nucleotidase in lymphoid blast crisis of chronic myeloid leukemia, *Blood*, 58, 1107, 1981.
31. Boss, G. R., Thompson, L. F., Spiegelberg, H. L., Pichler, W. J., and Seegmiller, E., Age-dependency of lymphocyte ecto '5'-nucleotidase activity, *J. Immunol.*, 125, 679, 1980.
32. Thompson, L. F., Saxon, A., and O'Connor, A. D., Ecto 5'-nucleotidase activity in human T-cell subsets. Decreased number of ecto 5'-nucleotidase positive cells from both OKT4[+] and OKT8[+] cells in patients with hypogammaglobulinemia, *J. Clin. Invest.*, 71, 892, 1983.
33. Conway, E. J. and Cook, R., The deaminases of adenosine and adenylic acid in blood and tissues, *Biochem. J.*, 33, 479, 1939.
34. Agarwal, R. P., Sagar, S. M., and Parks, R. E., Jr., Adenosine deaminase from human erythrocytes: purification and effects of adenosine analogs, *Biochem. Pharm.*, 24, 693, 1975.
35. Brady, T. G., Adenosine deaminase, *Biochem. J.*, 36, 478, 1942.
36. Brady, T. G. and O'Donovan, C. I., A study of the tissue distribution of adenosine deaminase in six mammal species, *Comp. Biochem. Physiol.*, 14, 101, 1965.
37. Hall, J. G., Adenosine deaminase activity in lymphoid cells during antibody production, *Am. J. Exp. Biol.*, 41, 93, 1963.
38. Koehler, L. H. and Benz, E. J., Serum adenosine deaminase: methodology and clinical application, *Clin. Chem.*, 8, 133, 1962.
39. Nishihara, H., Akedo, H., Okada, H., and Hattori, S., Multienzyme patterns of serum adnosine deaminase by agar gel electrophoresis, *Clin. Chim. Acta*, 30, 251, 1970.
40. Nishihara, H., Ishikawa, S., Shinkai, K., and Akedo, H., Multiple forms of human adenosine deaminase, *Biochem. Biophys. Acta*, 302, 429, 1973.
41. Sufrin, G., Tritsch, G. L., Mittleman, A., and Murphy, G. P., Adenosine deaminase activity in patients with carcinoma of the bladder, *J. Urol.*, 119, 343, 1978.
42. Formeister, J. F., Tritsch, G. L., and Mittleman, A., Adenosine deaminase levels in construction workers with asbestos contact dermatitis, *J. Med.*, 9, 285, 1978.
43. Scholar, E. M. and Calabresi, P., Identification of the enzymatic pathways of nucleotide metabolism in human lymphocytes and leukemic cells, *Cancer Res.*, 33, 94, 1973.
44. Dissing, J. and Knudsen, B., Adenosine deaminase deficiency and combined immunodeficiency syndrome, *Lancet*, 2, 1316, 1972.
45. Parkman, R. G., Gelfand, F. W., Rosen, F., Sanderson, A., and Hirschhorn, R., Severe combined immunodeficiency disease associated with adenosine deaminase deficiency, *N. Engl. J. Med.*, 292, 714, 1975.
46. Meuwissen, H. J., Pollara, B., and Pickering, R. J., Combined immunodeficiency disease associated with adenosine deaminase, *J. Pediatr.*, 86, 169, 1975.
47. Carson, D. A. and Seegmiller, J. E., Effect of adenosine deaminase inhibition upon human lymphocyte blastogenesis, *J. Clin. Invest.*, 57, 274, 1976.
48. Hovi, T., Smyth, J. F., Allison, A. C., and Williams, S. C., Role of adenosine deaminase in lymphocyte proliferation, *Clin. Exp. Immunol.*, 23, 395, 1976.
49. Fischer, D., Van der Weyden, M. B., Snyderman, R., and Kelley, W. N., A role of adenosine deaminase in human monocyte maturation, *J. Clin. Invest.*, 58, 399, 1976.
50. Agarwal, R. P., Spector, T. A., and Parks, R. E., Jr., Tight binding inhibitors. IV. Inhibition of adenosine deaminases by various inhibitors, *Biochem. Pharm.*, 26, 359, 1977.
51. Cha, S., Agarwal, R. P., and Parks, R. E. J., Tight-binding inhibitors. II. Non-steady state nature of inhibition of milk xanthine oxidase by allopurinal and alloxanthine and of human erythrocytic adenosine deaminase by coformycin, *Biochem. Pharm.*, 24, 2187, 1975.
52. Ballef, J. J., Insel, R., Merler, E., and Rosen, F. S., Inhibition of maturation of human precursor lymphocytes by coformycin, inhibitor of the enzyme adenosine deaminase, *J. Exp. Med.*, 143, 1271, 1976.
53. Wolberg, G. T., Zimmermann, T. P., Hiemstra, H., Winston, M., and Chu, L. C., Adenosine inhibition of lymphocyte mediated cytolysis: possible role of cyclic adenosine monophosphate, *Science*, 187, 957, 1975.

54. Smyth, J. F. and Harrap, K. R., Adenosine deaminase activity in leukemia, *Br. J. Cancer,* 31, 544, 1975.
55. Grever, M. R., Coleman, M. S., and Balerczak, S. P., Adenosine deaminase and terminal deoxynucleotidyl transferase: biochemical markers in the management of chronic myelogenous leukemia, *Cancer Res.,* 43, 1442, 1983.
56. Tritsch, G. L. and Minowada, J., Differences in purine metabolizing enzyme activities in human leukemia T-cell, B-cell and null cell lines: brief communication, *J. Natl. Cancer Inst.,* 60, 1301, 1978.
57. Tritsch, G. L. and Minowada, J., Adenosine deaminase activity during the growth cycle of T- and B-lymphoid cell lines, *Immunol. Commun.,* 6, 483, 1977.
58. Meier, J., Coleman, M. S., and Hutton, J. J., Adenosine deaminase activity in peripheral blood cells of patients with hematologic malignancies, *Br. J. Cancer,* 33, 312, 1976.
59. Coleman, M. S., Greenwood, M. F., Hutton, J. J., Holland, P., Lamplin, B., Krill, C., and Kastelic, J. E., Adenosine deaminase, terminal deoxynucleotidyl transferase (TdT), and cell surface markers in childhood acute leukemia, *Blood,* 52, 1125, 1978.
60. Sullivan, J. L., Osborne, W. R. A., and Wedgewood, R. J., Adenosine deaminase in lymphocytes, *Br. J. Haematol.,* 37, 157, 1977.
61. Ramot, B., Brok-simmoni, F., Barnea, N., Bank, I., and Holzmann, F., Adenosine deaminase (ADA) activity in lymphocytes of normal individuals and patients with chronic lymphatic leukemia, *Br. J. Haematol.,* 36, 67, 1977.
62. Ben-Bassat, I., Simoni, F., Holtzman, F., and Ramot, B., Adenosine deaminase activity of normal lymphocytes and leukemic cells, *Isr. J. Med. Sci.,* 15, 925, 1979.
63. Tung, R., Silber, R., Quagliata, F., Conklyn, M., Gottesman, J., and Hirshhorn, R., Adenosine deaminase activity in chronic lymphocytic leukemia, *J. Clin. Invest.,* 57, 756, 1976.
64. Zimmer, J., Khalkifa, A. S., and Lightbody, J. J., Decreased lymphocyte adenosine deaminase activity in acute lymphoblastic leukemia children and their parents, *Cancer Res.,* 35, 68, 1975.
65. Liso, L., Tursi, V., Speechia, G., Troccolli, G., Lovia, M. P., and Bonomo, L., Adenosine deaminase activity in acute lymphoblastic leukemia: cytochemical, immunological and clinical correlation, *Scand. J. Haematol.,* 21, 167, 1978.
66. Smyth, J. F., Poplack, D. G., Holiman, B. J., Leventhal, B. G., and Yabro, G., Correlation of adenosine deaminase activity with cell surface marker in acute lymphoblastic leukemia, *J. Clin. Invest.,* 62, 710, 1978.
67. Brouet, J. C. and Seligmann, M., The immunological classification of acute lymphoblastic leukemias, *Cancer,* 42, 817, 1978.
68. Hopkinson, D. A., Cook, P. J. L., and Harris, H., Further data on the adenosine deaminase (ADA) polymorphism and a report of a new phenotype, *Ann. Hum. Genet.,* 32, 361, 1969.
69. Wiginton, D. A., Coleman, M. S., and Hutton, J. J., Purification, characterization and radioimmunoassay of adenosine deaminase from human leukemic granulocytes, *Biochem. J.,* 195, 389, 1981.
70. Piras, M. A., Longinott, M., Ogiano, L., and Gakis, C., Serum adenosine deaminase activity in multiple myeloma and Hodgkin's disease, *I.R.C.S. Med. Sci.,* 9, 197, 1981.
71. Smyth, J. F., Chassin, M. M., Harrap, K. R., Adamson, R. H., and Johns, D. G., 2'-Deoxycoformycin, Phase I trial and clinical pharmacology, *Proc. Am. Assoc. Cancer Res.,* 20, 47, 1979.
72. Poplack, D. G., Sallan, S. E., Rivera, G., Holcenberg, J., Murphy, S. B., Blatt, J., Lipton, J. M., Venner, P., Glaubiger, D. L., Ungerleider, R., and Johns, D., Phase I study of 2'-deoxycoformycin in acute lymphoblastic leukemia, *Cancer Res.,* 41, 3343, 1981.
73. Major, P. P., Agarwal, R. P., and Kufe, D. W., Deoxycoformycin: neurological toxicity, *Cancer Chemother. Pharmacol.,* 5, 193, 1981.
74. Major, P. P., Agarwal, R. P., and Kufe, D. W., Clinical pharmacology of deoxycoformycin, *Blood,* 58, 91, 1981.
75. Major, P. P., Agarwal, R. P., and Kufe, D. W., Clinical pharmacology of arabinosyladenine in combination with deoxycoformycin, *Cancer Chemother. Pharmacol.,* 10, 125, 1983.
76. Agarwal, R. P., Blatt, J., Miser, J., Sallan, S., St. Lipton, J. M., Reaman, G. H., Holcenberg, J., and Poplack, D. G., Clinical pharmacology of adenine arabinoside in combination with deoxycoformycin, *Cancer Res.,* 42, 3884, 1982.
77. Koller, C. A., Mitchell, B. S., Grever, M. R., Mejias, E., Malspeis, L., and Metz, M. N., Treatment of acute lymphoblastic leukemia with 2'-deoxycoformycin: clinical and biochemical consequences of adenosine deaminase inhibition, *Cancer Treat. Rep.,* 63, 194, 1979.
78. Prentice, H. G., Gareshguru, K., Bradstock, K. F., Goldstone, A. H., Smyth, J. F., Wonke, B., Janossy, G., and Hoffbrand, A. V., Remission induction with adenosine deaminase inhibitor 2'-deoxycoformycin in thy-lymphoblastic leukemia, *Lancet,* 2, 170, 1980.
79. Kanofsky, J. R., Roth, D. G., Smyth, J. F., Bann, J. F., Sweet, D. L., and Uttman, J. E., Treatment of lymphoid malignancies with 2'-deoxycoformycin — a pilot study, *Am. J. Clin. Oncol.,* 5, 179, 1982.

80. Parks, R. E., Jr. and Agarwal, R. P., Purine nucleoside phosphorylase, *Enzymes,* 7, 483, 1972.
81. Biggar, W. D., Giblett, E. R., Ozerre, R. L., and Grover, B. D., A new form of nucleoside phosphorylase deficiency in two brothers with defective T-cell function, *J. Pediatr.,* 92, 354, 1978.
82. Dietz, A. A. and Czebotar, V., Purine metabolic cycle in normal and leukemic leukocytes, *Cancer Res.,* 37, 41, 1977.
83. Blatt, J., Simon, R., and Poplack, D., Purine nucleoside phosphorylase (PNP) and adenosine deaminase (ADA) in human lymphoid malignancies, *Proc. Am. Assoc. Cancer Res.,* 21, 229, 1980.
84. Borgers, M., Verhaegan, H., DeBrabander, M., et al., Purine nucleoside phosphorylase in chronic lymphocytic leukemia, *Blood,* 52, 886, 1978.
85. Carson, D. A., Kay, J., and Seegmiller, J. E., Lymphospecific toxicity in adenosine deaminase deficiency and purine nucleoside phsophorylase deficiency: possible role of nucleoside kinase(s), *Proc. Natl. Acad. Sci. U.S.A.,* 74, 5677, 1977.
86. Barton, R., Martinuik, F., Hirschhorn, R., and Goldschneider, I., Inverse relationship between adenosine deaminase and purine nucleoside phosphorylase in rat lymphocyte population, *Cellular Immun.,* 49, 208, 1980.
87. Dawson, D. M., Goodgriend, T. J., and Kala, N. O., Lactate hydrogenase: function of the two types, *Science,* 143, 929, 1964.
88. Papadopoulos, N. M. and Kintzios, J. A., Quantitative electrophoretic determination of lactate dehydrogenase isoenzymes, *Am. J. Clin. Pathol.,* 47, 96, 1967.
89. Wieme, R. J., Van Hove, W. Z., and Van Der Straeten, M. E., The influence of cytostatic treatment on serum LDH patterns of patients with bronchial carcinoma and its relation to tumor regression, *Ann. N.Y. Acad. Sci.,* 151, 213, 1968.
90. Plum, J. and Ringoir, S., A characterization of human B & T lymphocytes by their lactate dehydrogenase isoenzyme pattern, *Eur. J. Immunol.,* 5, 871, 1965.
91. Sabbe, X., et al., Cell marker studies in CLL with monoclonal OKT anti sera and lactic dehydrogenase isoenzyme, *Blut,* 46, 261, 1983.
92. Blatt, J., et al., Lactate dehydrogenase isoenzymes in normal and malignant human lymphoid cells, *Blood,* 60, 491, 1982.
93. Trenfiedl, K. and Masters, C., Patterns of synthesis and degradation of lactate dehydrogenase during the cell cycle of Burkitt's lymphoma cells, *Int. J. Biochem.,* 11, 55, 1979.
94. Plum, J. and Ringoir, S., Lactate dehydrogenase isoenzyme pattern as a measure of cellular differentiation in lymphocytic cells, *J. Reticuloendothel. Soc.,* 21, 225, 1977.
95. Blatt, J., Reaman, G., and Poplack, D. G., Biochemical markers in lymphoid malignancies, *N. Engl. J. Med.,* 303, 918, 1980.
96. Plum, J., Ringoir, S., and de Smedt, M., Lactic dehydrogenase activity: thymocyte populations, *Lancet,* 2, 721, 1977.
97. Ellis, R. B., et al., Expression of hexosaminidase isoenzymes in childhood leukemia, *N. Engl. J. Med.,* 298, 476, 1978.
98. Tanaka, T., Kobayashi, M., Saito, O., Kamada, N., Kuramoto, A., and Usui, T., Hexosaminidase isoenzyme profiles in leukemic cells, *Clin. Chim. Acta,* 128, 1, 19, 1983.
99. Dempsey, S. I., Crockard, A. D., and Bridges, J. M., An estimation of beta-glucuronidase and glucosaminidase activity in normal and chronic lymphocytic leukaemia lymphocytes, *Acta Haematol. (Basel),* 64(3), 141, 1980.
100. Crockard, A. D. and Morris, T. C., T Lysosomal enzyme activities in a case of T-cell chronic lymphocytic leukaemia, *Scand. J. Haematol.,* 25, 3, 226, 1980.
101. Invernizzi, R., Girino, M., and Nano, R., N-Acetyl-beta-glucosaminidase activity in normal and acute leukemia blood cells, *Basic Appl. Histochem.,* 25, 2, 121, 1981.
102. McCaffrey, R., Smoler, D. F., and Baltimare, D., Terminal deoxynucleotidyl transferase in a case of childhood acute lymphoblastic leukemia, *Proc. Natl.* 70, 521, 1973.
103. Greenwood, M. F., Coleman, M. D., Hutton, J. J., Lamplin, B., Krill, C., Bollum, F. J., and Holland, P., Terminal deoxynucleotidyl transferase distribution in neoplastic and hematopoietic cells, *J. Clin. Invest.,* 59, 889, 1977.
104. Coleman, M. A., Greenwood, M. D., Hutton, J. F., Bollum, F. J., Lapkin, B., and Holland, P., Serial observations on terminal deoxynucleotidyl transferase activity and lymphoblast surface markers in acute lymphoblastic leukemia, *Cancer Res.,* 36, 120, 1976.
105. McCaffrey, R., Lillquist, A., Sallan, S., Cohen, E., and Osband, M., Clinical utility of leukemia cell terminal transferase measurement, *Cancer Res.,* 41, 4814, 1981.
106. Canellos, G. P., DeVita, V. T., Whang-Peng, J., and Carbone, P. P., Hematologic and cytogenetic remission of blastic transformation in chronic granulocytic leukemia, *Blood,* 38, 671, 1971.
107. McCaffrey, R., Greaves, M., Harrison, T. A., et al., Biochemical and immunological evidence for lymphoblastic conversion in chronic myelogenous leukemia, *Blood,* 46, 1043, 1975.
108. Hoffbrand, A. V., Ganeshguru, K., Janossy, G., et al., Terminal deoxynucleotidyltransferase levels and membrane phenotypes in diagnosis of acute leukemia, *Lancet,* 2, 520, 1977.

109. Greaves, M. F., Cell surface characteristics of human leukaemic cells, *Essays Biochem.*, 15, 78, 1979.
110. Kung, P. C., Long, J. C., McCaffrey, R. P., Ratiliff, R. L., Harrison, T. A., and Baltimore, D., Terminal deoxynucleotidyl transferase in the diagnosis of leukemia and malignant lymphoma, *Am. J. Med.*, 64, 788, 1978.
111. Doinlon, J. A., Jaffe, E. S., and Braylan, R. C., Terminal deoxynucleotidyl transferase activity in malignant lymphoma, *N. Engl. J. Med.*, 286, 461, 1977.
112. Janossy, G., personal communication.
113. Bradstock, F., Papageorgiou, E. S., Janossy, G., Hoffbrand, A. V., Willoughby, M. L. Roberts, P. D., and Bollum, F. J., Detection of leukaemic lymphoblasts in CSF by immunofluorescence for terminal nucleotidyl transferase, *Lancet*, 1, 114, 1980.
114. Bollum, F. J., Terminal deoxynucleotidyl transferase as a hematopoietic cell marker, *Blood*, 54, 1203, 1979.
115. McCaffrey, R. P., Bell, R., Lillquist, A., Wright, G., and Baril, E., The Bollum enzyme in leukemia and lymphoma cells: the first decade, in *Terminal Transferase in Immunobiology and Leukemia*, Bertazzoni, U., Ed., Plenum Press, 1982, 221.
116. Janossy, G., Bollum, F. J., Bradstock, K. F., McMichael, A., Rapson, N., and Greaves, M. F., Terminal transferase positive human bone marrow cells exhibit the antigen phenotype of common acute lymphoblastic leukaemia, *J. Immunol.*, 12, 1252, 1979.
117. Froehlich, T. W., Buchanan, G. R., Cornet, J. M., Sartain, P. A., and Smith, R. G., Terminal deoxynucleotidyl transferase-containing cells in peripheral blood: implications for the surveillance of patients with lymphoblastic leukemia or lymphoma in remission, *Blood*, 58, 214, 1981.
118. Baltimore, D., Is terminal deoxynucleotidyl transferase a somatic mutagen in lymphocytes?, *Nature (London)*, 248, 409, 1974.
119. Alt, R. W. and Baltimore D., Joining of immunoglobulin heavy chain gene segments: implications from a chromosome with evidence of three D-$J_H$ fusions (recognition elements/Abelson murine leukemia virus/N gene segment/terminal deoxynucleotidyl transferase), *Proc. Nat. Acad. Sci. U.S.A.*, 79, 4118, 1982.

Chapter 8

# THE MAJOR HISTOCOMPATIBILITY COMPLEX AND LYMPHOMAS

## David Osoba

### TABLE OF CONTENTS

| | | |
|---|---|---|
| I. | Introduction | 168 |
| II. | Structure and Function | 168 |
| | A. H-2 | 168 |
| | B. HLA | 170 |
| III. | The MHC and Disease — Some General Considerations | 174 |
| IV. | H-2 and Leukemia in Mice | 175 |
| V. | HLA and the Lymphomas | 176 |
| | A. Problems and Pitfalls | 176 |
| | B. Specific Diseases | 179 |
| |     1. Hodgkin's Disease | 179 |
| |     2. Non-Hodgkin's Lymphomas | 183 |
| |     3. Burkitt's Lymphoma | 183 |
| |     4. Acute Leukemia | 184 |
| VI. | Summary and Conclusions | 184 |
| References | | 185 |

## I. INTRODUCTION

Originally, the major histocompatibility complex (MHC) in man was designated as histocompatibility locus A (HLA)[1] reflecting perhaps, the preoccupation of early workers with transplantation, but since the antigens of this genetic system are expressed on leukocytes and are usually detected in the tissue-typing laboratory by using lymphocytes, the term HLA is now used by most authors to refer to human leukocyte antigens. Also, with time, it has become clear that this system is the genetic basis not only for histocompatibility, but also for distinguishing between self and nonself in general. This belief is based partly on the strong similarities between HLA and the analogous system, histocompatibility-2 (H-2), in the mouse and partly on direct observations in man. In the mouse, there is ample evidence for genes within H-2 that govern immunological responsiveness to a wide variety of antigens and susceptibility or resistance to neoplasia. In man, the evidence for similar genes is less abundant. Although associations between certain HLA genes and some human diseases are strong; e.g., B27 and ankylosing spondylitis, DR2 and multiple sclerosis, DR3 and celiac disease (to mention only a few), the associations between HLA genes and malignant diseases seem much weaker, or perhaps, nonexistent. It must be asked, therefore, whether the failure to demonstrate strong associations in human malignant diseases represents a true difference in the two species, or whether the differences are more apparent than real. Also, it may be that the strong association of certain genes with diseases has made us concentrate primarily on searching for genes associated with susceptibility to malignant disease, whereas it may be more informative to look for associations of HLA genes with survival, or outcome.

The purpose of this selective review is to describe briefly the structure and functions of HLA and H-2 and to examine the rationale for seeking an association between HLA and malignant disease. Particular attention will be paid to the results of investigations in the lymphomas and leukemias.

## II. STRUCTURE AND FUNCTION

### A. H-2

Despite millenia of divergent evolution there are many striking similarities between the structure and function of the MHC of the mouse and the MHC of man. Thus, discoveries in one species have often led to similiar discoveries in the other. Only a brief description of the mouse MHC will be given here, and more detailed descriptions can be found in reviews by Klein[2] and Murphy.[3]

The MHC of the mouse is composed of multiple, tightly linked loci located on chromosome 17 (linkage group IX).[4,5] Through the study of informative H-2 recombinants in congenic lines of inbred mice, it has been possible to identify the position of several marker genes with respect to each other as well as to the centromere (Figure 1). The extreme ends of H-2 are marked by the K and D regions. The gene products of these regions have a molecular weight (mol wt) of 45,000 daltons,[6] and each is associated with $\beta$ 2 microglobulin (12,000 mol wt)[7-10] which is encoded by a locus on chromosome 2.[11]

The K and D region products are expressed as surface determinants on most, if not all, cells of the body.[12] There are multiple allelic forms of each gene product and several antibodies can be raised against the product of a single allele, thus indicating that there are more than one determinant on a single molecule. Some of these determinants are unique to a particular allelic product (private specificities) and some are shared by several allelic products (public specificities).[13]

The physiologic function of the allelic products of the K and D regions is still uncertain. Although it is known that they are recognized and serve as targets during the

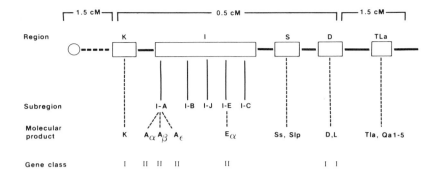

FIGURE 1. A schematic representation of a portion of the genetic map of the 17th murine chromosome. The circle represents the centromere and the rectangles are genetic regions. cM is the distance in centimorgans. See the text for a detailed explanation.

rejection of skin and tumor allografts,[14] in cell-mediated lympholysis (CML),[15] and as weak lymphocyte-activating determinants in the mixed leukocyte reaction (MLR),[16-18] these phenomena are not physiologic, in the sense that mice do not normally come into contact with foreign cells except in the hands of scientists in laboratories. Thus, the physiologic roles of these gene products must have some other function; they must have evolved and been retained as a result of natural selection, presumably because they confer a survival advantage. Since the gene products of these regions, even after induced mutations, are known to control the response of cytotoxic T ($T_c$) cells to virus-infected cells,[19] it seems that the natural function of these molecules is to guide T cells in their response to viruses. Also, since these gene products control the capacity of $T_c$ cells to react to chemically modified autologous lymphocytes,[20] they probably play a crucial role in the capacity of an organism to recognize its own tissues.

The I region is of great interest. It lies between the K and S regions[21] and contains at least four or five subregions, designated I-A, I-B, I-J, I-E, and I-C.[3,12,13] The gene products of the I-B, I-J, and I-C subregions have not been characterized as yet. Those of the I-A and I-E subregions consist of $\alpha$ chains with a 32,000 to 33,000 mol wt and $\beta$ chains of 28,000 mol wt.[22] They are designated $A_\alpha$, $A_\beta$, $A_\epsilon$, and $E_\alpha$. It is the $\beta$ chain which carries the polymorphic determinants. There is also a third chain with a molecular weight of 30,000 daltons which, at times, coprecipitates with the other two chains. These chains form dimers which integrate into the plasma membrane and are known as Ia (immune-region associated) antigens. Unlike the gene products of the K and D regions they are found mainly on lymphocytes, macrophages, and epidermal cells.[23]

The I-A, I-B, and I-E subregions contain loci that determine the capacity of a mouse to produce an immune reponse to a given antigen.[21,24,25] Hence these are known as Ir genes. Immune suppression (Is) genes are found in the I-A and I-C subregion[26,27] The I-J subregion is thought to contain genes coding for T suppressor ($T_s$) cell markers,[28] but this is still controversial. In addition, control of T-B cell cooperation and T helper ($T_h$) cell specificity, as well as allograft rejection, the MLR, and CML are encoded in the I-A and I-E subregions.[2,3,12] Again, however, only the control of T-B cell cooperation, $T_h$, and $T_s$ functions could be considered as physiologically relevant.

The S region is involved in controlling complement activity (C4).[29] Although complement is involved in immunological functions, the molecules of this region are strikingly different from those controlled by K, D, or I regions.

Recently, it has been shown that the TLa region located outside that which is bounded by K and D contains loci Qa 1-5 and TLa, that are involved in immune functions such as skin and tumor graft rejection, and CML.[30,31]

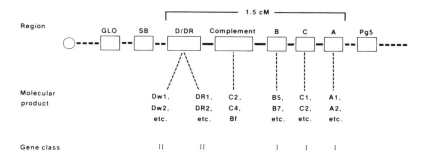

FIGURE 2. A schematic representation of a portion of the genetic map of the sixth human chromosome. The circle represents the centromere and the rectangles are genetic regions. cM is the distance in centimorgans, GLO is glycosylase and Pg5 is pepsinogen. The remaining terms are explained in the text.

It would seem, thus, that the MHC of the mouse is a highly complicated area of regions, subregions, loci, and multiple genes, but recently Klein et al.[32] have argued convincingly that the apparent complexity is primarily historical artifact. If only those functions considered to be natural (or physiological) are considered (and if some of the uncertainty regarding assignment of functions to new subregions is left in abeyance until definitive data is available)) it is possible to simplify the genetic map remarkably. In this simplified model there are only seven loci; namely K, $A_\alpha$, $A_\beta$, $E_\beta$, $E_\alpha$, D, and L, and each one may be considered as belonging to one or other of only two functional gene classes, I and II. Class I loci control $T_c$ cells, while class II loci control regulatory ($T_h$ and $T_s$) T cells. Qa and TLa loci should be included in the MHC since they resemble the class I loci. Klein et al.[32] conclude that all other traits attributed to H-2 molecules are a reflection of the basic need for T cells to distinguish between self and nonself. There seems much to recommend the adoption of this simplified view — perhaps the application of Occam's Razor is a sufficient reason by itself — and it also helps to make the analogies between the murine and human MHCs more clearly visible.

## B. HLA

The complex of genes making up HLA is located on the short arm of chromosome 6.[33,34] At least four main regions, or loci (A, B, C, and D/DR), are associated with immunological reactions and histocompatibility (Figure 2). As well there is a locus within the complex controlling components of the complement system (C2, C4, properidin or Bf) and one associated with the Chido and Rodgers blood groups (for detailed reviews and nomenclature see references 35 to 37). Recently, a locus denoted SB which is responsible for responses in the secondary MLR in individuals identical at the A, B, C, and D/DR loci,[38,39] as well as HLA-linked immune suppression genes, have been described.[40]

For several years the similarities between portions of H-2 and HLA have prompted speculations as to which regions in the two species are homologous. Until recently it had been assumed that HLA-B and H-2K were homologous as were HLA-A and H-2D, but Barnstable et al. noted that at least three sets of loci could be aligned; namely HLA-B, the complement loci and HLA-D/DR in HLA with H-2D, S and I in H-2[41] (Figure 3). Bodmer suggested that there is a parallel between HLA-C and H-2L, and that the gap between HLA-A and C might contain the equivalent of the TLa loci. Furthermore, if an intrachromosomal, unequal, double crossover event is postulated, one can complete the transition from HLA to H-2 in one step.[42] (Alternatives to this postulate are also reviewed by Bodmer in Reference 43).

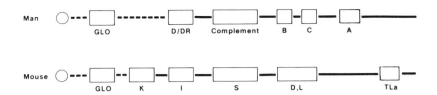

FIGURE 3. A schematic comparison of the genetic maps of the analogous portions of H-2 in the mouse and HLA in man.

The nomenclature that has evolved for this complex is now straightforward.[37] Gene products of the A, B, C, and D/DR regions are denoted by the letter for the locus and a number, e.g., A1, A2, etc., B5, B7, etc., DR1, DR2, etc. When there is insufficient evidence to give a specificity a definitive number, the small letter w, which denotes workshop status, is used, as in Aw19, Bw44, Cw1, DRw4, etc. When sufficient agreement among workers in the field is reached as to a given specificity, the w designation is removed.

Over the years as more and more antisera were developed and tested, it was found that some specificities were really composed of more than one specificity and, therefore were "split", e.g., A10 into A10, A25, and A26.

The genes in each of the loci are inherited codominantly and segregate independently. Since the number of known allelic forms at each locus is large, e.g., 20 at A, more than 40 at B, 8 at C, 12 at D, and 10 at DR[37] (more about the peculiarities of D and DR later), and since two different alleles may be expressed for a given locus on each of the two chromosomes in anyone individual, the chance of two unrelated individuals being completely identical at HLA has been estimated to be less than one in 300 million.[36] Thus, it seems that almost every individual is unique for this portion of the chromosome except for individuals within a family where the possibility of complete identity at HLA between siblings is one in four.

The linear array of genes on any one of the two chromosomes is known as a haplotype. Each individual inherits one maternal and one paternal haplotype and these together are the genotype. The expressed characteristics encoded in the genotype make up the phenotype. Since it is possible to determine only the phenotype by direct testing, family studies are necessary to determine the genotype.

The reason for the extreme polymorphism, greater than that known for any other genetic region (with the possible exception of the immunoglobulin loci), in this relatively short segment of chromosomal material is unknown. The development and retention through evolution of heterozygosity and polymorphism suggests that such a state is associated with a survival advantage. Perhaps the accumulation in a population of genes with deleterious effects may be offset by the concomitant presence of other genes that provide beneficial effects.[44] At present there is no direct evidence for such a model of "balanced polymorphism", but the observation of a nonrandom association between two genes on one haplotype suggests such a speculation. This is known as linkage disequilibrium and is seen most clearly in the unexpectedly frequent association of A1 with B8 and DR3, A3 with B7 and DR2, and A2 with B12 and DRw7.[36,44] The concepts of linkage disequilibrium and linked genes are of importance in the consideration of the association of HLA with disease,[36] and will be discussed later.

The gene products, or HLA antigens, encoded by the A, B, and C loci are found on all cells of the body except mature erythrocytes, sperm, and trophoblast.[45] These antigens are detected by antibodies that either have been raised deliberately, particularly as monoclonal antibodies, or are present in the sera of multiparous women. Crossreactivity between A-locus antigens or B-locus antigens is frequent.[35,46]

The D/DR locus gene products are expressed on B lymphocytes and their precursors, and on monocytes and macrophages.[47,48] Initially, they were detected by MLRs between individuals identical at the A and B (and presumably C) loci.[49] This led to the concept that D locus genes controlled lymphocyte-activating determinants, but more recently antisera have been found that react either with D region gene products or with the gene products of a closely related, hence DR, chromosomal locus.[50] The DR determinants have a similar tissue distribution as do D determinants.[50,51] It has not been possible as yet to conclude with certainty whether the D and DR loci are identical, albeit detectable by different methods, i.e., that lymphocytes in the MLR and DR antisera detect different determinants on the same gene product, or whether each is a separate locus responsible for closely related gene products.[35,43]

The biochemistry of the HLA gene products is remarkably similar to that of H-2 gene products. The A, B, and C gene products (class I genes) consist of glycosylated polypeptides with a molecular weight of 43,000 to 46,000 daltons associated with $\beta2$ microglobulin (12,000 mol wt). The amino acid sequence for the $\beta2$ microglobulin and for some of the heavy HLA chains has been found to have a significant degree of homology with immunoglobulin constant regions. Class II gene products, encoded by D/DR genes, also are composed of at least two polypeptide chains (33,000 and 28,000 mol wt), but recently a third chain having an intermediate molecular weight of 30,000 daltons which coprecipitates with the other two chains has been described both in man[52-54] and mouse.[55] Apparently, it is the light chain, i.e., 28,000 mol wt, that carries the polymorphic determinants.[43,53]

It is of interest that in both mouse and man the MHC contains within its borders a region or locus coding for complement components.[55] Although the location of these genes does not necessarily imply that their products are involved intimately with other gene products of the MHC in common functions, it has led to speculation that HLA-A, B and C, or DR products behave like complement components on the cell surface and interact with the T cell receptor once it has interacted with antigen.[43] This model of T cell receptor-antigen-HLA gene product interaction parallels the antibody-antigen-complement interaction in classic immunological reactions, and has been proposed as an alternative explanation to the dual recognition or altered-self models proposed by Doherty and Zinkernagel[19] as a means of explaining H-2 and HLA restriction.

Whether any of the above speculations are correct or not, it is clear that the functions of class I and class II gene products are related to recognition of self and non-self.[57,58] As in the mouse, human class I (A,B,C) gene products are targets for cell-mediated lympholysis[59] while class II gene products are involved in recognition both of allogeneic differences[49] and of autologous cells.[60-62] Thus, it is possible to see a proliferative response in an autologous MLR between partially purified responding T cells and stimulating B cells, but this proliferative response does not lead to a cytotoxic response as is normally seen in allogeneic MLRs.

Unlike the situation in the mouse, the evidence in man for immune response genes associated with the HLA region is still largely circumstantial and indirect. Some studies, based on a survey of populations, have been interpreted as suggesting that genes in the HLA region may be associated with the outcome of infectious disease. For example, the HLA phenotypes of the descendants of Dutch immigrants to Surinam who survived epidemics of typhoid fever and yellow fever are different with respect to C3, Gm, HLA-B, and GLO markers than are the phenotypes of a randomly selected Dutch population.[63] However, these results really do not distinguish between whether those immigrants who survived did so because immune response genes in the MHC of infected individuals enabled them to react immunologically to the biological agents and thereby develop immunity rapidly enough to recover (the *outcome* hypothesis), or whether they survived because they were resistant to the agents and did not become infected to begin with (the *susceptibility* hypothesis). Either situation, Ir gene differences or disease-susceptibility (Ds) gene differences, may be reflected in HLA phenotype differences if there is a strong linkage disequilibrium between the class I genes and the Ir or Ds genes. In order to distinguish between these two different but not mutually exclusive hypotheses, it is necessary to know both the proportion of individuals who become infected (resulting in either clinical or subclinical disease), as well as the proportion of individuals who recover from the infection. The former gives a measurement of susceptibility in the population in question, while the latter gives a measurement of the outcome in the susceptible subgroup.

Similarly, the studies of Piazza et al., who found a difference in the frequency of HLA-B antigens in coastal populations as compared to mountain populations of Sardinians,[64] are subject to more than one interpretation. The coastal population had been exposed to endemic malaria while the mountain population had been free of malaria for centuries. Although differences in the HLA-B phenotypes of these populations likely were due to selection by malaria, it is not possible to distinguish between selection based on susceptibility as compared to selection based on outcome in susceptible individuals. Since malaria in the coastal populations has been eradicated since World War II it is no longer possible to answer this question.

An attempt to deal with this problem in a somewhat different manner was made by Osoba et al., who estimated the proportion of eastern Tanzanians exposed to falciparum malaria by determining their antibody levels.[65] The highest titers were most frequently found in individuals who possessed both HLA-AW30 and A2. These results suggested that individuals with this phenotype may also carry linked genes enabling a strong immune response to malaria antigens, but other interpretations, such as the temporal relationship to the infection are also possible. Although the association of the highest titers with the presence of two genes is a possibility suggested by studies in the mouse,[55] in the case of the results reported by Osoba et al., another apparent problem is that the class I genes were both in the A region, whereas, by analogy with the mouse, the putative closely-linked Ir genes would more likely be in the D region and therefore, more likely to be associated with B rather than A region genes. However, this result may not be as aberrant as it seems in the light of the suggestions that the A region in man is really the homologue of the TLa region in the mouse.[41-43] This latter region now has been shown to be involved intimately with many immune functions, including the production of cell surface molecules with a 43,000 to 45,000 mol wt associated with a $\beta$2-microglobulin subcomponent and possible Ir-like genes.[30,31] Thus, linkage disequilibrium between A region genes and Ir genes in man is a distinct possibility. If the analogy with the mouse is correct, human studies should be directed towards searching for association between immune responses and either D/DR-region genes or A-region genes. However, it must be borne in mind that a strong immune response, as shown by antibody titers or by cellular reactions, does not necessarily predispose to a favorable disease outcome and a survival advantage. For example, in mice the immune response to infection with *Schistosoma mansoni* is under the control of H-2, but mice with the strongest response also have the highest mortality.[66]

It should be noted at this point that if a disease can exert a selective pressure on populations that might be reflected by a loss or gain of certain HLA genes in subsequent generations, this will be detected only if the disease produces a high mortality among affected individuals before they reach sexual maturity. Clearly, such a selective pressure would not be exerted by diseases that affect populations after the reproductive stage of life has passed. Since epidemics of most infectious diseases often do produce a high mortality rate in the very young, it can be seen why the idea of infectious disease exerting a selective pressure has so much appeal. However, the results of population studies have not yet provided a clear answer to the question of whether the HLA complex contains Ir genes controlling the immune response to infectious agents, but some of these results are in keeping with such a hypothesis.

Somewhat more direct evidence for Ir genes in the HLA region comes from attempts to immunize individuals and determine if there is an association between HLA gene products and a high vs. a low or no response to the immunizing agent.[67-78] As in the mouse,[73] there is some evidence in man that genes governing the response to virus-infected cells are associated with HLA,[74,75] although such a restriction has not been demonstrated universally.[76] Only one study, however, has included the necessary analysis of family studies to determine the mode of inheritance of immune responsiveness.[40] Sasazuki et al., used streptococcal cell wall (SCW) antigen (since all the population studied would have been exposed previously to this antigen) and found that a single dominant gene appears to control *low* responsiveness to this antigen.[40] In a pedigree analysis the low responsiveness to SCW antigen always traveled with a particular HLA haplotype in each family. A linkage analysis implied that the recombination fraction, and hence the distance, between genes coding for the class I gene products and the gene coding for low response to SCW was extremely small.

It is surprising, perhaps, that a dominantly inherited gene is associated with a weak immune response rather than a strong response. However, it is possible to rationalize how this might result in a survival advantage, since a strong response might conceivably be associated with an increased mortality in the era before the availability of penicillin. Thus, a weak response may have been advantageous for survival with respect to the sequelae of streptococcal infection.

## III. THE MHC AND DISEASE — SOME GENERAL CONSIDERATIONS

Some comments about the role of the MHC in infectious diseases with particular reference to evidence for Ir genes in man have been made in the preceding section. A detailed discussion of the statistically significant associations between many other diseases and HLA would be out of place here (see references 79 and 80 for examples), but these associations do raise some general points for consideration.[81] With only a few exceptions (e.g., B27 and ankylosing spondylitis, A3 and hemochromatosis), the described associations are strongest between a given disease and D/DR region gene products; e.g., Dw/DR2 and multiple sclerosis, Dw/DR3 and insulin-dependent diabetes (as well as many other endocrinopathies that may have an autoimmune basis), and Dw/DR3 and autoimmune diseases not affecting endocrine organs (reviewed in Reference 82).

Since D/DR-region genes are thought most likely to be closely associated with Ir genes it seems reasonable to assume that these diseases have a common etiologic basis related to Ir genes. In the case of the D/DR associations, Bodmer has suggested that these diseases may have in common the production of autoantibody, as is the case in myasthenia gravis where autoantibody to the acetylcholine receptor exists, whereas in those diseases associated with B27, it would seem that T cell autoimmunity may be involved.[43,83]

Despite the appeal of the Ir-gene hypothesis as an explanation for susceptibility through autoimmune reactivity, it does not explain what leads to such reactivity in the first place. Is it possible that autoimmune reactivity is a common feature during life, but normally is suppressed by immune-suppression (Is) genes? If so, the absence or nonexpression of Is genes would result in the production of autoantibody or autoreactive cells in only a minority of the population. The demonstration of virtually universal T cell autoreactivity against autologous B cell components in autologous MLRs suggests that autoreactivity is indeed the norm.

Explanations other than the Ir and Is gene hypotheses may also be relevant and must be considered. These include the possibility of mimicry between infectious agents and self-determinants so that infectious agents are not recognized as nonself,[84] and the possibility that some HLA specificities resemble certain ligand receptors resulting in a modification of end-organ susceptibility.[85] Such hypotheses have only scanty support as yet, and there is some evidence to the contrary so far as the mimicry hypothesis is concerned.[83] (Other possible explanations and mechanisms are discussed in References 86 and 87).

It is important at this juncture to make note of some further important considerations. One of these is that the causation and development of a disease is usually multifactorial. Whether or not a host is affected may in part be dependent upon HLA-associated genes, but determinants not linked to HLA may also be involved. Thus, in multiple sclerosis, susceptibility is related to determinants tightly linked to DR2 haplotypes as well as to other determinants (which may include family environment) that are unlinked, but interact to simulate a loose linkage.[88] Indeed, similar explanations seem reasonable to account for the lack of a strong association between HLA determinants and disease, since even in the case of HLA-B27 and ankylosing spondylitis, where the relative risk of carriers of B27 developing the disease is the highest yet found, not all individuals carrying B27 will develop the disease. In some associations the relative risk for carriers of a particular specificity may be only three to four times that for noncarriers. Thus, other factors must also be of importance, and in many situations perhaps of more importance than the HLA genotype. Recently, Green has reviewed the fundamental principles and measures which must be considered in measuring association strength between HLA and disease.[89,90] Since it seems reasonable to assume that HLA factors are probably not the causal factors but only correlated to the causal factors, and since the causal factors are probably heterogeneous, one can appreciate difficulties inherent in proposing a simple hypothesis that will explain the observed associations.

Another consideration has been alluded to earlier. Susceptibility to the *development* of a disease may not necessarily be dependent upon the same factors as is the *outcome* of the disease once it has developed. Thus, it is possible to visualize that the development of a disease may arise as a consequence of T cell recognition of nonself, but survival may be dependent upon the capacity to produce antibody, a B cell function which is encoded in a different portion of the genome. Furthermore, of the proportion of a population exposed to the disease-producing factors it is likely that only a subgroup will express the clinical manifestations of the disease whereas some members of the exposed population will show evidence of exposure; e.g., development of antibodies (in the case of some infectious diseases), but not become clinically ill. Although the outcome in the latter group can be considered universally favorable and is of great importance, this population may not be examined by investigators unless screening methods are used that can detect this population.

Finally, the success of immunization in preventing epidemics caused by communicable disease and of antibiotics in combating infection, and the improvement of treatment that prolongs life or even cures some malignancies, may have a profound effect on studies of the association of HLA genes and disease. It is only in recent history that medicine has made a significant impact on survival in these situations. Therefore, natural selection may no longer be dependent on the same factors, e.g., the MHC, in those populations having access to modern preventive medicine and medical care, as it does in populations without such access.

## IV. H-2 AND LEUKEMIA IN MICE

In mice, genes in H-2 have a major effect on the outcome of infection by a number of oncogenic viruses, including Gross,[91-93] Friend,[94-100] Balb/Tennant,[101] radiation leukemia,[102,103] and mammary tumor viruses.[104] Resistance and susceptibility to Gross leukemia virus is determined primarily by Rgv-1. In crosses between H-$2^k$ and H-$2^b$ mice, the homozygous H-$2^k$ offspring have a greater than 90% incidence of the leukemia, while heterozygous and homozygous H-$2^b$ mice have a lower incidence (30% to 50%), as well as a delayed onset. Rgv-1 maps towards the K region of H-2, probably within the I region. Thus, Rgv-1 confers resistance and is dominant, whereas susceptibility is a recessive trait in the development of Gross virus leukemia. However, in animals infected with Friend leukemia virus, Rgv-1 does not influence initial susceptibility, but instead governs the outcome of the disease by governing recovery from virus-induced splenomegaly thus leading to decreased mortality.[96] The mechanism by which Rgv-1 influences the outcome of Friend leukemia is uncertain, although experiments in Gross virus leukemia indicate that mice carrying Rgv-1 regularly develop detectable antibodies to Gross virus antigen, whereas those lacking Rgv-1 do not, suggesting that the development of an immune response to viral antigen may be of importance.[105,106]

In contrast to the situation in Gross virus leukemia, resistance to Friend leukemia and radiation virus leukemia map in the D region of H-2. The genes Rfv-1 and Rrv-1 confer resistance, but again the mechanisms are unclear.[99,100] In the case of Friend leukemia, Blank et al. suggest that resistant animals are capable of a cell-mediated response to the tumor cells, while susceptible animals are not.[107] However, Chesebro et al. were unable to demonstrate an immune response associated with infection,[97,98] but as pointed out by Meruelo and McDevitt, the infecting dose of virus was so small that a strong immune response may not have been induced.[108]

The gene responsible for resistance to radiation leukemia virus seems not to have an effect so much on initial infection as it does on a later stage of disease, thereby influencing recovery from the disease.[108]

Thus, although the precise mechanisms are uncertain, it seems that both the I and D regions of H-2 are associated with the outcome of leukemia virus infection. It is of interest that resistance conferred by the genes in these regions is in each case a dominant trait. Also, it should be noted that genes on chromosomes other than chromosome 17 influence the efficiency of initial virus infection by Friend virus (Fv-1 on chromosome 4) and the initial expression of virus in AKR mice (Akv-1 on chromosome 7), indicating that susceptibility and resistance to leukemia viruses are not solely H-2-associated functions (for a detailed review see References 108 and 109).

## V. HLA AND THE LYMPHOMAS

### A. Problems and Pitfalls

In the preceding sections the striking similarities between the MHCs of mouse as well as man and the association between murine leukemias/lymphomas and genes in the MHC have been emphasized. Therefore, it seems reasonable to think that there may be analogous genes in man that control susceptibility and resistance to the development and outcome of leukemia and lymphomas. However, before embarking on a review of the work that has been done in the area of HLA associations with leukemias and lymphomas, certain problems and pitfalls should be noted.

The similarities between human and murine leukemia/lymphoma may not be as close as they appear to be at first thought. The murine leukemias studied most extensively and about which, therefore, the most is known are all virus-induced diseases in highly inbred strains of laboratory mice, as opposed to diseases occurring naturally in wild mice. Therefore, it may be asked whether the results of such studies, although of great interest and importance for our understanding of the genetic control of virus-induced diseases, nevertheless may be over-emphasizing only a small fraction of the "real-life" situation outside the laboratory. For example, it has been pointed out that spontaneous tumors occurring in wild mice do not seem to result in the development of anti-tumor antibodies whereas anti-tumor responses can be demonstrated with regularity in laboratory strains of mice.[110] Furthermore, although many leukemias and lymphomas in mice are known to be caused by viruses, there is not a single human leukemia or lymphoma for which a viral cause has been fully established. Perhaps Burkitt's lymphoma is the most likely candidate, but even in this situation it is still not definite that the Epstein-Barr virus is the primary etiologic agent. Therefore, for human leukemias and lymphomas the appropriate murine model may be that of spontaneous tumors in wild mice rather than virus-induced tumors in laboratory strains of mice.

Another problem in the search for associations between HLA and lymphomas relates to methodology. In early studies there was an obvious need for standardization of reagents, i.e., the HLA antisera, and this has been met in recent years. However, as more recent antisera are found or developed, e.g., monoclonal antisera and DR antisera, or as more specificities detected by antisera are split into more and more antigenic determinants, the need for repeating older studies using the newer reagents becomes necessary. In addition, rapid changes in technology and new information have required frequent revisions and additions to the nomenclature and terminology in this field,[37] thereby causing frustration and confusion for all but the workers directly involved in this area.

Problems which result from the rapid expansion of research activity and knowledge are unavoidable, but certain other methodological problems can be avoided. Two examples of avoidable problems are (1) inadequate sampling of the population to be studied resulting in a multitude of reports each containing results from only a small number of patients and (2) selective sampling of patients presenting to an institution resulting in the possibility that certain subgroups of patients are not proportionately represented and the results are skewed. An excellent example of the first problem, inadequate sampling, is provided by attempts to study HLA associations in the non-Hodgkin's lymphomas. Depending upon which classification system one prefers, there may be a dozen or more histological varieties of non-Hodgkin's lymphoma,[111,112] or stated another way, a dozen different diseases, all having some similarity to each other but each having a different prognosis and possibly a different etiologic cause or host response. Therefore, if one accepts this view, each histological variety should be represented by an adequate sample size. With more than 90 distinguishable HLA specificities being detectable, and some of these occurring only infrequently, it is clear each sample size must be very large if hope of distinguishing differences between the disease and the normal population or differences between the varieties of the disease are to be detected. Also, the sample size should be determined by the magnitude of the difference one wishes to demonstrate between the disease population and the disease-free population. Since the frequency of many of the histological varieties of non-Hodgkin's lymphoma is very low, it is virtually impossible to obtain samples of sufficient size unless multicenter cooperative groups (perhaps international in scope) are involved. Such an approach then raises new problems; i.e., the variability in disease patterns in different populations and the difficulties of reaching agreement on the histological variety of disease. One way of avoiding these difficulties is to narrow the scope of the question being asked, e.g., is there an association between known DR specificities and a particular disease subgroup? This approach simplifies matters to some degree, but of course leads to the difficulty that associations between the subgroup of the disease in question and a genetic locus other than DR would be missed as would associations between other subgroups and DR or other loci.

A second problem related to sampling has to do with selection of only certain individuals out of the total population afflicted with the disease. It also applies to the selection of only certain individuals in the normal, or disease-free control population. If testing of all consecutively presenting individuals with a given disease is not strictly adhered to, then inadvertent selection of certain subpopulations will occur. Thus, if patients who are readily available to the experimental laboratory, such as hospitalized patients, are the only ones tested then these will be over-represented, while those who are ambulatory and attending the outpatient clinic only will be under-represented. Also, sampling of all patients, whether hospitalized or ambulatory, in a tertiary referral center such as a university teaching hospital or a hospital specialized in the treatment of a particular disease, will still miss those patients who are not thought to be ill enough or of insufficient medical interest to be referred to that center. Finally, disease-free individuals drawn for the control group often are not representative of the disease-free population at large. The selected individuals may come from among hospital and laboratory staff, in which case they may be representative only of individuals employed in a health-related occupation (further selection may occur from subpopulations of interested health-care workers, i.e., laboratory technicians, nurses, and physicians, with exclusion of other health-care workers), or from families of patients who are potential recipients of kidney or bone marrow transplants (in which case relatives of individuals with certain diseases are over-represented), or from blood donors in blood donor clinics. While the last example represents a better sample that the other examples mentioned, it still is obviously selected for individuals with a particular interest, i.e., giving blood, and does not truly represent the large proportion of the population that are not blood donors.

All of the above examples can lead to the inadvertent selection of subpopulations and, therefore, a loss or skewing of data. The safest course in these difficult waters is for researchers to report exactly how the studied sample was selected, citing as well the number of individuals who were not available for study or who were available but were not selected. The citing of such denominators allows the reader to interpret the data appropriately.

Another difficulty has to do with interpretation rather than selection. There may be natural variation between different populations which are studied. It is known that HLA phenotypes can vary from one ethnic group to another; e.g., A2 occurs much more frequently in indigenous African blacks than in Scandinavian caucasoids. Individuals either derived or descended from these populations are represented in almost every major urban center in Europe and North America, as well as elsewhere. Therefore, it is of importance to provide information, at least in a broad way, as to the ethnic composition of both disease and disease-free samples.

A statistical problem relating to interpretation is that of determining whether an association between a given HLA specificity or haplotype and a disease is of significance, statistically or otherwise. This question has been dealt with by others,[113-115] and will only be touched upon here. First, the statistical significance of an association is dependent upon disproving the null hypothesis, i.e., that an observed association is really a chance event. It is common to accept that if an association of events is such that the probability of the associations occurring by chance alone is less than 1 in 20, i.e., less than 5% of the time (hence, $p = < 0.05$), then the null hypothesis is disproven. However, when an investigator attempts to detect one specificity as a marker out of a large number of specificities (more than 90), the possibility of chance associations in the order of 1 in 20 will lead to misinterpretations of the results in the population of individuals tested. Therefore, it has become common practice to multiply the $p$ value obtained by the number of specificities being detected in order to try to approximate the true probability. Thus, if the $p$ value obtained was 0.001 and the number of specificities being detected is 66, then the $p$ value becomes 0.066, and would probably not be regarded as significant.

Another problem related to statistics is the difficulty of determining a true decrease of a particular specificity in a sample of the disease population if that specificity is relatively infrequent in the normal population. For example, if a specificity occurs in 3% of a normal population (frequency = 0.03) it is difficult to be certain, unless the sample size is adequately large, if an observed frequency of 0.015 in the disease sample is significant. Yet, a decreased frequency of a particular specificity in a given disease could mean that the specificity in question is linked with a disease-resistance gene.

Even if statistically significant associations indicating either susceptibility or resistance are found, how much significance do they really have in practical terms?[116] The strong association between B27 and ankylosing spondylitis may help in the differential diagnosis of an atypical presentation of this disease, but not all individuals having B27 also have ankylosing spondylitis. Yet, this is the strongest known association between an HLA specificity and a disease. In other situations where the associations are much weaker, much more attention needs to be paid to subgroups of patients with a given disease, as in the example of multiple sclerosis given earlier.[88]

It should also be noted that the efficacy of modern therapy may change the outcome of a disease, thereby apparently altering the results of current studies as compared with earlier studies. The modern therapy of Hodgkin's disease, which has changed survival significantly over the past 10 to 15 years, might obscure any HLA associations having an effect on survival and thereby give rise to different results than those obtained earlier in untreated or ineffectively treated patients.

B. Specific Diseases

The role of the HLA complex in lymphomas and leukemias may be considered from two perspectives. The first is that genes in the HLA region may determine susceptibility or resistance to the development of the disease, and the second is that HLA genes may determine outcome or survival in individuals who already have the disease. These need not be mutually exclusive possibilities, nor is either one of them necessarily true despite the fact that most workers in this field have tended to favor one or the other.

The suggestion that HLA genes govern susceptibility or resistance requires the demonstration of either an increased or decreased frequency of a particular specificity or specificities in patients with the disease, as compared to its frequency in a disease-free population, whereas association with survival requires that the frequency of a particular specificity be increased in long-term survivors or decreased in patients who die early in the course of the disease as compared to the frequency of that specificity in the disease population at the time of diagnosis.

*1. Hodgkin's Disease*

In 1967 Amiel reported a nearly twofold increase in the frequency of the compound specificity then known as 4C in a group of 41 patients with Hodgkin's disease.[117] This initial report of an apparent association of HLA with a disease was instrumental in launching a large number of investigations dealing with HLA and disease.[115] Initially these dealt frequently with Hodgkin's disease, since the possibility that Hodgkin's disease has a viral etiology (reviewed in reference 118), and the analogy with Gross leukemia in mice was uppermost in investigators minds.

Soon after Amiel's report the compound specificity 4C was split into four specificities now known as B5, B15, B18, and Bw35. Several subsequent reports[119-129] seemed to confirm Amiel's original observation, showing increased frequencies of one or another of these four specificities (reviewed by Bodmer[130]). The fact that not all reports found an increased frequency of exactly the same specificity initially was not worrisome since these are highly cross-reacting specificities and slight variations in the detecting antisera from one laboratory to another could account for the discrepancies. In addition, some of the early studies also showed an increased frequency of A1 and B8, two specificities that frequently occur together on the same haplotype.[127,131-133] The apparent problem posed by this observation, i.e., that two loci were involved, could be resolved by the interpretation that only one of these two specificities is increased in patients with Hodgkin's disease, and other is also present because of the known linkage disequilibrium between these two loci.

It was soon found in studies of the families of patients that all of these specificities were inherited in the expected manner,[127,128] thus excluding the possibility that they were disease determinants present in patients with Hodgkin's disease which cross-react with actual HLA specificities. This set the stage for the postulate that the HLA gene products are not themselves involved in susceptibility to the disease, but are merely markers for other genes, termed disease-susceptibility genes by Bodmer,[130] and that these genes are in linkage disequilibrium with detectable HLA genes in a manner analogous to the linkage disequilibrium between the genes encoding A1 and B8. It also led to the suggestion that the extreme polymorphism seen in the HLA system is a balance resulting from natural selection, with genes having a survival advantage compensating for disease-susceptibility genes.

Since that early period (1967 to 1972) several important developments have taken place. The need for a cooperative effort, to pool antisera and results, resulted in collaboration by many workers who came together periodically to exchange information in "Histocompatibility Workshops". HLA antisera were standardized and more and more specificities demonstrated, many of the "new" ones being in reality splits of old ones. Currently, the specificity called B5 consists of B5, Bw51, and Bw52, whereas B15 has been split into B15, Bw62, and Bw63.[111] Therefore, the specificity 4C now consists to the above six specificities plus B18 and Bw35. Whether this list comprises the final situation, only the future will reveal.

Conceptual advances have been as important as technical ones. As more studies were done, failure to confirm earlier results become more frequent. For example, Falk and Osoba, in their initial report, agreed with the suggestion that B5 was increased in frequency in patients with Hodgkin's disease,[127] but subsequently when they studied a series of consecutive patients, all tested within a year of the onset of their disease, the earlier result could not be confirmed.[131] This led them to suggest that since the initial series of patients studied did not include all available patients presenting to the hospital within a given period of time, there may have been an inadvertent sampling bias introduced into their own as well as other studies. The bias may have been in favor of those patients readily available for testing, perhaps because they were already in-hospital or lived close by, thus excluding patients who were relatively well and came for less frequent follow-up, or who had been seen in consultation only and now were being followed away from the Center where the HLA phenotyping was being done. Furthermore, such patients might not represent a true cohort, since they would in reality be a mixture of patients with respect to duration of disease, some of them having been phenotyped soon after the onset of disease and others several years or even decades after the onset of disease. Therefore, patients who had died after relatively short survival times might not be proportionately represented. Although it is likely that both types of sampling errors were present in early studies it is not possible to conclude with certainty that they account entirely or even in part for the differences in observations reported. It is also possible that some of the other errors discussed earlier, e.g., nonrandom control samples or ethnic differences also were present.

The sampling bias in early studies was also recognized by Kissmeyer-Nielsen et al. who, in 1971, began to phenotype all new patients with Hodgkin's disease included in the Danish Hodgkin's disease project LYGRA.[132,133] The data from the prospective Canadian and Danish studies, numbering 280 patients,[131,133] as well as from combined material on 523 patients studied during the fifth workshop on histocompatibility testing,[134] did not confirm the previously suggested evidence for an increase in the 4C related antigens in the patients taken as a whole, i.e., without regard to possible subgroups. However, increases in A1 and B8 were present in the Danish series as well as in the material from the workshop.

The possibility of an increased frequency of any HLA antigen in Hodgkin's disease is surprising, since an increased frequency implies increased susceptibility. Yet, if the analogy with leukemia and H-2 in the mouse is to be considered, the H-2 genes detected thus far are associated with increased resistance; e.g., mice with Rgv-1 are not as susceptible to developing Gross leukemia as are mice without this gene. Therefore, in the case of Hodgkin's disease, it would be expected that any HLA genes serving as markers for disease-resistance genes should be decreased in frequency. However, only some of the available data seems to support this possibility. Falk and Osoba reported a decreased frequency of A3 and A11 (two cross-reacting specificities) in two groups of patients, both of which were phenotyped within a year of onset of disease,[127,131] but this result has not been confirmed by other studies. Although the reason is unknown, it must be pointed out that it is extremely difficult, from a statistical point of view, to show a significant decrease in frequency of a specificity or specificities that are somewhat low in frequency in the normal population unless the decrease is dramatic, or very large numbers of patients are studied. Also, it is possible that resistance is not absolute, similar to the results in mouse Gross leukemia studies where 30 to 50% of resistant mice still develop the disease as compared to 100% of susceptible mice. Also, resistance may be dependent on more than one gene, only one of which is in the HLA region.

A further concept introduced into studies after 1971 was the need to examine subgroups of patients with Hodgkin's disease.[127] This would be of particular importance if it is true that the clinical entity diagnosed as Hodgkin's disease is really two or more etiological entities that result in closely related clinical pictures. Some of the factors that have been examined in subgroups of patients include the age and sex of the patients and the histological varieties of disease. Age has been considered of importance because the peculiar bimodal age distribution and epidemiological data suggest that the disease seen in younger individuals (under 40 years) may be due to an infectious agent, whereas that seen in older individuals may be a true neoplasm.[118,135] However, no consistent relationship between the sex or age of patients at onset of disease and HLA antigens has been found.

The attempts to relate histological variety of disease to HLA antigen frequencies introduced another complication. There was frequent disagreement (particularly in the 1960s) among pathologists as to the most appropriate histological classification, but even after most adopted the Rye classification[136] there still may be frequent interpathologist variation in the opinions given. (In fact a single pathologist may give a different opinion some years later when asked to review material previously examined by himself). This complication is probably responsible for the variation from one study to another in the proportion of patients reported with each histological variety. Even if reports of series containing only consecutively presenting patients and using the same histological classification system are considered,[131,133,137] it is apparent that the proportion of patients with any one histological variety differs from study to study. The proportion of patients with the nodular sclerosis variety in the Falk and Osoba series[131] is similar to that usually reported in North American caucasoids,[118,135,138] in that it is the most common variety, whereas in the two Scandinavian series[133,137] there is a higher proportion of the mixed cellularity and lymphocyte predominance types. It is unknown whether these differences are the result of differing assignment because of interpathologist variation or whether a true difference exists in the populations studied. Nevertheless, the failure to show consistent relationships between histological variety of disease and HLA phenotype may be explained by one or both of these possibilities.

It has been known for some time that there appears to be an increased risk, estimated at three- to sevenfold, for close relatives of a patient with the disease to develop the disease as compared to the risk in families without an affected member.[131-141] Therefore, another approach, used in more recent years, has been to determine the HLA genotypes of siblings and other relatives in families where two or more members have developed Hodgkin's disease and to compare the genotypes of the affected members with those of unaffected members in the same family (reviewed by Hors et al.[142]). If there is a multigenic influence on susceptibility this may be better detected when the entire genotpye is used as the marker for disease susceptibility or resistance genes rather using a single gene marker. When the available combined data given in the report by Hors et al.[142] as well as other reports[143,144] are considered together, the observed frequency of identical HLA genotypes present among affected siblings is from two of three times higher than expected. In 21 affected siblings, the observed number of HLA-identical siblings was 13, whereas the expected number is only 5 or 6. These data suggest that susceptibility genes for Hodgkin's disease may be associated with the MHC complex and, in addition, suggest that susceptibility may be a recessive trait, as is known to be the case in murine leukemia (reviewed in an earlier section). However, as pointed out by Hors et al.,[142] it is unlikely that all affected siblings who have been HLA genotyped have been reported. Therefore, they suggest that an international registry is required for such data. In addition, it would be important to ascertain that genotyping be done whenever possible on a world-wide basis, since selected sampling may be misleading.

Thus, despite the enormous effort put forth into searching for associations between the MHC of man and Hodgkin's disease that might suggest susceptibility (by 1975 Svejgaard et al.[145] had registered nearly 1500 patients — albeit most were phenotyped retrospectively without regard to duration of disease), no strong associations have been proven in either entire populations or in subpopulations of patients. Only the results of a small number of family studies suggest such an association, but these are also suspect because of possibly selective reporting.

The idea that survival of patients with Hodgkin's disease may be influenced by genes in the MHC (analogous to the influence of Rgv-1 on splenomegaly due to Friend leukemic virus in mice) was first suggested by Falk and Osoba.[127,131] In two separate retrospective studies, including a total of 73 patients who were phenotyped after they had already survived more than 5 years, the median being 9.8 years, the frequency of B8 was found to be significantly increased. However, since these were retrospective studies they are subject to the same kinds of sampling errors discussed earlier. Only the results of prospective studies in which the patients are followed without significant loss to follow-up for a sufficient time, probably 10 years, can be considered as giving valid information. Thus far, there are no reports of studies with follow-up periods of that length, but such studies are in progress. Thus, the question of whether the MHC influences long-term survival and whether this is detectable by studying HLA marker genes remains to be resolved.

In one of the ongoing prospective studies, it has been found that patients carrying the compound specificity Aw19 (now known to be composed of Aw19, A29, Aw30, Aw31, Aw32, and Aw33) have a shorter survival time than do other patients in the cohort.[146,147] Even when disease parameters known to be of prognostic value for survival,[148] such as age, stage of disease, and histology were taken together, the presence or absence of Aw19 provided additional prognostic information.[147] Thus, carriers of Aw19 who were more than 40 years of age and had either Stage III or IV lymphocyte depletion or mixed cellularity disease had a significantly poorer survival (a median of

2 years) than did patients with the same prognostic factors who do not have Aw19 (median survival not yet reached after 7 years of follow-up). In the patients in whom the non-HLA prognostic factors were favorable to begin with, i.e., less than 40 years of age and either Stage I or II nodular sclerosis or lymphocyte predominance disease, the presence or absence of Aw19 did not influence the outcome of the disease and the median survival for both these groups has not yet been reached after 7 years of follow-up.

The presence of B5 at the onset of disease may be an additional indicator of a poor prognosis, since an earlier analysis of the same group of 79 patients, within 3 years of diagnosis, showed an excess frequency of B5 in the patients who had died.[146] It was suggested, therefore, that B5 might also serve as a marker for disease with a poor prognosis. Also, this finding could account for the increased frequency of B5 in retrospective studies, since patients with B5 may have been in-hospital frequently either because of rapid progression of their disease or for more treatment than non-B5 patients. Thus, they would have been readily availble for study and may have been over-represented. As discussed earlier, this explanation would also account for the failure of prospective studies to find an increased frequency of B5 at the onset of the disease. At present, however, the role of B5 in Hodgkin's disease is uncertain.

Another question that remains unresolved is whether associations between HLA genes and Hodgkin's disease or any of the other lymphomas might be best detected by typing for D/DR region gene products rather than for A, B, and C region gene products.

### 2. Non-Hodgkin's Lymphomas

Although at least two early studies[149,150] seemed to indicate an increased frequency of B12 in association with non-Hodgkin's lymphomas, particularly of the follicular variety,[151] later studies have not been confirmatory. Whether the multitude of histological varieties of non-Hodgkin's lymphomas represents a multitude of etiological factors or whether this is an expression of only one or a few factors is unknown. There has been much disagreement as to the appropriate histological classification and only recently has some international consensus been reached.[112] However, the new cytomorphic and immunological approaches to classification have resulted in a large variety of phenotypes and, if HLA associations with each phenotype are to be sought, the number of patients studied will need to be very large. It is likely that only cooperative group efforts would be successful. Thus, data on HLA associations with non-Hodgkin's lymphomas are inconclusive and data on associations with survival are not available.

### 3. Burkitt's Lymphoma

The rationale for attempting to demonstrate associations between the MHC and Burkitt's lymphoma lies in the possibility that this disease has a viral etiology[152] modified by immunological factors resulting from chronic malarial infection.[153-155] Also, since it is primarily a malignancy of childhood and is usually fatal, if untreated, it might be expected to exert some selection pressure on the population in which it occurs. Thus, associations of HLA with susceptibility or resistance and with outcome of disease are of great interest. However, it must be borne in mind that if malaria does play a role in the development of the disease, then it would be necessary to separate associations of HLA with susceptibility and outcome to the Epstein-Barr viral component from associations with susceptibility and outcome to the malarial component.

Although three earlier studies involving 106 patients and 169 controls failed to reveal an association between any HLA phenotype and Burkitt's lymphoma,[156-158] even when the data were pooled and analyzed as a group,[159] a recent survey of 78 patients did reveal an increased relative risk in patients having DR7, A1, and B12 (Bw44).[160] The relative risk for DR7 was 3.3, and the associated increased risk for B12 (Bw44) is probably the result of a linkage disequilibrium between B12 and DR7. These results await confirmation. None of these four studies was prospective and included both previously treated as well as newly diagnosed cases. Thus, no data are available on HLA associations with survival.

*4. Acute Leukemia*

The acute leukemias, strictly speaking, are not lymphomas, but there is a strong suspicion that they may be caused by viruses. Therefore, brief consideration will be given here to associations of HLA genes with acute myeloblastic (AML) and acute lymphoblastic (ALL) leukemia.

In AML, one prospective study of 146 patients provides the major evidence against any association of HLA genes with the disease at the time of presentation.[161] However, when these patients were followed throughout the course of the disease, a progressive rise in the frequency of survivors with B12 was seen.[161,162] Similar observations, albeit not in prospectively studied patients, were made by Oliver et al.[163] and von Fliedner et al.[164]

A similar situation pertains to ALL, where no consistent association has been found between HLA antigens and the disease. It seems that no prospective studies have been done, all studies containing patients phenotyped at various stages in the course of the disease.[162,164,165] In some of these, A2 has been increased in frequency, but these results have not always been confirmed. A more consistent observation has been the increased frequency of A9 associated with improved survival.[162] The improvement in survival is accounted for by an increased length of first remission, particularly in patients with the null cell variety of ALL.[165] Once patients with A9 suffer a relapse after first remission, their survival is similar to that of patients who do not have A9. The absence of consistently effective treatment for relapse may be a contributing factor in this result.

Although it is premature to conclude that HLA genes govern survival in ALL, confirmation of the above results would indicate that the gene(s) influencing survival is in linkage disequilibrium with A9, a gene in the A region, rather than with a gene in the B or DR region. This would mean that genes influencing the outcome of ALL can be located in an area of the chromosome that Bodmer[43] suggested is analogous to the TLa region in the mouse. TLa genes play a role in determining certain leukemic cell surface determinants that, when expressed, may be recognized by the host's immune system.[30,31] Thus, an increase in survival may be mediated by an immunological mechanism. If the immune response is controlled by Ir genes, this would be another way in which the MHC may influence the course of a disease.

Another observation of interest in both AML and ALL is the apparently increased frequency of homozygosity for certain DR specificities in patients with these diseases.[166] In a study of 89 patients, the only study reported thus far in which DR phenotyping has been done, an excesss of phenotypes showing only one identifiable DR antigen was present. Within such phenotypes DRw3 was significantly increased in AML, whereas DRw6 may be increased in adult ALL, and DRw7 in childhood ALL. The best explanation for these findings is an excess of homozygotes for those antigens. Such an explanation is in keeping with the view that leukemia susceptibility genes in man are inherited in a recessive fashion, similar to the inheritance of susceptibility genes for virus-induced leukemia in mice.

## VI. SUMMARY AND CONCLUSIONS

The MHCs of mouse and man have many similarities. Both are highly polymorphic, yet occupy relatively short lengths of their respective chromosomes. Thus, the recombination rate with the complex is relatively low and the genetic material is highly conserved during evolution. The gene products (molecules) of each MHC have similar structures and are associated with $\beta$-2 microglobulin. Class I gene products, encoded in the K, D, or L regions in the mouse and in the A, B, and C regions in man, are found as surface structures on most, if not all cells of the body, and serve as targets for cell-mediated lympholysis, graft-rejection, and, most notably, recognition of virus-infected cells. Class II gene products, encoded in the I region of the mouse and the D/DR region of man, are found primarily on cells of the immune system (B cells, T cells, and macrophages). They are thought to serve as guides for T cells, enabling them to distinguish between self and nonself, as exemplified in the mixed leukocyte reaction between either allogencic or autologous cells. Thus, class I and II gene products enable cells in the immunological system to recognize foreign and self-antigens and also each other, thereby allowing both for immunological responses to foreign antigens and for cell-to-cell cooperation during these responses.

In the inbred laboratory mouse the MHC also has been shown to contain genes that impart resistance to the development of virus-induced leukemia. They also play a role in determining the outcome of the disease once it has developed. Thus, a search has been made in the leukemias and lymphomas of man for genes with similar properties. The methodological difficulties that beset investigators attempting genetic studies in an outbred population are extreme and progress has been slow. In addition, most data have been collected in retrospective studies without regard to duration of disease or consecutive sampling of patients, thus leading to incomplete and biased information. Since, at present, disease susceptibility or resistance genes can be deduced only from linkage with detectable HLA gene products, the latter only serve as markers for the gene being sought. If the linkage is weak, the marker genes may not be seen to be associated with the disease. Also, if several genes are involved in susceptibility and resistance, some of which may be on chromosomes different from the one bearing the MHC, the effect of MHC genes may be obscured. Finally, environmental factors also play an important role in the multifactorial etiology of malignant disease and must be integrated into the picture derived from genetic studies.

To date there is no proven association of a particular HLA marker with leukemia or lymphoma in man. There are tantalizing suggestions from family studies that recessive HLA-linked genes may be involved with susceptibility to acute leukemia and Hodgkin's disease but the evidence is still insufficient to be convincing. Similarily, there are suggestions that survival in acute leukemia and Hodgkin's disease may depend, in part, on HLA-linked genes, but much remains to be done before this conclusion can be fully accepted.

# REFERENCES

1. Amos, D. B., Human histocompatibility locus HL-A, *Science,* 159, 659, 1968.
2. Klein, J., H-2 mutations: their genetics and effect on immune functions, *Adv. Immunol.,* 26, 55, 1978.
3. Murphy, D. B., Genetic fine structure of the H-2 gene complex, in *The Role of the Major Histocompatibility Complex in Immunobiology,* Dorf, M. E., Ed., Garland STPM Press, New York, 1981, 1.
4. Gorer, P. A. and O'Gorman, P., The cytotoxic activity of isoantibodies in mice, *Transplant. Bull.,* 3, 142, 1956.
5. Klein, J., Cytological identification of the chromosome carrying the IXth linkage (including H-2) in the house mouse, *Proc Natl. Acad. Sci. U.S.A.,* 68, 1954, 1971.
6. Nathenson, S. G. and Cullen, S. E., Biochemical properties and immunochemical genetic relationships of mouse H-2 alloantigens, *Biochem. Biophys. Acta,* 344, 1, 1974.

7. Rask, L., Lindbolm, J. B., and Peterson, P. A., Subunit structure of H-2 alloantigens, *Nature (London)*, 249, 833, 1974.
8. Sliver, J. and Hood, L., Detergent-solubilised H-2 alloantigen is associated with a small molecular weight polypeptide, *Nature (London),*. 249, 764, 1974.
9. Silver, J. and Hood, L., Structure and evolution of transplantation antigens: partial amino-acid sequences of H-2K and H-2D alloantigens, *Proc. Natl. Acad. Sci. U.S.A.*, 73, 599, 1976.
10. Strominger, J. L., Engelhard, V. H., Fuks, A., Guild, B. C., Hyafil, F., Kaufman, J. F., Korman, A. J., Kostyk, T. G., Krangel, M. S., Lancet, D., Lopez, X., de Castro, J. A., Mann, D. L., Orr, H. T., Parham, P. R., Parker, K. C., Ploegh, H. L., Pober, J. S., Robb, R. J., and Shackleford, D. A., Biochemical analysis of products of the MHC, in *The Role of the Major Histocompatibility Complex in Immunobiology*, Dorf, M. E., Ed., Garland, STPM Press, New York, 1981, 115.
11. Michaelson, J., Genetic polymorphism of $\beta$ 2-microglobulin ($\beta$ 2M) maps to the H-3 region of chromosome 2, *Immunogenetics*, 13, 167, 1981.
12. Shreffler, D. C. and David, C. S., The H-2 major histocompatibility complex and the I immune response region: genetic variation, function and organization, *Adv. Immunol.*, 20, 125, 1974.
13. Klein, J., Flaherty, L., VandeBerg, J. L., and Shreffler, D. C., H-2 haplotypes, genes, regions and antigens: first listing, *Immunogenetics*, 6, 489, 1978.
14. Stimpfling, J. H. and Reichert, A. E., Strain C57BL/10ScSn and its congeneic resistant sublines, *Transplant. Proc.*, 2, 39, 1970.
15. Klein, J., Genetics of cell-mediated lymphocytoxicity in the mouse, *Springer Semin. Immunopathol.*, 1, 31, 1978.
16. Klein, J., Widmer, M. B., Segall, M., and Bach, F. H., Mixed lymphocyte culture reactivity and H-2 histocompatibility loci differences, *Cell Immunol.*, 4, 442, 1972.
17. Okuda, K., David, C. S., and Shreffler, D. C., The role of gene products of the I-J subregion in mixed lymphocytic reactions, *J. Exp. Med.*, 146, 1561, 1977.
18. Lonai, P. and McDevitt, H. O., The expression of I-Region gene products on lymphocytes. II. Genetic localization and cellular distribution of MLR determinants, *Immunogenetics*, 4, 33, 1977.
19. Zinkernagel, R. M. and Doherty, P. C., Restriction in *in vitro* T cell-mediated cytotoxicity in lymphocytic choriomeningitis within a syngeneic or semiallogeneic system, *Nature (London)*, 248, 701, 1974.
20. Shearer, G. M., Rehn, T. G., and Schmitt-Verhulst, A. M., Role of the murine major histocompatibility complex in the specificity of *in vitro* T-cell-mediated lympholysis against chemically-modified autologous lymphocytes, *Transplant. Rev.*, 29, 222, 1976.
21. McDevitt, H. O., Deak, B. D., Shreffler, D. C., Klein, J., Stimpfling, J. H., and Snell, D. G., Genetic control of the immune response. Mapping of the Ir-1 locus, *J. Exp. Med.*, 135, 1259, 1972.
22. Uhr, J. W., Capra, J. D., Vitetta, E. S., and Cook, R. G., Organization of the immune response genes, *Science*, 206, 292, 1979.
23. Hammerling, G. J., Mauve, G., and Goldberg, E., Tissue distribution of Ia antigens. Ia on spermatozoa, macrophages, and epidermal cells, *Immunogenetics*, 1, 428, 1975.
24. Benacerraf, B. and McDevitt, H. O., Histocompatibility-linked immune response genes, *Science*, 175, 273, 1972.
25. Zaleski, M. and Klein, J., H-2 mutation affecting immune response to THY-1 antigen, *J. Exp. Med.*, 145, 1602, 1977.
26. Kapp, J. A., Pierce, C. W., Schlossman, S., and Benacerraf, B., Genetic control of immune responses *in vitro*. V. Stimulation of suppressor T cells in nonresponder mice by the terpolymer L-glutamic acid$^{60}$-L-alanine$^{30}$-L-tyrosine$^{10}$(GAT), *J. Exp. Med.*, 140, 648, 1974.
27. Benacerraf, B. and Dorf, M. E., Genetic control of specific immune responses and immune suppression by I-region genes, *Cold Spring Harbor Symp. Quant. Biol.*, 41, 465, 1977.
28. Murphy, D. B., Herzenberg, L. A., Okamura, K., Herzenberg, L. A., and McDevitt, H. O., A new I subregion (I-J) marked by a locus (Ia-4) controlling surface determinants on suppressor T lymphocytes, *J. Exp. Med.*, 144, 699, 1976.
29. Roos, M. H., Atkinson, J. P., and Shreffler, D. C., Molecular characterization of the Ss and Slp (C4) proteins of the mouse H-2 complex: subunit composition, chain size polymorphism, and an intracellular (PRO-S) precursor, *J. Immunol.*, 121, 1106, 1978.
30. Flaherty, L., The TLa region of the mouse: identification of a new serologically defined locus, Qa-2, *Immunogentics*, 3, 533, 1976.
31. Flaherty, L., TLa region antigens, in *The Role of the Major Histocompatibility Complex in Immunobiology*, Dorf, M. E., Ed., Garland STPM Press, New York, 1981, 33.
32. Klein, J., Juretic, A., Baxevanis, C. N., and Nagy, Z. A., The traditional and a new version of the mouse *H-2* complex, *Nature (London)*, 291, 455, 1981.
33. Lamm, L. U., Freidrich, U., Peterson, G. B., Jorgensen, J., Nielsen, J., Therkelsen, A. J., and Kissmeyer-Nielsen, F., Assignment of the major histocompatibility complex to chromosome No. 6 in a family with a pericentric inversion, *Hum. Hered.*, 24, 273, 1974.

34. Francke, U. and Pellegrino, M. A., Assignment of the major histocompatibility complex to a region of the short arm of human chromosome 6, *Proc. Natl. Acad. Sci. U.S.A.*, 74, 1147, 1977.
35. Van Rood, J. J., DeVries, R. R. P., and Bradley, B. A., Genetics and biology of the HLA system, in *The Role of the Major Histocompatibility Complex in Immunobiology*, Dorf, M. E., Ed., Garland STPM Press, New York, 1981, 59.
36. Bodmer, W. F. and Bodmer, J. G., Evolution and function of the HLA system, *Br. Med. Bull.*, 34, 309, 1978.
37. Albert, E., Amos, D. B., Bodmer, W. F., Ceppelini, R., Dausset, J., Kissmeyer-Nielsen, F., Mayr, W., Payne, R., Van Rood, J. J., Terasaki, P. I., and Walford, R. L., Nomenclature for factors of the HLA system 1980, *Immunobiology*, 158, 307, 1981.
38. Shaw, S., Kavathas, P., Pollack, M. S., Charmot, D., and Mawas, C., Family studies define a new histocompatibility locus, SB, between HLA-DR and GLO, *Nature (London)*, 293, 745, 1981.
39. Kavathas, P., DeMars, R., Bach, F. H., and Shaw, S., SB: a new HLA-linked human histocompatibility gene defined using HLA-mutant cell lines, *Nature (London)*, 293, 747, 1981.
40. Sasazuki, T., Kaneoka, H., Nishimura, Y., Kaneoka, R., Hayama, M., and Ohkuni, H., An HLA-linked immune suppression gene in man, *J. Exp. Med.*, 152, 2975, 1980.
41. Barnstable, C. J., Jones, E. A., and Bodmer, W. F., The genetic structure of major histocompatibility regions, in defence and recognition. II.A. Cellular aspects, *International Reviews in Biochemistry* Vol. 22, Lennox, E., Ed., University Park Press, Baltimore, 1979, 151.
42. Bodmer, W. F., The major histocompatibility gene clusters of man and mouse, in *Mammalian Genetics and Cancer: The Jackson Laboratory Fiftieth Anniversary Symposium, Progress in Clinical and Biological Research*, Vol. 45, Russell, E. S., Ed., Alan R. Liss, New York, 1981, 213.
43. Bodmer, W. F., HLA structures and functions a contemporary view, *Tissue Antigens*, 17, 9, 1981.
44. Welsh, K. I., Amlot, P., and Batchelor, J. R., Do alleles in linkage disequilibrium compensate for each other's disadvantageous effects? *Tissue Antigens*, 17, 91, 1981.
45. Brodsky, F. M., Parham, P., Barnstable, C. J., Crumpton, M. J., and Bodmer, W. F., Monoclonal antibodies for the analysis of the HLA system, *Immunol. Rev.*, 47, 3, 1979.
46. Joyce, V. C. and Wolf, E., HLA-A and -B and -C antigens, their serology and cross-reactions, *Br. Med. Bull.*, 34, 217, 1978.
47. Thorsby, E., Albrechtsen, D., Hirschberg, H., Kaakinen, A., and Solheim, B. G., MLC-activating HLA-D determinanta: identification, tissue distribution, and significance, *Transplant. Proc.*, 9, 393, 1977.
48. Festenstein, H. and Halim, K., HLA-D locus determinants detected by perm-lymphocyte culture, *Transplant. Proc.*, 9, 1239, 1977.
49. Eijsvoogel, V. P., Van Rood, J. J., du Toit, E. D., and Schellekens, P. T. A., Position of a locus determining mixed lymphocyte reaction distinct from the known HL-A loci, *Eur. J. Immunol.*, 2, 413, 1972.
50. Bodmer, J. G., Ia antigens. Definition of the HLA-DRw specificities, *Br. Med. Bull.*, 34, 233, 1978.
51. van Leeuwen, A., Winchester, R. J., and van Rood, J. J., Serotyping for MLC. II. Technical aspects, *Ann. N.Y. Acad. Sci.*, 254, 289, 1975.
52. Charron, D.J. and McDevitt, H. O., Analysis of HLA-D region associated molecules with monoclonal antibody, *Proc. Natl. Acad. Sci. U.S.A.*, 76, 6567, 1979.
53. Shackleford, D. A. and Strominger, J. L., Demonstration of structural polymorphism among HLA-DR lightchains by two-dimensional gel electrophoresis, *J. Exp. Med.*, 151, 144, 1980.
54. Lee, J. S., Trosdale, J., and Bodmer, W. F., Synthesis of HLA antigens from membrane-associated messenger RNA. II, *J. Exp. Med.*, 152, 3, 1980.
55. Jones, P. P., Murphy, D. B., and McDevitt, H. O., Two-gene control of the expression of a murine Ia antigen, *J. Exp. Med.*, 148, 925, 1978.
56. Lachman, P. J. and Hobart, M. J., Complement genetics in relation to HLA, *Br. Med. Bull.*, 34, 247, 1978.
57. Bodmer, W. F., Evolutionary significance of the HL-A system, *Nature (London)*, 237, 139, 1972.
58. Dausset, J. and Contu, L., MHC in general biologic recognition: its theoretical implications in transplantation, *Transplant. Proc.*, 13, 895, 1981.
59. Eijsvoogel, V. P., Schellekens, P. T. A., du Bois, M. J. G., and Zeijlemaker, W. P., Human cytotoxic lymphocytes after alloimmunization in vitro, *Transplant, Rev.*, 29, 125, 1976.
60. Opelz, G., Kiuchi, M., Takasugi, M., and Terasaki, P. I., Autologous stimulation of human lymphocyte subpopulations, *J. Exp. Med.*, 142, 1327, 1975.
61. Kuntz, M. M., Innes, J. B., and Weksler, M. E., Lymphocyte transformation induced by autologous cells. IV. Human T-lymphocyte proliferation induced by autologous or allogeneic non-T lymphocytes, *J. Exp. Med.*, 143, 1042, 1976.
62. Hausman, P. B. and Stobo, J. D., Specificity and function of a human autologous reactive T cell, *J. Exp. Med.*, 149, 1537, 1979.

63. de Vries, R. R. P., Meera-Khan, P., Bernini, L. F., van Loghem, E., and van Rood, J. J., Genetic control of survival in epidemics, *J. Immunologenet.*, 6, 271, 1979.
64. Piazza, A., Belvedere, M. C., Bernoco, D., Conighi, C., Contu, L., Cutroni, E. S., Mattiuz, P. L., Mayr, W., Richiardi, P., Schudeller, G., and Ceppellini R., HL-A variation in four Sardinian villages under differential selective pressure by malaria, in *Histocompatibility Testing 1972*, Dausset, J. and Colombani, J., Eds., Munksgaard, Copenhagen, 1973, 73.
65. Osoba, D., Dick, H., Voller, A., Goosen, T. J., Goosen, T., Draper, C. C., and de The, G., Role of the HLA complex in the antibody response to malaria under natural conditions, *Immunogenetics*, 8, 323, 1979.
66. Claas, F. H. J. and Dulder, A. M., H-2 linked immune response to murine experimental *Schistosoma mansoni* infections, *J. Immunogenet.*, 6, 167, 1969.
67. Levine, B. B., Stember, R. H., and Fotino, M., Ragweed hay fever: genetic control and linkage to HL-A haplotypes, *Science*, 178, 1201, 1972.
68. Blumenthal, M., Noreen, H., Amos, D. B., and Yunis, E., Genetic mapping of Ir gene in man. Linkage with second locus of HL-A, *J. Allerg., Clin. Immunol.*, 53, 93, 1974.
69. March, D. G., Bias, W. B., and Hsu, S. H., Association of the HL-A7 cross-reacting group with a specific reaginic antibody response in allergic man, *Science*, 179, 691, 1973.
70. Greensberg, L. J., Gray, E. D., and Yunis, E. J., Association of HL-A5 and immune responsiveness in vitro to streptococcal antigens, *J. Exp. Med.*, 141, 935, 1975.
71. Spencer, M. J., Cherry, J. D., and Terasaki, P. I., HL-A antigen and antibody response after influenza A vaccination: decreased response associated with H1-A type w16, *N. Engl. J. Med.*, 294, 13, 1976.
72. De Vries, R. R. P., Kreeftenberg, H. G., Loggen, H. G., and van Rood, J. J., In vitro immune responsiveness to vaccinia virus and HLA, *N. Engl. J. Med,*. 297, 692, 1977.
73. Buckley, C. E., III, Dorsey, F. C., Corley, R. B., Ralph, W. B., Woodbury, M. A., and Amos, D. B., HL-A linked immune-response genes, *Proc. Natl. Acad. Sci U.S.A.*, 70, 2157, 1973.
74. Doherty, P. C., Blanden, R. U., and Zinkernagel, R. M., Specificity of virus-immune effector T cells for H-2K or H-2D compatible for H-antigen diversity, *Transplant. Rev.*, 29, 89, 1976.
75. McMichael, A. J., Ting, A., Zweermik, H. J., and Askonas, B. A., HLA restriction of cell-mediated lysis of influenza-virus infected human cells, *Nature (London)*, 270, 524, 1977.
76. Shaw, S., Biddison, W. E., Pichler, W. J., and Shearer, G. M., HLA restriction of human influenza cytotoxic T cells, *Transplant Proc.*, 11, 1845, 1979.
77. Jondal, M., Svedmyr, E., Klein, E., and Singh, S., Killer T cells in a Burkitt's lymphoma biopsy, *Nature (London)*, 255, 405, 1975.
78. Sasazuki, T., Kohno, Y., Iwamoto, I., Tanimura, M., and Naito, S., Association between an HLA haplotype and low responsiveness to tetanus toxoid in man, *Nature (London)*, 272, 359, 1978.
79. Dausset, J. and Svejgaard, A., Eds., *HLA and disease*, Munksgaard, Copenhagen, 1977.
80. Ryder, L. P., Anderson, E., and Svejgaard, A., Eds., *Third Report of HLA and Disease Registry*, Munksgaard, Copenhagen, 1979.
81. Dick, H. M., HLA and disease: introductory review, in the HLA system, Bodmer, W. F., Ed., *Br. Med. Bull.*, 34, 271, 1978.
82. Cudworth, A. G. and Wolf, E., The HLA system and disease, *Clin. Sci.*, 61, 1, 1981.
83. Bodmer, W. F., Models and mechanisms for HLA and disease associations, *J. Exp. Med.*, 152, 353, 1980.
84. Geczy, A. F., Alexander, K., Bashir, H. V., and Edmonds, J., A factor(s) in Klebsiella culture filtrates specifically modifies an HLA-B27-associated cell-surface component, *Nature (London)*, 283, 782, 1980.
85. Svejgaard, A. and Ryder, L. P., Interaction of HLA molecules with non-immunological ligands as an explanation of HLA and disease associations, *Lancet*, 2, 547, 1976.
86. Amos, D. B. and Ward, F. E., Theoretical consideration in the association between HLA and disease, in *HLA and Disease*, Dausset, J. and Svejgaard, A., Eds., Munksgaard, Copenhagen, 1977, 269.
87. Zinkernagel, R. M. and Doherty, P. C., Possible mechanisms of disease susceptibility association with major transplantation antigens, in *HLA and Disease*, Dauset, J. and Svejgaard, A., Eds., Munksgaard, Copenhagen, 1977, 256.
88. Ho, H.-Z., Tiwari, J. L., Haile, R. W., Terasaki, P. I., and Morton, N. E., HLA-linked and unlinked determinants of multiple sclerosis, *Immunogenetics*, 15, 509, 1982.
89. Green, A., Epidemiologic considerations on studies of HLA and disease associations. I. The basic measures, concepts and estimation procedures, *Tissue Antigens*, 19, 245, 1982.
90. Green, A., The epidemiologic approach to studies of association between HLA and disease. II. Estimation of absolute risks, etiologic and preventive fraction, *Tissue Antigen*, 19, 259, 1982.
91. Lilly, F., The inheritance of susceptibility to Gross leukemia virus in mice, *Genetics*, 53, 529, 1966.
92. Lilly, F., The role of genetics in Gross virus leukemogenesis, in *Comparative Leukemia Research 1969, Bibl. Hematology*, No. 36, Dutcher, R. M., Ed., Karger, New York, 1970.

93. Lilly, F., Boyse, E. A., and Old, L. J., Genetic basis of susceptibility to viral leukemogenesis, *Lancet*, 2, 1207, 1964.
94. Lilly, F., Susceptibility to two strains of Friends leukemia virus in mice, *Science*, 155, 461, 1967.
95. Lilly, F., The effect of histocompatibility-2 type on response to the Friend leukemia virus in mice, *J. Exp. Med.*, 127, 465, 1968.
96. Lilly, F. and Pincus, T., Genetic control of murine viral leukemogenesis, *Adv. Cancer Res.*, 17, 231, 1973.
97. Chesebro, B. and Wehrly, K., Studies on the role of the host immune response in recovery from Friend virus leukemia. I. Antiviral and antileukemia cell antibody, *J. Exp. Med.*, 143, 73, 1976.
98. Chesebro, B. and Wehrly, K., Studies on the role of the host immune response in recovery from Friend virus leukemia. II. Cell-mediated immunity, *J. Exp. Med.*, 143, 85, 1976.
99. Chesebro, B. and Wehrly, K., *Rfv-1* and *Rfv-2*, two H-2 associated genes which influence recovery from Friend leukemia virus-induced splenomegaly, *J. Immunol.*, 120, 1081, 1978.
100. Chesebro, B., Wehrly, K., and Stimpfling, J., Host genetic control of recovery from Friend leukemia virus-induced splenomegaly. Mapping of a gene within the major histocompatibility complex, *J. Exp. Med.*, 140, 1457, 1974.
101. Tennant, J. and Snell, G. D., The H-2 locus and viral leukemogenesis as studied in congeneic strains of mice, *J. Natl. Cancer Inst.*, 41, 597, 1968.
102. Meruelo, D., Lieberman, M., Ginzton, N., Deak, B., and McDevitt, H. O., Genetic control of radiation leukemia virus-induced tumorigenesis. I. Role of the major murine histocompatibility complex, H-2, *J. Exp. Med.*, 146, 1079, 1977.
103. Meruelo, D., Deak, B., and McDevitt, H. O., Genetic control of cell-mediated responsiveness to an AKR tumour-associated antigen. Mapping of the locus involved to the I region of the H-2 complex, *J. Exp. Med.*, 146, 1367, 1977.
104. Mühlbock, O. and Dux, A., Histocompatibility genes and susceptibility to mammary tumour virus (MTV) in mice, *Transplant. Proc.*, 3, 1247, 1971.
105. Aoki, T., Boyse, E. A., and Old, L. J., Occurrence of natural antibody to the G (Gross) Leukemia antigen in mice, *Cancer Res.*, 26, 1415, 1966.
106. Sato, H., Boyse, E. A., Aoki, T., Iritani, C., and Old, L. J., Leukemia-associated transplantation antigens related to murine leukemia virus. The X. I system: immune response controlled by a locus linked to H-2, *J. Exp. Med.*, 138, 593, 1973.
107. Blank, K. K., Freedman, J. A., and Lilly, F., T lymphocyte response to Friend virus induced tumour cell lines in mice of strains congeneic at H-2, *Nature (London)*, 260, 150, 1976.
108. Meruelo, D. and McDevitt, H. O., Recent studies on the role of the immune response in resistance to virus-induced leukemias and lymphomas, *Semin. Hematol.*, 15, 399, 1978.
109. Klein, G., Mouse histocompatibility genetics and tumour immunology, in *Mammalian Genetics and Cancer: The Jackson Laboratory Fiftieth Anniversary Symposium, Progress in Clinical and Biological Research*, Vol. 45, Russell, E. S., Ed., Alan R. Liss, New York, 1981, 197.
110. Klein, G. and Klein, E., Rejectability of virus-induced tumors and non-rejectability of spontaneous tumours — a lesson in contrasts, *Transplant. Proc.*, 9, 1095, 1977.
111. Lukes, R. J. and Collins, R. D., Immunological characterization of human malignant lymphomas, *Cancer*, 34, 1488, 1974.
112. National Cancer Institute sponsored study of classifications of non-Hodgkin's lymphomas, Summary and description of a working formation for clinical usage, *Cancer*, 49, 2112, 1982.
113. Kaslow, R. A. and Shaw, S., The role of histocompatibility antigens (HLA) in infection, *Epidemiol. Rev.*, 3, 90, 1981.
114. Tiilikainen, A., On the way to understanding the pathogenesis of HLA disease, *Med. Biol.*, 58, 53, 1980.
115. Svejgaard, A. and Ryder, L. P., Associations between HLA and disease in *HLA and Disease*, Dausset, J. and Svejgaard, A., Eds., Munksgaard, Copenhagen, 1977, 46.
116. Tiilikainen, A., Is there biological relevance in the statistically significant association between the HLA system and disease?, *Med. Biol.*, 58, 241, 1980.
117. Amiel, J. L., Study of the leucocyte phenotypes in Hodgkin's disease in *Histocompatibility Testing 1967*, Curtoni, E. S., Mattiuz, P. L., and Tosi, R. M., Eds., Munksgaard, Copenhagen, 1967, 79.
118. Vianna, N. J., Epidemiology of Hodgkin's disease: review and etiologic leads, in *CRC Crit. Rev. Clin. Lab. Sci.*, 5, (3), 1975, 245.
119. Zervas, J. D., Delamore, I. W., and Israels, M. C. G., Leukocyte phenotypes in Hodgkin's disease, *Lancet*, 2, 634, 1970.
120. Forbes, J. F. and Morris, P. J., Leucocyte antigens in Hodgkin's disease, *Lancet*, 2, 849, 1970.
121. Morris, P. J. and Forbes, J. F., HL-A and Hodgkin's disease, *Transplant. Proc.*, 3, 1275, 1971.
122. Thorsby, E., Falk, J., Engeseth, A., and Osoba, D., HL-A antigens in Hodgkin's disease, *Transplant. Proc.*, 3, 1279, 1971.

123. Coukell, A., Bodmer, J. G., and Bodmer, W. F., HL-A types in 44 Hodgkin's patients, *Transplant Proc.*, 3, 1291, 1971.
124. van Rood, J. J. and van Leeuwen, A., HL-A and the group 5 system in Hodgkin's disease, *Transplant. Proc.*, 3, 1283, 1971.
125. Kissmeyer-Nielsen, F., Jensen, K. B., Ferrara, G. B., Kjerbye, K. E., and Svejgaard, A., HL-A phenotypes in Hodgkin's disease. Preliminary report, *Transplant. Proc.*, 3, 1287, 1971.
126. Bertrams, J., Kuwerst, E., Bohme, U., Reis, H. E., Gallmeier, W. M., Wetter, O., and Schmidt, C. G., Antigens in Hodgkin's disease and multiple myeloma. Increased frequency of W18 in both diseases, *Tissue Antigens*, 2, 41, 1972.
127. Falk, J. and Osoba, D., HL-A antigens and survival in Hodgkin's disease, *Lancet*, 2, 1118, 1971.
128. Forbes, J. F. and Morris, P. J., Analysis of HL-A antigens in patients with Hodgkin's disease and their families, *J. Clin. Invest.*, 51, 1156, 1972.
129. Jeannet, M. and Magnin, C., HL-A antigens in malignant disease, *Transplant. Proc.*, 3, 1301, 1971.
130. Bodmer, W. F., Genetic factors in Hodgkin's disease: association with a disease-susceptibility locus (DSA) in the HL-A region, *Natl. Cancer Inst. Monogr.*, 36, 127, 1973.
131. Falk, J. and Osoba, D., The association of the human histocompatibility system with Hodgkin's disease, *J. Immunogenet.*, 1, 53, 1974.
132. Kissmeyer-Nielsen, F., Lamm, L. U. Kjerbye, K. E., Jensen, K. B., Nordentoft, A. M., Thorling, K., and Hastrup, J., HL-A phenotypes in Hodgkin's disease, in *Histocompatibility Testing 1972*, Munksgaard, Copenhagen, 1973, 593.
133. Kissmeyer-Nielsen, F., Kjerbye, K. E., and Lamm, U., HL-A in Hodgkin's disease. III. A prospective study, *Transplant. Rev.*, 22, 168, 1975.
134. Morris, P. J., Lawler, S. D., and Oliver, R. T., HL-A and Hodgkin's disease, in *Histocompatibility Testing 1972*, Munksgaard, Copenhagen, 1973, 669.
135. MacMahon, B., Epidemiology of Hodgkin's disease, *Cancer Res.*, 26, 1189, 1966.
136. Lukes, R. J., Craver, L. F., Hall, T. C., Rappaport, H., and Rubin, T., Report of the nomenclature committee, *Cancer Res.*, 26, 1311, 1966.
137. Björkholm, M., Holm, G., Johansson, B., Mellstedt, H., and Moller, E., A prospective study of HL-A antigen phenotypes and lymphocyte abnormalities in Hodgkin's disease, *Tissue Antigens*, 6, 247, 1975.
138. O'Conor, G. T., Correa, P., Christine, B., Axtell, L., and Myers, M., Hodgkin's disease in Connecticut: histology and age distribution, *Natl. Cancer Inst. Monogr.*, 36, 3, 1973.
139. Devore, J. W. and Doan, C. A., Studies in Hodgkin's syndrome. XII. Hereditary and epidemiologic aspects, *Ann. Int. Med.*, 47, 300, 1957.
140. Razis, D. V., Diamond, H. D., and Crauer, L. F., Familial Hodgkin's disease, *Ann. Int. Med.*, 51, 933, 1959.
141. Grufferman, S., Cole, P., Smith, P. G., and Lukes, R. J., Hodgkin's disease in siblings, *N. Engl. J. Med.*, 296, 248, 1977.
142. Hors, J., Steinberg, G., Andrieu, J. M., Jacquillat, G., Minev, M., Messerschmitt, J., Malvinaud, G., Fumerson, F., Dausset, J., and Bernard, J., HLA genotypes in familial Hodgkin's disease. Excess of HLA identical affected siblings, *Eur. J. Cancer*, 16, 809, 1980.
143. Nagel, G. A., Nagel-Studer, E., Seiler, W., and Hofer, O., Malignant lymphoma is four or five siblings, *Int. J. Cancer*, 22, 675, 1978.
144. Chrobak, L., Radochova, D., and Erbenova, E., Incidence of Hodgkin's disease in siblings, *Hradci Kralove*, 19, 1, 1976.
145. Svejgaard, A., Platz, P., Ryder, L. P., Nielsen, L. S., and Thomsen, M., HL-A and disease associations. A survey, *Transplant. Rev.*, 22, 3, 1975.
146. Falk, J. and Osoba, D., The HLA system and survival in malignant disease: Hodgkin's disease and carcinoma of the breast, in *HLA and Malignancy*, Murphy, G. P., Ed., Alan R. Liss, New York, 1977, 205.
147. Osoba, D., Balk, J. A., Sousan, P., Ciampi, A., and Till, J. E., The prognostic value of HLA phenotypes in Hodgkin's disease, *Cancer*, 46, 1825, 1980.
148. Rosencweig, M., Kenis, Y., and Staquet, M., Hodgkin's disease: prognostic factors and clinical evaluation, in *Cancer Therapy: Prognostic Factors and Criteria of Response*, Staquet, M. J., Ed., Raven Press, New York, 1975, 49.
149. Forbes, J. F. and Morris, P. J., Transplantation antigens and malignant lymphomas in man: follicular lymphoma, reticulum cell sarcoma and lymphosarcoma, *Tissue Antigens*, 1, 265, 1971.
150. Dick, F. R., Fortuny, I., Theoglides, A., Greally, J., Wood, N., and Yunis, E. J., HL-A and lymphoid tumours, *Cancer Res.*, 32, 2608, 1972.
151. Van den Twell, J. G., Dugas, D. J., and Loon, J., The biology of the HL-A system and the association with malignant lymphomas, *Am. J. Clin. Pathol.*, 72, 732, 1979.
152. Epstein, M. A., Achong, B. G., and Barr, Y. M., Virus particles in cultured lymphoblasts from Burkitt's lymphoma, *Lancet*, 1, 702, 1964.

153. Biggar, R. J. and Nkrumah, F. K., Burkitt's lymphoma in Ghana: urban-rural distribution, time-space clustering and seasonality, *Int. J. Cancer*, 23, 330, 1979.
154. Magrath, I. T., Immunosuppression in Burkitt's lymphoma. I. Cutaneous reactivity to recall antigens: alterations induced by a tumour burden and by BCG administration, *Int. J. Cancer*, 13, 839, 1974.
155. Nkrumah, F. K., Herberman, R., Biggar, R., and Perkins, I. H., Sequential evaluation of cutaneous delayed hypersensitivity responses to recall and to lymphoid cell line antigens in Burkitt's lymphoma, *Int. J. Cancer*, 20, 6, 1977.
156. Dausset, J., Singh, S., Gournad, J. L., Degos, L., Solal, C., and Klein, G., HL-A and Burkitt's disease, *Tissue Antigens*, 5, 48, 1975.
157. Dick, H., Steel, C. M., Levin, A. G., and Henderson, N., Burkitt's lymphoma and HL-A antigens, *Tissue Antigens*, 5, 52, 1975.
158. Bodmer, J. G., Bodmer, W. F., Ziegler, J., and Magrath, I. T., HL-A and Burkitt's tumour — a study in Uganda, *Tissue Antigens*, 5, 59, 1975.
159. Bodmer, J. G., Bodmer, W. F., Pickbourne, P., Degos, L., Dausset, J., and Dick, H. M., Combined analysis of three studies of patients with Burkitt's lymphoma, *Tissue Antigens*, 5, 63, 1975.
160. Jones, E. H., Bigger, R. J., Nkrummah, F. K., and Lawler, S. D., Study of the HLA system in Burkitt's lymphoma, *Hum. Immunol.*, 3, 207, 1980.
161. Harris, R., Zuhrie, S. R., Freeman, C. B., Taylor, G. M., MacIver, J. E., Geary, C. G., Delamore, I. W., Hull, P. J., and Tooth, J. A., Active immunotherapy in acute myelogenous leukemia and the induction of second and subsequent remissions, *Br. J. Cancer*, 37, 282, 1978.
162. Harris, R., Lawler, S. D., and Oliver, R. T. D., The HLA system in acute leukemia and Hodgkin's disease, *Br. Med. Bull.*, 34, 301, 1978.
163. Oliver, R. T. D., Pillai, A., Klouda, P. T., and Lawler, S. D., HLA-linked resistance factors and survival in acute myelogenous leukemia, *Cancer*, 39, 2937, 1977.
164. VonFliedner, V. E., Sultan-Khan, Z., and Jeannet, M., HLA-A and HLA-B antigens in acute leukemia: A2-B12 phenotypes correlate with longer survival in acute myelogenous leukemia, *Acta Haematol.*, 65, 73, 1981.
165. Davey, F. R., Lachant, N. A., Dock, N. L., Hubbell, C., Stockman, J. A., III, and Henry, J. B., HLA antigens and childhood acute lymphocytic leukemia, *Br. J. Haematol.*, 47, 211, 1981.
166. VonFliedner, V. E., Sultan-Khan, Z., and Jeannet, M., HLA-DRw antigens associated with acute leukemia, *Tissue Antigens*, 16, 399, 1980.

# INDEX

## A

Acute lymphoblastic leukemia, see Leukemia, acute lymphoblastic (ALL)
Acute nonlymphocytic leukemia, see Leukemia, acute nonlymphocytic (ANLL)
ADA, see Adenosine deaminase
ADCC, see Antibody-dependent cell-mediated cytotoxicity
Adenosine deaminase (ADA), 155—157
Adherent cells in HD, 8, 9, 11
Adult T cell leukemia, see Leukemia, adult T cell (ATL)
AIHA, see Anemia, autoimmune hemolytic
ALL, see Leukemia, acute lymphoblastic
AMLR, see Lymphocyte reaction, autologous mixed
Anemia, autoimmune hemolytic (AIHA), 13, 14
Angioimmunoblastic lymphadenopathy, see Lymphadenopathy, immunoblastic
ANLL, see Leukemia, acute nonlymphocytic
Antibodies, monoclonal
  advantages, 110
  autologous bone marrow transplantation treatment, 120—121
  binding, 109, 112
  detection of lymphocytes and, 138
  diagnostic aid in ALL and ANLL, 114, 115
  disadvantages, 110—112
    binding specificity, 110—112, 114
  drug-antibody conjugates and, 121
  HD and, 56
  hybridoma method for production, 109—111
  identification
    B cell antigens, 115—116
    malignant T cells, 115, 135—136
    tumor specific, 116—117
  serotherapy treatment, 117—120
    antigenic heterogeneity and, 119, 121
    problems with, 118—120
  treatment of NHL, 99
  usefulness, 121—122
Antibodies, polyclonal, see also Serum immunoglobulins
  anti-idiotypic, in treatment of NHL, 99
  B cell production of, 108, 111
  binding, 108, 112
  diagnostic aid in ALL, 113—114
  effects of immunization on production of, 108—109
  response of
    in HD, 5
    in NHL, 94
    synthesis, in HD, 11
Antibody-dependent cell-mediated cytotoxicity (ADCC)
  in HD, 10
  in NHL, 85

Antigenic modulation, 119
Antigens, see also specific antigens
  detection of, 171—172
  disease-susceptibility genes and, 180—181
  lymphocyte response to, see Lymphocyte response to antigens and mitogens
  similarities of human type to mouse H-2, 172, 185
  T cell receptor interaction, 172
ATL, see Leukemia, adult T cell
Autoimmune disease, see specific diseases
Autoimmune hemolytic anemia, see Anemia, autoimmune hemolytic (AIHA)
Autologous mixed lymphocyte reaction, see Lymphocyte reaction, autologous mixed (AMLR)

## B

B cells, see B lymphocytes
Binding specificity, 108, 110—112
Biochemical markers, see also specific markers, 154
  clinical utility, 161
  phenotypic differences between normal and neoplastic cells and, 161
B lymphocytes
  ADA activity in, 155—156
  CLL and, 95—98, 145
  counts, see also Lymphocyte counts, 84, 138
  development, 35
  distribution, 68
  HD and
    changes of, 38
    clumping, 42
    monocytes and, 47—48
    peripheral blood, 52
    tissue, 47—50
  identification of antigens of with monoclonal antibodies, 115—116
  LDH in, 157
  NHL and, 86, 97, 98
  5'-NT activity and, 154
  organization of in lymph node cortex, 36
  organization of in spleen, 36
  PNP activity, 156—157
  reduction of antibodies and, 108, 111
  transformation of as basis of classification, 68
  types, 35
Bone marrow
  autologous transplantation of and monoclonal antibodies, 120—121
  Ig production and, 98
  transplantation in HD, 4
  transplantation in NHL, 99
Brill-Symmers disease, 66

British National Lymphoma Investigation Classification, 69—71
Burkitt's lymphoma, 17, 67
  HLA phenotypes and, 183—184

## C

Cancer, see Malignancies; specific diseases
Cell-mediated immunity, see Immunity, cell-mediated (CMI)
Chromosome 14, 16—17
Chronic lymphocytic leukemia, see Leukemia, chronic lymphocytic (CLL)
Classification, of non-Hodgkin's lymphomas, 114—115
  by cell type and transformation (Lukes and Collins), 67—69
  by clinical correlations (NCI), 73, 74
  comparison of systems of, 75—76
  confusion in, 72—73
  by cytologic category (Rappaport), 67, 73
  by cytologic features (Kiel), 69, 70
  differentiation of lymphoid system as basis of, 136
  by follicular pattern (British), 69—71
  by follicular pattern (Dorfman), 71—72
  phenotyping as technique for, 139
  prognosis and, 82—83, 99
  WHO, 72
CLL, see Leukemia, chronic lymphocytic
Clonality
  as concept in lymphomas, 39—40
  in Hodgkin's disease vs. other lymphomas, 41
CMI, see Immunity, cell-mediated (CMI)
Coomb's-positive hemolytic anemia, see Anemia, autoimmune hemolytic (AIHA)
CTCL, see Lymphoma, cutaneous T cell
Cutaneous T cell lymphomas, see Lymphomas, cutaneous T cell (CTCL)

## D

Defense mechanisms, nonimmune, 94—95
Delayed hypersensitivity, see Hypersensitivity, delayed (DTH)
2'-Deoxycoformycin (DCF), 156
Dermatomyositis and malignancy, 13
DNA, 17
  prognosis and, 6
Dorfman classification, 71—72
DTH, see Hypersensitivity, delayed
Duncan's disease, and response to EBV, 41

## E

EBV, see Epstein-Barr virus
Ecto-5' nucleotidase, see 5'-Nucleotidase
Epstein-Barr virus (EBV)
  Burkitt's lymphoma and, 44, 67
  Duncan's disease and, 41
  HD and, 43, 44
E rosettes, see Rosetting

## F

FCC, see Lymphomas, non-Hodgkin's, follicular center cell (FCC) type
Ferritin, as antigen in Hodgkin's disease, 44—45
Ficoll®-Hypaque technique, 135

## G

Graft versus host disease, 4, 120, 138

## H

HD, see Hodgkin's disease
Herpes zoster and Hodgkin's disease, 54
Hexosaminidase, as biochemical marker, 157—158
Histocompatibility complex, major (HHC)
  autoimmune reactivity hypothesis and, 174
  causation vs. correlation issue, 175
  coding for complement components, 172
  D/DR-region genes and, 174
  development of vs. outcome of disease, 175, 179
  HD survival and, 182—183
  linkage disequilibrium and, 171, 173, 174, 180, 184
  in mice, 168—170
    similarities to human systems of, 170, 172, 184—185
    simplified view of, 170
  mimicry hypothesis and, 175
  nomenclature for, 171
  susceptibility genes for Hodgkin's disease and, 182
Histocompatibility locus A (HLA)
  Burkitt's lymphoma and, 183—184
  gene products of, see Antigens, human
  genetic maps, 171
  HD and, 179—183
  immune response genes and, see Immune response genes
  leukemias and, 184
  lymphomas and, 177—179
  malignancies and, 168
  methodological problems with, 177—179, 185
  polymorphism and, 171
  regions of, 170—171
  similarities to H-2 regions, 170, 172, 184—185
Histocompatibility-2 (H-2), 168—170
  genetic maps, 171
  leukemia in mice and, 175—176
  similarities to HLA, 170, 172, 184—185

Hodgkin cells, 38
Hodgkin's disease (HD), 66
   autoimmune neutropenia and, 14
   B lymphocytes and, see B lymphocytes, in HD
   bone marrow transplantation and, 4
   cell biological questions of, 34
   cell-mediated immunity in, 2—11, 19—20, 50—53
      tests of, see specific tests
   characteristics, 38
   classification, 39
   coexisting malignancies and, 18—19
   compared to NHL, 38—42
      clonality, 41—42
      histology, 38—39
      immunohistology, 39—41
      in vitro analyses, 41
      lymph node characteristics, 40
      phenotyping, 40—41
   etiology, 2, 57
   histological variety in and research results, 181—182
   homograft rejection and, 4
   humoral immunity and, 5—6, 45—50
   immune mechanisms in, see Immune mechanisms, in Hodgkin's disease
   immunodeficiency in, see Immunodeficiency, acquired
   infection and, 2—3
   ITP and, 13
   lymphocyte transfer and, 4
   macrophage function and, 10
   MHC and, 182—183
   MLA and, 179—183
   models, 11
   multigenic influences as factor in, 182
   nephrotic syndrome and, 14—15
   predicting prognosis, 46
   relationship to malignancies, research in
      epidemiological data, 56—57
      monoclonal antibodies in, 56
      tissue cell focus of, 56
   second malignancy in, 19
   Sjogren's syndrome and, 12
   SLE and, 12
   therapeutic approach to, 37—38
   T lymphocytes and, see T lymphocytes
   treatment effects, 55—56
Homograft rejection, 4
HTLV, see Human T cell leukemia virus
H-2, see Histocompatibility-2
Human T cell leukemia virus (HTLV), 145, 147
Humoral immunity, see Immunity, humoral
Hypersensitivity, delayed (DTH)
   in CLL, 96
   in HD, 3—4, 54
   in NHL, 84, 86—88
      disadvantages, 85
      relationship to stage, 87—88

# I

Ia antigen antiserum, 135
IgA, deficiency and malignancy, 16
Immune function tests, see also specific tests, 83—85
Immune mechanisms, in Hodgkin's disease, 42—45
   cell interactions as evidence for, 42, 45
   clumping and, 42
   ecotaxopathy theory, 45
   epidemiology as evidence for, 43
   ferritin as antigen in, 44—45
   pathogenesis as evidence for, 44
   T lymphocyte activation and, 44
   virology as evidence for, 43—44
Immune modulation, 4—5
Immune response genes, 172—174
Immune thrombocytopenic purpura (ITP)
   AIHA and, 14
   HD and, 13
Immunity, cell-mediated (CMI)
   antibody-dependent cytotoxicity and, see Antibody-dependent cell-mediated cytotoxicity (ADCC)
   CLL and, 96, 97, 99
   delayed hypersensitivity, see Hypersensitivity, delayed (DTH)
   HD and, see also Immunodeficiency, 2—11, 19—20, 50—53
   lymphocyte counts and, see Lymphocyte counts
   lymphocyte proliferation and, see Lymphocyte response to antigens and mitogens
   lymphocyte reactions and, see Lymphocyte reaction, autologous mixed (AMLR); Lymphocyte reaction, mixed (MLR)
   lymphokine production and, see Lymphokine production
   natural killing and, see Natural killing (NK)
   NHL and, 85—88, 97, 99
   tests for, see specific tests
Immunity, humoral
   antibody response and, see Antibodies, polyclonal
   CLL and, 96—99
   HD and, 5—6, 45—50
   NHL and, 88—94, 97, 99
   serum immunoglobulins and, see Serum immunoglobulins
   tests for, see also specific tests, 88
Immunoblastic lymphadenopathy, 146—147
Immunodeficiency, acquired
   histology, 53—54
   as precedent for neoplasia, 20
   prognosis and, 6
   Hodgkin's disease and, 2, 53—55
   lymphomas and
      chromosome defects as explanation for, 16—17

chronic antigen stimulation as explanation for, 18
impaired immunoregulation as explanation for, 17
viruses as explanation for, 17
malignancies and, 16—18
NHL and, 97, 99
etiology, 97—99
frequency, 82
Immunodeficiency, primary, 16
Immunoglobulins, see Serum immunoglobulins
Immunoglobulin synthesis, in HD, 11
Immunosuppressive therapy, effects of, 16
Infections
in HD, 2—3, 54
in NHL
as cause of death, 82
nonimmune host defense mechanisms and, 94—95
Infectious mononucleosis and HD, 43
Interdigitating cell, see Reticulum interdigitating cell
Interferon, production of in Hodgkin's disease, 51
ITP, see Immune thrombocytopenic purpura

## K

Kaposi's sarcoma
acquired immunodeficiency and, 16
disease pattern of, 43
HD and, 18, 19
Kidney transplantation, see Organ transplantation
Kiel classification, 69, 70
comparison with other systems of, 75—76

## L

Lactate dehydrogenase, as biochemical marker, 157
LDH, see Lactate dehydrogenase
Lennert's lymphoma, see Lymphoma, Lennert's
Leukemia, acute lymphoblastic (ALL), 148
clinical progression, 144, 148
monoclonal antibodies and
as diagnostic aid, 114, 115
serotherapy treatment of, 117—120
polyclonal antibodies as diagnostic aid in, 113—114
Leukemia, acute nonlymphocytic (ANLL), 114
Leukemia, adult T cell (ATL), 144—145
clinical progression, 144—145
CTCL and, 147
DCF in treatment of, 156
HTLV and, 145, 147
monoclonal antibodies and
as diagnostic aid, 114
in serotherapy treatment, 118

Leukemia, chronic lymphocytic (CLL), 95—97, 148
cell-mediated immunity in, 96, 97, 99
characteristics, 95
classification, 145
etiology, 97—98
evidence of monoclonality, 95
humoral immunity in, 96—99
serotherapy treatment of B cell variant of with monoclonal antibodies, 118
T cell origin, 146
Leukemias, see also specific diseases
association with HD, 18, 19
association with HLA genes, 184
hexosaminidase as biochemical marker in, 158
TdT as biochemical marker in, 158—160
Leukocyte reactions, see Lymphocyte reaction, autologous mixed (AMLR); Lymphocyte reaction, mixed (MLR)
Lukes-Collins classification, 67—69
comparison with other systems of, 75—76
Lymphadenopathy, immunoblastic, 146—147
Lymph nodes
distribution of lymphocytes in, 36
HD compared to NHL, 40
Lymphoblastic lymphoma, 77
Lymphocyte counts
HD peripheral blood, 6, 20, 50—53
B lymphocytes, 52
lymphopenia, 50
monocytes, 52—53
prognosis, 6
T lymphocytes, 50—52
HD tissue, 6—7
NHL, 83—86
relationship to stage and subgroup, 86
Lymphocyte proliferation, see Lymphocyte response to antigens and mitogens
Lymphocyte reaction, autologous mixed (AMLR)
in HD, 8—10
Lymphocyte reaction, mixed (MLR)
in HD, 8—10
in NHL, 85
Lymphocyte response to antigens and mitogens
in CLL, 96
in HD, 7—8, 20
in NHL, 88
Lymphocytes
B cell, see B lymphocytes
identification process, 134—135
immunoperoxidase and biotin-avidin complexes in identification of, 136
measurements of functional characteristics, 139
measurements of with intact tissues, 139
natural killer cells, 36
null cells, 36
prognostic index in HD, 46
reactive role in HD, 66
T cell and B cell systems of, 67—68
T cells, see T lymphocytes
Lymphocyte transfer, 4

Lymphoid tissue, normal structure of, 34
Lymphokine production
　in HD, 8, 51
　in NHL, 84
Lymphoma, cutaneous T cell, 140—144
　ATL and, 147
　classification, 142—143, 147
　clinical progression, 143—144, 147
　HD and, 147—148
　lymphomatoid papulosis and, 143
　mycosis fungoides, see Mycosis fungoides
　relationship among variants of, 141—142
　serotherapy treatment of with monoclonal antibodies, 118
　Sézary's syndrome, see Sézary's syndrome
Lymphoma, Hodgkin's disease, see Hodgkin's disease (HD)
Lymphoma, Lennert's, 146—147
Lymphomas, non-Hodgkin's (NHL), see also Hodgkin's disease; Leukemias; specific lymphomas, 55, 68
　analysis, 147
　B cell variants, 118
　biochemical markers for
　　ADA, 155—157
　　hexosaminidase, 157—158
　　LDH, 157
　　5'-NT, 154—155
　　PNP, 157
　　TdT, 158—161
　cell-mediated immunity in, 85—88, 97, 99
　　preservation of, 99
　　tests for, 83—85
　classification, see Classification, of non-Hodgkin's lymphomas
　clinicopathological features, 86
　　in GCC group, 90—91
　　in group with monoclonal Ig protein and depression of Ig, 92—93
　　in high grade group, 90
　　in lymphocytic group, 91—92
　clonality and, 39—40
　compared to Hodgkin's disease, see Hodgkin's disease (HD)
　follicular types, 66
　　center cell (FCC) type, 68, 77
　histiocytic, 77
　histocompatibility research and, 183
　history of research on, 66—67
　humoral immunity in, 88—94, 97, 99
　immunodeficiency in, see Immunodeficiency, acquired
　immunologic identification, 73, 77
　infection in, see Infections, in NHL
　monoclonal antibodies and, see Antibodies, monoclonal
　monoclonal origin, 83
　naming, 66—67
　nephrotic syndrome and, 14—15
　nonimmune host defense mechanisms and, 94—95
　organ transplantation and, 16—18
　phenotypic characteristics, 83, 138
　prognosis
　　cell type and, 73
　　Dorfman classification and, 71—72
　　follicular pattern and, 73, 77
　　Kiel classification and, 69
　　Lukes and Collins classification and, 68
　　Rappaport classification and, 67
　similarities of human and mouse response to, 176—177
　SLE and, 12
　T cell variants of, 17, 77, 139—140
　therapeutic strategies for, 99
　　2'-deoxycoformycin (DCF), 156
　　drug-antibody conjugates, 121
　T lymphocytes and, see T lymphocytes, in NHL
　variety of surface phenotypes in, 115
Lymphomatoid papulosis, 141, 143
Lymphoreticular malignancies
　acquired immunodeficiency and, 16
　primary immunodeficiency and, 16
　Sjogren's syndrome and, 12

# M

Macrophage function, 10
Malignancies, see also specific types of malignancy
　acquired immunodeficiency and, 16
　cell-specific antigens, 117
　characteristics, 37
　clonal origin, 115—116
　definition, 37
　HD and, 18—19, 55
　myositis and, 13
　relationship of to host, 37
　tumor-specific antigens and, 116—117
MHC, see Histocompatibility complex, major
Mitogen response, see Lymphocyte response to antigens and mitogens
Mixed lymphocyte reaction, see Lymphocyte reaction, mixed (MLR)
Modulation, antigenic, 119
Monoclonal antibodies, see Antibodies, monoclonal
Monocytes
　characteristics, 36
　definition, 34
　difficulty in separation techniques, 135
　enumeration, 138
　HD and, 46—47
　HD peripheral blood cells and, 52—53
　HD tissue and, 50
　B lymphocytes, 47—48
　histochemical identification, 47
　mediation of suppression of lymphoproliferation and, 9
　promonocytic form of and NK cells, 36
Multiple myeloma (MM), etiology, 98

Mycosis fungoides, 77, 140
    DCF in treatment of, 156
    lymphomatoid papulosis and, 143
    relationship of to Sezary's syndrome, 141—142

## N

National Cancer Institute (NCI) classification, 73, 74
    comparison with other systems, 75—76
Natural killing (NK)
    HD, 10
    NHL, 85
Neoplasms, see Leukemia; Lymphomas; Malignancies
Nephrotic syndrome
    HD and, 14
    immunological basis for development, 15
    lipoid, 15
    lymphoma and, 14—15
Neutropenia, autoimmune, and HD, 14
NHL, see Lymphomas, non-Hodgkin's
Nicotinamide adenine dinucleotide, as cofactor with LDH, 157
NK, see Natural killing
Non-Hodgkin's lymphoma, see Lymphomas, non-Hodgkin's (NHL)
Nonimmune host defense mechanisms, 94—95
5'-Nucleotidase (5'-NT), as biochemical marker, 154—155

## O

Organ transplantation
    malignancies and, 16
    T lymphocyte alterations with, 138

## P

Pautrier's abscesses, 145, 147
    mycosis fungoides, 141
    Sezary's syndrome, 141
Peripheral blood lymphocytes, see Lymphocyte counts
PHA response, see Lymphocyte response to antigens and mitogens
Phenotyping, see Antibodies, monoclonal
*Pneumocystis carinii*, HD and, 54
PNP, see Purine nucleoside phosphorylase
Polymyositis, see also Dermatomyositis; Myositis, 13
Pooling, monoclonal antibodies, 112
Pseudolymphoma, and Sjogren's syndrome, 12
Purine nucleoside phosphorylase (PNP)
    as biochemical marker, 156—157
    relationship to ADA activity, 156, 157

## R

Rappaport classification, 67, 73
    comparison with other systems of, 75—76
Reed-Sternberg (R-S) cells, 7
    clumping, 42
    effects, 38
    HD and
        characteristic of, 66
        mixed cellularity form, 39
        necrosis in tissue, 46
        nodular sclerosing form, 47
    immunohistology, 40
    interdigitating reticulum cell and, 20, 42
    lymphocytes and, 44
    presence, 38, 45
    source, 52—53
Renal transplants, see Organ transplantation
Reticulum cell sarcoma, see Lymphoreticular malignancies
Reticulum interdigitating cell, 7, 11
    R-S cell and, 20, 42
Rosetting
    ALL classification and, 144
    forms, 42
    HD tissue and, 48—49
    identification of T lymphocyte subsets, 51, 84, 135, 145
    inhibition, 138
    NK cells, 36
    phenotyping lymphomas, 138—139
    process of, 134—136, 139
    technical problems, 50
    treatment effects and, 55
R-S cell, see Reed-Sternberg (R-S) cell

## S

St. Bartholomew's Hospital, patients managed at, 82—99
Serotherapy, 117—120
Serum immunoglobulins
    CLL and, 96—97
        as measure of remission, 97
    measurement, 83—84
    NHL and, 88—94
        clinicopathological characteristics, 91—92
        comparative results, 93—94
        in group with monoclonal Ig protein and depression of Ig, 92—93
        relationship to Ig class, 88—89
        relationship to subtype, 88—90
Sezary's syndrome, 77, 141—142, 156
    mycosis fungoides and, 141—142
Sjogren's syndrome and lymphoreticular disorders, 12
Skin cancers, see also Lymphomas, cutaneous T cell (CTCL)
    HD and, 18, 19

Skin tests, see Hypersensitivity, delayed (DTH)
SLE, see Systemic lupus erythematosus
Socioeconomic factors, in incidence of HD, 43
Spleen
 distribution of lymphocytes in, 36
 peripheralization process in, 35
Splenectomy
 AIHA treatment and, 14
 antibody response in HD and, 5
 association of with ITP and, 13, 14
Systemic candidiasis and HD, 54
Systemic lupus erythematosus (SLE), 15
 lymphoma and, 12

## T

T11 antiserum, 135
T cell chronic lymphocytic leukemia, see Leukemia, chronic lymphocytic, of T cell origin
T cell lymphoma, see Lymphomas, T cell
T cells, see T lymphocytes
TdT, see Terminal deoxynucleotidyl transferase
Terminal deoxynucleotidyl transferase (TdT)
 as biochemical marker, 156, 158—161
 physiological function, 161
 treatment of blast crisis, 159—160
Thrombocytopenic purpura, immune, see Immune thrombocytopenic purpura (ITP)
Tissue, in Hodgkin's disease, 45—50
 composition, 49—50
  B lymphocytes, 49—50
  monocytes, 50
  T lymphocytes, 49
 histology, 46—47
  lymphocytes, 46
  monocytes, 46—47
 immunohistology, 47—48
  monocyte and B lymphocyte differences, 47—48
  pattern of Reed-Sternberg T lymphocytes, 47
  T lymphocyte predominance, 47
 in vitro analysis of, 48—49
  antibody production, 49
  E rosetting cells, 48—49
  immunoglobulin, 48, 49
  lymphocyte response, 48
  monocytes, 49
  T lymphocyte redistribution, 48
Tissue lymphocytes, see Lymphocyte counts
T lymphocytes
 activation of and neoplastic transformation in Hodgkin's disease, 44, 45
 ADA activity, 155—156
 alteration in transplantation, 138
 antigenic markers for, 136—137
 antigens on, 137—138
 autoantibodies to, 138
 B-CLL and, 96
 CLL and, 95, 98, 145
 clumping and, 42
 development, 35
 differentiation, 136—137
 distribution, 68
 enumeration by E rosette formation, 135
 HD and
  changes of, 38
  thymic processing, 51
 HD peripheral blood cells and, 50—52
  abnormalities in, 53
  adoptive transfer capacity, 51—52
  in vitro response, 51
  rosetting and, 51
  synthesis of lymphokines in, 51
 HD tissue and, 49
  predominance, 47
  redistribution, 48
 helper/inducer set, 35
 helper vs. suppressor type in leukemia, 144
 humoral immunity and, 134
 identification of
  antisera and, 135
  monoclonal antibodies and, 115, 135—136
  in tumor masses, 136
 IgMEA receptors in Hodgkin's disease tissue, 47
 LDH in, 157
 malignancies and, 138
 measurement, 83—84
 neutral, 35
 NHL and, 86, 97, 98
 5′-NT activity, 154, 155
 organization in lymph node paracortical region, 36
 organization in spleen, 36
 PNP activity, 156—157
 proportion in lymphomas, 40
 quantitation, 139
 Reed-Sternberg cells and, 44
 separation, 139
 suppressor/cytotoxic set, 35
 transformation as basis of classification, 68
Transferrin receptors, identification in Hodgkin's disease, 45
Treatment effects, in Hodgkin's disease, 55
Tuberculosis, 2
Tumors, see also Lymphomas; specific malignancies

## U

U cell, 68

## V

Viruses
 HTLV, 145, 147
 interaction with immunodeficiency and lymphoma, 17
 role in HD, 43—44

## W

Waldenstrom's macroglobulinemia and Sjogren's syndrome, 12
World Health Organization (WHO) Classification, 72

## X

X-linked hypogammaglobulinemia and malignancies, 16

Skin tests, see Hypersensitivity, delayed (DTH)
SLE, see Systemic lupus erythematosus
Socioeconomic factors, in incidence of HD, 43
Spleen
    distribution of lymphocytes in, 36
    peripheralization process in, 35
Splenectomy
    AIHA treatment and, 14
    antibody response in HD and, 5
    association of with ITP and, 13, 14
Systemic candidiasis and HD, 54
Systemic lupus erythematosus (SLE), 15
    lymphoma and, 12

## T

T11 antiserum, 135
T cell chronic lymphocytic leukemia, see Leukemia, chronic lymphocytic, of T cell origin
T cell lymphoma, see Lymphomas, T cell
T cells, see T lymphocytes
TdT, see Terminal deoxynucleotidyl transferase
Terminal deoxynucleotidyl transferase (TdT)
    as biochemical marker, 156, 158—161
    physiological function, 161
    treatment of blast crisis, 159—160
Thrombocytopenic purpura, immune, see Immune thrombocytopenic purpura (ITP)
Tissue, in Hodgkin's disease, 45—50
    composition, 49—50
        B lymphocytes, 49—50
        monocytes, 50
        T lymphocytes, 49
    histology, 46—47
        lymphocytes, 46
        monocytes, 46—47
    immunohistology, 47—48
        monocyte and B lymphocyte differences, 47—48
        pattern of Reed-Sternberg T lymphocytes, 47
        T lymphocyte predominance, 47
    in vitro analysis of, 48—49
        antibody production, 49
        E rosetting cells, 48—49
        immunoglobulin, 48, 49
        lymphocyte response, 48
        monocytes, 49
        T lymphocyte redistribution, 48
Tissue lymphocytes, see Lymphocyte counts
T lymphocytes
    activation of and neoplastic transformation in Hodgkin's disease, 44, 45
    ADA activity, 155—156
    alteration in transplantation, 138
    antigenic markers for, 136—137
    antigens on, 137—138
    autoantibodies to, 138
    B-CLL and, 96
    CLL and, 95, 98, 145
    clumping and, 42
    development, 35
    differentiation, 136—137
    distribution, 68
    enumeration by E rosette formation, 135
    HD and
        changes of, 38
        thymic processing, 51
    HD peripheral blood cells and, 50—52
        abnormalities in, 53
        adoptive transfer capacity, 51—52
        in vitro response, 51
        rosetting and, 51
        synthesis of lymphokines in, 51
    HD tissue and, 49
        predominance, 47
        redistribution, 48
    helper/inducer set, 35
    helper vs. suppressor type in leukemia, 144
    humoral immunity and, 134
    identification of
        antisera and, 135
        monoclonal antibodies and, 115, 135—136
        in tumor masses, 136
    IgMEA receptors in Hodgkin's disease tissue, 47
    LDH in, 157
    malignancies and, 138
    measurement, 83—84
    neutral, 35
    NHL and, 86, 97, 98
    5'-NT activity, 154, 155
    organization in lymph node paracortical region, 36
    organization in spleen, 36
    PNP activity, 156—157
    proportion in lymphomas, 40
    quantitation, 139
    Reed-Sternberg cells and, 44
    separation, 139
    suppressor/cytotoxic set, 35
    transformation as basis of classification, 68
Transferrin receptors, identification in Hodgkin's disease, 45
Treatment effects, in Hodgkin's disease, 55
Tuberculosis, 2
Tumors, see also Lymphomas; specific malignancies

## U

U cell, 68

## V

Viruses
    HTLV, 145, 147
    interaction with immunodeficiency and lymphoma, 17
    role in HD, 43—44

## W

Waldenstrom's macroglobulinemia and Sjogren's syndrome, 12
World Health Organization (WHO) Classification, 72

## X

X-linked hypogammaglobulinemia and malignancies, 16

THE LIBRARY
UNIVERSITY OF CALIFORNIA
San Francisco
666-2334

**THIS BOOK IS DUE ON THE LAST DATE STAMPED BELOW**

Books not returned on time are subject to fines according to the Library Lending Code. A renewal may be made on certain materials. For details consult Lending Code.

14 DAY
MAR 13 1986
**RETURNED**
MAR 13 1986
14 DAY
JUN 28 1986
RETURNED
JUN 29 1986
**14 DAY**
MAR 26 1993
RETURNED
MAR 22

Series 4128